MRI of the Liver

Guest Editor

ALIYA QAYYUM, MD

MAGNETIC RESONANCE IMAGING CLINICS OF NORTH AMERICA

www.mri.theclinics.com

Consulting Editors
VIVIAN S. LEE, MD, PhD, MBA
LYNNE STEINBACH, MD
SURESH MUKHERJI, MD

August 2010 • Volume 18 • Number 3

SAUNDERS an imprint of ELSEVIER, Inc.

W.B. SAUNDERS COMPANY
A Division of Elsevier Inc.

1600 John F. Kennedy Boulevard ● Suite 1800 ● Philadelphia, Pennsylvania 19103-2899

http://www.theclinics.com

MRI CLINICS OF NORTH AMERICA Volume 18, Number 3
August 2010 ISSN 1064-9689, ISBN 13: 978-1-4377-2691-6

Editor: Joanne Husovski
Developmental Editor: Donald Mumford

Magnetic Resonance Imaging Clinics of North America (ISSN 1064-9689) is published quarterly by Elsevier Inc., 360 Park Avenue South, New York, NY 10010-1710. Months of issue are February, May, August, and November. Business and Editorial Offices: 1600 John F. Kennedy Blvd., Ste. 1800, Philadelphia, PA 19103-2899. Customer Service Office: 3251 Riverport Lane, Maryland Heights, MO 63043. Periodicals postage paid at New York, NY and additional mailing offices. Subscription prices are $309.00 per year (domestic individuals), $455.00 per year (domestic institutions), $150.00 per year (domestic students/residents), $345.00 per year (Canadian individuals), $571.00 per year (Canadian institutions), $448.00 per year (international individuals), $571.00 per year (international institutions), and $217.00 per year (international and Canadian students/residents). International air speed delivery is included in all *Clinics* subscription prices. All prices are subject to change without notice. **POSTMASTER:** Send address changes to *Magnetic Resonance Imaging Clinics*, Elsevier Health Sciences Division, Subscription Customer Service, 3251 Riverport Lane, Maryland Heights, MO 63043. Customer Service (orders, claims, online, change of address): Elsevier Health Sciences Division, Subscription Customer Service, 3251 Riverport Lane, Maryland Heights, MO 63043. Tel:1-800-654-2452 (U.S. and Canada); 314-447-8871 (outside U.S. and Canada). Fax: 314-447-8029. E-mail: journalscustomerservice-usa@elsevier.com (for print support); journalsonlinesupport-usa@elsevier.com (for online support).

Reprints. For copies of 100 or more of articles in this publication, please contact the Commercial Reprints Department, Elsevier Inc., 360 Park Avenue South, New York, NY 10010-1710. Tel.: 212-633-3812; Fax: 212-462-1935; E-mail: reprints@elsevier.com.

Magnetic Resonance Imaging Clinics of North America is covered in the *RSNA Index of Imaging Literature, MEDLINE/PubMed (Index Medicus),* and *EMBASE/Excerpta Medica.*

Printed in the United States of America.

GOAL STATEMENT

The goal of *Magnetic Resonance Imaging Clinics of North America* is to keep practicing physicians up to date with current clinical practice by providing timely articles reviewing the state of the art in patient care.

ACCREDITATION

The *Magnetic Resonance Imaging Clinics of North America* is planned and implemented in accordance with the Essential Areas and Policies of the Accreditation Council for Continuing Medical Education (ACCME) through the joint sponsorship of the University of Virginia School of Medicine and Elsevier. The University of Virginia School of Medicine is accredited by the ACCME to provide continuing medical education for physicians.

The University of Virginia School of Medicine designates this educational activity for a maximum of 15 *AMA PRA Category 1 Credits*™ for each issue, 60 credits per year. Physicians should only claim credit commensurate with the extent of their participation in the activity.

The American Medical Association has determined that physicians not licensed in the US who participate in this CME activity are eligible for a maximum of 15 *AMA PRA Category 1 Credits*™ for each issue, 60 credits per year.

Credit can be earned by reading the text material, taking the CME examination online at http://www.theclinics.com/home/cme, and completing the evaluation. After taking the test, you will be required to review any and all incorrect answers. Following completion of the test and evaluation, your credit will be awarded and you may print your certificate.

FACULTY DISCLOSURE/CONFLICT OF INTEREST

The University of Virginia School of Medicine, as an ACCME accredited provider, endorses and strives to comply with the Accreditation Council for Continuing Medical Education (ACCME) Standards of Commercial Support, Commonwealth of Virginia statutes, University of Virginia policies and procedures, and associated federal and private regulations and guidelines on the need for disclosure and monitoring of proprietary and financial interests that may affect the scientific integrity and balance of content delivered in continuing medical education activities under our auspices.

The University of Virginia School of Medicine requires that all CME activities accredited through this institution be developed independently and be scientifically rigorous, balanced and objective in the presentation/discussion of its content, theories and practices.

All authors/editors participating in an accredited CME activity are expected to disclose to the readers relevant financial relationships with commercial entities occurring within the past 12 months (such as grants or research support, employee, consultant, stock holder, member of speakers bureau, etc.). The University of Virginia School of Medicine will employ appropriate mechanisms to resolve potential conflicts of interest to maintain the standards of fair and balanced education to the reader. Questions about specific strategies can be directed to the Office of Continuing Medical Education, University of Virginia School of Medicine, Charlottesville, Virginia.

The faculty and staff of the University of Virginia Office of Continuing Medical Education have no financial affiliations to disclose.

The authors/editors listed below have identified no professional or financial affiliations for themselves or their spouse/partner:
Maria Antonieta Bali, MD; Susanne Baroud, MD; Ahmed Ba-Ssalamah, MD; Nina Bastati, MD; Hersh Chandarana, MD; Eduard de Lange, MD (Test Author); Farzin A. Farhadi, MD; Kiminori Fujimoto, MD, PhD; Joanne Husovski (Acquisitions Editor); Gaurav Khatri, MD; Dow-Mu Koh, MD, MRCP, FRCR; Grant E. Lattin, Jr., MD; Vivian S. Lee, MD, PhD, MBA (Consulting Editor); Angela D. Levy, MD; Rachel B. Lewis, MD; Hala R. Makhlouf, MD, PhD; Celso Matos, MD; Laura Merrick, BA; Frank H. Miller, MD; Laurent Milot, MD; Anwar R. Padhani, FRCP, FRCR; Priya D. Prabhakar, MD, MPH; Anand M. Prabhakar, MD; Hima B. Prabhakar, MD; Aliya Qayyum, MD, MRCP, FRCR (Guest Editor); Eva Serrao, MD; Lynne Steinbach, MD (Consulting Editor); Bachir Taouli, MD; and Tatsuyuki Tonan, MD.

The authors/editors listed below identified the following professional or financial affiliations for themselves or their spouse/partner:
Rizwan Aslam, MD, ChB is an industry funded research/investigator for Bayer Pharmaceuticals.
Daniel T. Boll, MD is an industry funded research/investigator for Siemens Medical Solutions, Philips Healthcare, and Bracco Diagnostic.
Masoom A. Haider, MD is on the Advisory Committee/Board for Bayer and Siemens, and is a consultant for Bayer.
John R. Leyendecker, MD is on the Speakers' Bureau for Bayer Healthcare and Bracco Diagnostics, and is a consultant and is on the Advisory Committee/Board for Bayer Healthcare.
Elmar M. Merkle, MD is a consultant and is on the Speakers' Bureau for General Electric, Siemens Health Care, Philips Medical Systems, and Bayer Pharmaceuticals; is on the Advisory Committee/Board for General Electric, Siemens Health Care, and Bayer Pharmaceuticals; owns stock in General Electric; and is an industry funded research/investigator for Siemens Health Care.
Suresh Mukherji, MD (Consulting Editor) is a consultant for Philips.
Scott B. Reeder, MD, PhD is a consultant for GE Healthcare and Bracco; is on the Advisory Committee/Board for Bayer; and spouse is employed by and owns stock in GE Healthcare.
Duyshant Sahani, MD is an industry funded research/investigator for GE Healthcare, and is a consultant and is on the Advisory Committee/Board for Bracco Diagnostic.
Claude B. Sirlin, MD is an industry funded research/investigator for GE, Bayer, Bracco, Merck, ISIS, and Siemens (contract pending for Siemens); is a consultant for Bayer, Merck, and ISIS; is on the Advisory Committee/Board for GE and Bayer; and is on the Speakers' Bureau for Bayer.
Geoffrey E. Wile, MD is on the Speakers' Bureau and the Advisory Committee/Board for Bayer Healthcare.
Judy Yee, MD is an industry funded research/investigator for GE Healthcare.
Benjamin M. Yeh, MD is an industry funded research/investigator for General Electric Healthcare, MEDRAD, and Bayer.

Disclosure of Discussion of non-FDA approved uses for pharmaceutical products and/or medical devices:
The University of Virginia School of Medicine, as an ACCME provider, requires that all faculty presenters identify and disclose any "off label" uses for pharmaceutical and medical device products. The University of Virginia School of Medicine recommends that each physician fully review all the available data on new products or procedures prior to instituting them with patients.

TO ENROLL

To enroll in the Magnetic Resonance Imaging Clinics of North America Continuing Medical Education program, call customer service at 1-800-654-2452 or visit us online at www.theclinics.com/home/cme. The CME program is available to subscribers for an additional fee of $196.00.

Contributors

CONSULTING EDITORS

VIVIAN S. LEE, MD, PhD, MBA
Professor of Radiology, Physiology, and
Neurosciences; Vice-Dean for Science; and
Senior Vice-President and Chief Scientific
Officer at New York University Langone
Medical Center, New York, New York

LYNNE STEINBACH, MD
Professor of Clinical Radiology and
Orthopaedic Surgery at the University
of California, San Francisco, San Francisco,
California

SURESH MUKHERJI, MD
Professor and Chief of Neuroradiology and
Head and Neck Radiology; Professor of
Radiology, Otolaryngology Head Neck
Surgery, Radiation Oncology, Oral Medicine,
and Periodontics at the University of Michigan
Health System, Ann Arbor, Michigan

GUEST EDITOR

ALIYA QAYYUM, MD
Professor, Department of Radiology and
Biomedical Imaging, University of California,
San Francisco, San Francisco, California

AUTHORS

MARIA ANTONIETA BALI, MD
MR Imaging Division, Department
of Radiology, Cliniques Universitaires de
Bruxelles, Hôpital Erasme,
Université Libre de Bruxelles, Bruxelles, Belgium

RIZWAN ASLAM, MB ChB
Associate Clinical Professor of Radiology,
Department of Radiology and Biomedical
Imaging, University of California, San
Francisco, School of Medicine; Department
of Radiology, San Francisco Veterans Affairs
Medical Center, San Francisco, California

SUSANNE BAROUD, MD
Department of Radiology, Medical University
of Vienna, Vienna, Austria

NINA BASTATI, MD
Department of Radiology, Medical University
of Vienna, Vienna, Austria

AHMED BA-SSALAMAH, MD
Department of Radiology, Medical University
of Vienna, Vienna, Austria

DANIEL T. BOLL, MD
Department of Radiology, Duke University
Medical Center, Durham, North Carolina

HERSH CHANDARANA, MD
Department of Radiology, New York
University Langone Medical Center,
New York, New York

FARZIN A. FARHADI, MD
Clinical Research Fellow, Joint Department
of Medical Imaging, University Health
Network and Mount Sinai Hospital,
University of Toronto, Toronto, Ontario,
Canada

KIMINORI FUJIMOTO, MD, PhD
Associate Professor, Department of Radiology,
Kurume University School of Medicine;
Department of Radiology, Center for
Diagnostic Imaging, Kurume University
Hospital, Kurume, Japan

MASOOM A. HAIDER, MD
Professor of Radiology, Head of Abdominal
MRI, Joint Department of Medical Imaging,
University Health Network and Mount Sinai
Hospital; Department of Medical Imaging,
Sunnybrook Health Sciences Center,
University of Toronto, Toronto, Ontario,
Canada

GAURAV KHATRI, MD
Body Imaging Fellow, Department of
Radiology, Northwestern University
Feinberg School of Medicine,
Chicago, Illinois

DOW-MU KOH, MD, MRCP, FRCR
Department of Radiology, Royal Marsden
Hospital, Sutton, United Kingdom

MAJ GRANT E. LATTIN Jr, MD, USAF, MC
Department of Radiologic Pathology,
Armed Forces Institute of Pathology,
Washington, DC; Department of Radiology
and Nuclear Medicine, Uniformed Services
University of the Health Sciences, Bethesda,
Maryland

ANGELA D. LEVY, MD
Department of Radiology, Georgetown
University Hospital, Washington, DC

LCDR RACHEL B. LEWIS, MD, MC, USN
Department of Radiologic Pathology,
Armed Forces Institute of Pathology,
Washington, DC; Department of Radiology,
National Naval Medical Center; Department
of Radiology and Nuclear Medicine,
Uniformed Services University of the Health
Sciences, Bethesda, Maryland

JOHN R. LEYENDECKER, MD
Associate Professor, Abdominal Imaging
Section; Clinical Director of MRI, Department
of Radiology, Wake Forest University School
of Medicine, Winston-Salem, North Carolina

HALA R. MAKHLOUF, MD, PhD
Division of Hepatic and Gastrointestinal
Pathology, Armed Forces Institute of
Pathology, Washington, DC

CELSO MATOS, MD
MR Imaging Division, Department of
Radiology, Cliniques Universitaires de
Bruxelles, Hôpital Erasme, Université Libre de
Bruxelles, Belgium

ELMAR M. MERKLE, MD
Department of Radiology, Duke University
Medical Center, Durham, North Carolina

LAURA MERRICK, BA
Department of Radiology, Northwestern
University Feinberg School of Medicine,
Chicago, Illinois

FRANK H. MILLER, MD
Director of Body Imaging Section and
Fellowship Program; Professor, Department
of Radiology, Northwestern University
Feinberg School of Medicine; Chief,
Gastrointestinal Radiology; Medical Director
MR Imaging, Northwestern Memorial Hospital,
Chicago, Illinois

LAURENT MILOT, MD
Assistant Professor of Radiology, Department
of Medical Imaging, Sunnybrook Health
Sciences Center, Toronto, Ontario, Canada

ANWAR R. PADHANI, FRCP, FRCR
Paul Strickland MRI Center, Mount Vernon
Hospital, Northwood, Middlesex,
United Kingdom

ANAND M. PRABHAKAR, MD
Clinical Fellow in Abdominal Imaging,
Department of Radiology, Division of
Abdominal Imaging & Intervention,
Massachusetts General Hospital, Boston,
Massachusetts

HIMA B. PRABHAKAR, MD
Staff Radiologist, South Texas Radiology,
San Antonio, Texas

PRIYA D. PRABHAKAR, MD, MPH
Staff Radiologist, Wilmington Veterans
Administration Hospital, Wilmington, Delaware

ALIYA QAYYUM, MD
Professor, Department of Radiology and
Biomedical Imaging, University of California,
San Francisco, San Francisco, California

SCOTT B. REEDER, MD, PhD
Liver Imaging Research Program,
Departments of Radiology, Medical Physics,
Biomedical Engineering, and Medicine,
University of Wisconsin, Madison,
Wisconsin

DUYSHANT SAHANI, MD
Department of Radiology, Division of
Abdominal Imaging and Intervention,
Massachusetts General Hospital,
Boston, Massachusetts

EVA SERRAO, MD
MR Imaging Division, Department of
Radiology, Cliniques Universitaires de
Bruxelles, Hôpital Erasme, Université Libre de
Bruxelles, Belgium

CLAUDE B. SIRLIN, MD
Liver Imaging Group, Department of
Radiology, University of California San Diego,
San Diego, California

BACHIR TAOULI, MD
Department of Radiology, Mount Sinai School
of Medicine, New York, New York

TATSUYUKI TONAN, MD
Assistant Professor, Department of Radiology,
Kurume University School of Medicine,
Kurume, Japan

GEOFFREY E. WILE, MD
Assistant Professor, Body Imaging Section,
Department of Radiology, Vanderbilt
University Medical Center, Nashville,
Tennessee

JUDY YEE, MD
Professor and Vice-Chair of Radiology,
Department of Radiology, San Francisco
Veterans Affairs Medical Center,
San Francisco, California

BENJAMIN M. YEH, MD
Associate Professor, Department of Radiology
and Biomedical Imaging, University of
California, San Francisco, School of Medicine;
Department of Radiology, San Francisco
Veterans Affairs Medical Center,
San Francisco, California

Contents

Intracellular fat accumulation is common feature of liver disease. Intracellular fat (steatosis) is the histologic hallmark of nonalcoholic fatty liver disease but also may occur with alcohol abuse, viral hepatitis, HIV and genetic lipodystrophies, and chemotherapy. This article reviews emerging MR imaging techniques that attempt to quantify liver fat. The content provides an overview of fatty liver disease and diseases where fat is an important disease feature. Also discussed is the current use and limitation of nontargeted biopsy in diffuse liver disease and why quantitative noninvasive biomarkers of liver fat would be beneficial.

Iron overload is the histologic hallmark of hereditary hemochromatosis and transfusional hemosiderosis but also may occur in chronic hepatopathies. This article provides an overview of iron deposition and diseases where liver iron overload is clinically relevant. Next, this article reviews why quantitative noninvasive biomarkers of liver iron would be beneficial. Finally, we describe current state-of-the-art methods for quantifying iron with MR imaging and review remaining challenges and unsolved problems.

This article focuses on the current role of magnetic resonance imaging in the detection and characterization of chronic hepatitis and cirrhosis. In particular, the characteristic MR imaging features of morphologic changes and focal manifestations of chronic liver disease are highlighted.

MRI has become the most important imaging modality for detecting and characterizing focal liver lesions. The introduction of high-field-strengths, such as 3 Tesla MR imaging, in combination with the parallel imaging technique, has led to significant improvements in spatial and temporal resolution and has established this technique as a valuable asset in daily clinical practice. New techniques, such as diffusion-weighted imaging, may improve MR imaging sensitivity and specificity in the diagnostic workup of focal liver lesions. The tailored administration of various nonspecific and liver-specific contrast agents enables clinicians to increase the detection rate and improve the characterization of the different focal liver lesions. This article describes the usefulness of these imaging techniques in detecting and characterizing the most common benign focal liver lesions.

Hepatocellular carcinoma (HCC) is a common malignancy typically associated with chronic liver disease and is a leading cause of mortality among these patients. Prognosis is improved when detected early. MRI is the best imaging examination for accurate diagnosis. Although arterial enhancement with delayed washout, increased T2-weighted signal intensity, delayed capsular enhancement, restricted diffusion, and tumor thrombus are typical features, not all lesions demonstrate these findings. The radiologist must be familiar with these typical imaging characteristics, and less common appearances and associated findings of HCC, and must be able to differentiate them from those of lesions that mimic HCC. Knowledge of therapeutic options and how those are related to imaging findings is imperative to assist clinicians in managing these patients.

Liver metastases are the most frequently encountered malignant liver lesions in the Western countries. Accurate diagnosis of liver metastases is essential for appropriate management of these patients. Multiple imaging modalities, including ultrasound, CT, positron emission tomography, and MRI, are available for the evaluation of patients with suspected or known liver metastases. Contrast-enhanced MRI has a high accuracy for detection and characterization of liver lesions. Additionally, diffusion-weighted MRI (DWI) has been gaining increasing attention. It is a noncontrast technique that is easy to perform, could be incorporated in routine clinical protocols, and has the potential to provide tissue characterization. This article discusses the basic principles of DWI and discusses its emerging role in the detection of liver metastases in patients with extrahepatic malignancies.

Hepatic perfusion imaging with magnetic resonance (MR) imaging is an emerging technique for quantitative assessment of diffuse hepatic disease and hepatic lesion blood flow. The principal method that has been used is based on T1 dynamic contrast-enhanced MR imaging. Perfusion imaging shows promise in the assessment of tumor therapy response, staging of liver fibrosis, and evaluation of hepatocellular carcinoma. The future standardization of imaging protocols and MR imaging pulse sequences will allow for broader clinical applications.

This article presents current magnetic resonance imaging techniques for the diagnosis of biliary tumors. It emphasizes the need for a comprehensive protocol, combining imaging sequences of the liver parenchyma and soft tissues with magnetic resonance cholangiopancreatography and magnetic resonance angiography to detect and stage biliary malignancies. Imaging characteristics that may indicate a specific diagnosis are discussed. The potential role of diffusion-weighted imaging in diagnosing the cause of biliary obstruction and detecting unsuspected nodal disease and peritoneal seeding is emphasized and illustrated.

Priya D. Prabhakar, Anand M. Prabhakar, Hima B. Prabhakar, and Duyshant Sahani

Magnetic resonance cholangiopancreatography (MRCP) is an elegant MR technique for noninvasively delineating the biliary system. Technologic advances in MRCP acquisition and processing and the routine availability of three-dimensional sequences have facilitated detailed assessment of biliary anatomy and pathologic or congenital processes; therefore, invasive endoscopic retrograde cholangiopancreatography is rarely needed for establishing a diagnosis. MRCP can be combined with contrast-enhanced MR imaging to enable concurrent evaluation of organs such as the liver and pancreas in addition to functional biliary imaging. This review focuses on the current use of MRCP to evaluate nonmalignant processes affecting the biliary system.

Rizwan Aslam, Benjamin M. Yeh, and Judy Yee

Assessment of the hepatic vasculature is essential for tumor staging, surgical planning, and understanding of liver disease. Technological advances have made contrast-enhanced magnetic resonance (MR) imaging comparable to multidetector-row computed tomography for diagnostic vascular imaging with respect to spatial resolution. Unenhanced MR angiographic sequences enable reasonable clinical assessment of vessels without contrast agents in patients with contraindications or renal insufficiency. Furthermore, MR angiography may be used to provide directional information through manipulation of the signal intensity of flowing blood. A major limitation to consistent contrast-enhanced MR angiography is the timing of MR image acquisition with arrival of the contrast bolus in the structures of interest. In this article, the authors discuss currently available techniques for imaging of the hepatic vasculature.

Geoffrey E. Wile and John R. Leyendecker

The liver is one of the most challenging organs of the body to image with magnetic resonance because it is large and mobile, receives a dual blood supply, and is surrounded by organs and structures that contribute to artifacts from flow and susceptibility. Recent advances in imaging hardware, in addition to improvements in temporal resolution and development of hepatocyte-specific contrast agents, make imaging of the liver more approachable than in the past; however, it remains a complex process that requires compromise. In this article the authors discuss development and optimization of a liver imaging protocol at 1.5 T, with common variations in each element of the protocol, as well as the strengths and weaknesses associated with the relevant sequences.

Daniel T. Boll and Elmar M. Merkle

Clinical hepatobiliary magnetic resonance (MR) imaging continues to evolve at a fast rate. However, three basic requirements must still be satisfied if novel high-field MR imaging techniques are to be included in the hepatobiliary imaging routine: improvement of parenchymal contrast, suppression of respiratory motion artifact, and anatomic coverage of the entire hepatobiliary system. This article outlines the various arenas involved in MR imaging of the hepatobiliary system at 3 Tesla (T) compared with 1.5 T by (1) highlighting magnetic field–dependent MR contrast phenomena that contribute to the overall appearance of high-field hepatobiliary imaging; (2) summarizing the biodistributions of different gadolinium chelates used as MR contrast agents and their effectiveness regarding the static magnetic field; (3) showing the implementation of advanced imaging techniques such as three-dimensional acquisition schemes and parallel acceleration techniques used in T1-, T2-, and diffusion-weighted hepatobiliary imaging; and (4) addressing artifact mechanisms exacerbated by, or originating from, increase of the static magnetic field.

There is growing interest in exploring and using functional imaging techniques to provide additional information on structural alterations in the liver, which often occur late in the disease process. This article presents a summary of the different functional MR imaging techniques currently in use, focusing on dynamic contrast-enhanced MR imaging, diffusion-weighted MR imaging, MR spectroscopy, in- and oppose-phase MR imaging, and T2*-weighted imaging. For each technique, the biologic underpinning for the technique is explained, the clinical applications surveyed, and the challenges for their application enumerated. Developing and less frequently used techniques such as MR elastography, blood oxygenation level dependent imaging, dynamic susceptibility contrast-enhanced MR imaging, and diffusion-tensor imaging are reviewed. The challenges widespread adoption of functional MR imaging and the translation of such techniques to high field strengths are also discussed.

Primary tumors of the liver can be classified pathologically based on their cell of origin into epithelial tumors, arising from hepatocytes or biliary epithelium, and non-epithelial tumors, including mesenchymal tumors and lymphoma. Characteristic findings on MR imaging can be seen in many cases. This article reviews the MR imaging appearance of these tumors with pathologic correlation.

Magnetic Resonance Imaging Clinics of North America

THE CLINICS ARE NOW AVAILABLE ONLINE!

Access your subscription at:
www.theclinics.com

Preface

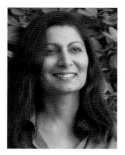

Aliya Qayyum, MD, MRCP, FRCR
Guest Editor

This issue of the *Magnetic Resonance Imaging Clinics of North America* brings together the most recent developments in liver MR imaging which have occurred over the last decade. Stronger gradients and faster sequences enable more robust imaging of abdominal organs. The combination of functional data acquisition with the drive towards obtaining more accurate and objective measures of disease continues to push the envelope in MR research.

Topics chosen in this issue review not only current interpretations of focal and diffuse liver disease morphology, but also novel techniques which assess microstructure *and* composition of tissue. Although many challenges remain, new solutions are continually developed furthering optimization and consistency of MR imaging. The discussion of focal benign and malignant liver lesions goes beyond the conventional T1- and T2-weighted and extracellular contrast enhanced imaging to include diffusion and perfusion applications, and liver-specific contrast agents. Considerable interest has also developed in the detection and staging of diffuse liver disease. More accurate estimation of liver and fat along with improving detection and characterization of focal lesions in cirrhosis has closely mirrored the unraveling of the complex patho-physiologic processes of diffuse liver disease, their interactions and the potential therapeutic interventions, *often based upon improved imaging methods*.

Liver imaging has been of particular interest to me for many years and the opportunity to work and share this mutual area of interest with these wonderful collaborators has indeed been a pleasure. I would like to thank the contributors for their hard work and excellent articles which comprise this *comprehensive* review of the current status of liver MR imaging.

I would also like to especially thank my UCSF colleague Alastair Martin, PhD for his advice and guidance, and my chairman at UCSF, Ronald Arenson, MD, for his mentorship and tremendous support.

Aliya Qayyum, MD, MRCP, FRCR
Department of Radiology and Biomedical Imaging
University of California San Francisco
505 Parnassus Avenue, Room L-307, Box 0628
San Francisco, CA 94143, USA

E-mail address:
aliya.qayyum@ucsf.edu

Magn Reson Imaging Clin N Am 18 (2010) xv
doi:10.1016/j.mric.2010.10.001

Quantification of Liver Fat with Magnetic Resonance Imaging

Scott B. Reeder, MD, PhD[a],*, Claude B. Sirlin, MD[b]

KEYWORDS

- Fat quantification • Magnetic resonance imaging
- Hepatic steatosis • Quantitative biomarkers

Fat deposition is a common condition of the liver. Fat is the histologic hallmark of nonalcoholic fatty liver disease (NAFLD) but also may occur with alcohol abuse, viral hepatitis, HIV and genetic lipodystrophies, and chemotherapy. This article reviews emerging MR imaging techniques that attempt to quantify liver fat. The content is divided into the following sections:

- Overview of fatty liver disease and diseases where fat is an important disease feature
- Review of the current use and limitation of nontargeted biopsy in diffuse liver disease and why quantitative noninvasive biomarkers of liver fat and iron would be beneficial
- Description of current state-of-the-art methods for quantifying fat with MR imaging, including remaining challenges and unsolved problems.

After reading this content, readers should understand the scope of diffuse liver disease in regards to hepatic steatosis and the limitations of biopsy, and be familiar with emerging quantitative MR imaging methods for measuring liver fat.

INTRACELLULAR FAT (HEPATIC STEATOSIS)
Steatosis Is an Important Feature of Liver Disease

Hepatic steatosis is the abnormal and excessive intracellular accumulation of fat in hepatocytes, primarily as triglycerides. Long considered an incidental consequence of other conditions, such as diabetes or obesity, steatosis is now recognized as having a causative role in important hepatic and systemic disorders.[1–11]

For example, NAFLD is present in 20 to 80 million Americans and is the most common chronic liver disease in the United States.[12–14] Steatosis is the instigating process in NAFLD and can lead to cirrhosis.[8,15–17] Free fatty acids, the substrate for triglyceride formation, trigger cell death by inducing oxidative stress, provoking production of cytokines and reactive oxygen species, and activating apoptosis, potentially resulting in progressive hepatic disease. Studies have shown that 5% to 15% of patients with NAFLD present with established cirrhosis on liver biopsy[8,16,17] and that 4% to 5% of individuals with isolated steatosis eventually developed cirrhosis.[8,11] Steatosis has also been shown to worsen the course of viral liver disease; in chronic hepatitis C infection, steatosis may reduce the efficacy of antiviral therapy and accelerate disease progression.[6,7] Furthermore, steatosis reduces hepatocellular functional reserve and contributes to postoperative hepatic failure after liver transplantation or resection.[18–20]

Emerging evidence suggests that hepatic steatosis increases risk of malignancy. The risk of hepatocellular carcinoma (HCC) is particularly high; 7% of patients with NAFLD-related cirrhosis developed HCC over a 10-year timeframe.[10]

[a] Liver Imaging Research Program, Departments of Radiology, Medical Physics, Biomedical Engineering, and Medicine, University of Wisconsin, E1/374 CSC, 600 Highland Avenue, Madison, WI 53792-3252, USA
[b] Liver Imaging Group, Department of Radiology, University of California San Diego, 408 Dickinson Street, San Diego, CA 92103-8226, USA
* Corresponding author. Liver Imaging Research Program, Department of Radiology, University of Wisconsin, E1/374 CSC, 600 Highland Avenue, Madison, WI 53792-3252.
E-mail address: sreeder@wisc.edu

Magn Reson Imaging Clin N Am 18 (2010) 337–357
doi:10.1016/j.mric.2010.08.013

Because of the high prevalence of NAFLD in the general population, it is possible that more than 50,000 Americans will eventually develop NAFLD-related HCC.[9] Recent reports describe HCC in patients with NAFLD without fibrosis or cirrhosis,[21] suggesting that hepatic fat may have direct carcinogenic effects.

Hepatic steatosis may have a causative effect and contribute to the development of diabetes through interference with insulin signaling and may be the pathogenic link between obesity and its metabolic complications.[3,4] In separate studies, 20% to 50% of individuals with steatosis subsequently became diabetic.[2,11] Furthermore, cardiovascular disease is the most common cause of morbidity and death in patients with NAFLD.[3,9,22,23] This association has previously been attributed to comorbidities of NAFLD (obesity, dyslipidemia, hypertension, and diabetes) rather than NAFLD itself,[9,22] but new data show that NAFLD is as an independent risk factor for cardiovascular mortality.[22] Of particular concern is that the increased cardiovascular mortality associated with NAFLD begins at age 45.[3]

Treatment of Fatty Liver Disease

Liver fat is a meaningful marker of, and a contributor to, both hepatic and systemic morbidity and mortality. Hepatic steatosis is not a benign process and has important implications for many important diseases, including cancer, diabetes, and cardiovascular disease. Fortunately, steatosis can be reversible with intervention, and reduction in liver fat may diminish many of its associated risks.

Weight loss, through exercise and diet, is central to improvement of obesity-related fatty liver disease although the precise nature of the relationship between weight loss and liver steatosis is poorly understood. Moreover, most NAFLD patients are unsuccessful at achieving sufficient weight loss and often other means are necessary. Laparoscopic gastric banding (LAGB), for example, has been demonstrated to be an effective surgical treatment of obesity and has been shown to reduce liver fat.[24,25]

New pharmacologic treatments of NAFLD that target its underlying insulin resistance have recently emerged. Lin and colleagues[26] demonstrated a marked decrease in steatosis in ob/ob mice, a leptin-deficient mouse model of steatosis and insulin resistance, when treated with metformin, a member of the biguanide drug class known to improve insulin sensitivity. Recently, Bugianesi and colleagues[27] demonstrated a significant decrease in hepatic steatosis in patients treated

with metformin. In addition, it has been shown recently that NAFLD patients treated with pioglitazone show improved hepatic steatosis.[28,29] Pioglitazone is a member of the thiazolidinedione drug class and, like metformin, improves insulin sensitivity.

Based on results such as these, the National Institute of Diabetes and Digestive and Kidney Diseases Clinical Research Network in Nonalcoholic Steatohepatitis (NASH) has two trials nearing completion for assessment of new treatments of NAFLD. The PIVENS[30] trial compares the efficacy of pioglitazone (vs vitamin E or placebo) in adults, whereas the TONIC[31] trial evaluates the efficacy of metformin (vs vitamin E or placebo) in children. Assessment of steatosis relies on biopsy, limited to the beginning and end of these trials due to the expense and risks associated with biopsy. Accurate measurement of steatosis with a quantitative imaging–based method in these studies would have permitted frequent evaluation with a greatly improved safety profile and reduced expense, tracking the time course of steatosis during each trial. Such methods could potentially transform the translation of new therapies from experimental drugs into clinical practice.

Quantification of Liver Fat Is Important

Because hepatic steatosis is a pathogenic, potentially reversible condition even in severe cases, there is an urgent need, in both clinical and research arenas, to detect its presence and to assess its severity.

Assessment of hepatic steatosis for clinical care requires not only diagnosis but also grading of severity. The relevant classification threshold depends on the clinical context and may vary widely, from the standard 5% steatosis threshold often used for defining hepatic steatosis to the 30% threshold for exclusion of liver transplantation donors.[32] Moreover, accurate quantification is necessary for grading steatosis and for longitudinal monitoring of patients.

In patients with known or suspected NAFLD, physicians often recommend weight loss to prevent the harmful consequences of hepatic steatosis. The amount of weight loss required to resolve NAFLD is unknown, however. The American Gastroenterological Association recommends a 5% to 10% reduction in body weight for obesity-related NAFLD.[33] This recommendation is based on reductions in indirect variables, however, such as cholesterol and blood pressure, not on reduction in liver fat. There is no solid evidence showing that 5% to 10% weight loss effectively treats NAFLD because there have been no prospective studies using accurate quantitative measurements to answer this fundamental question. Accurate and precise quantification of liver fat is required to guide treatment of NAFLD by evidenced-based weight loss.

Liver fat is also a highly active topic of investigative interest. The National Institute of Health's Research Portfolio Online Reporting Tools (http://projectreporter.nih.gov/reporter.cfm) lists 122 grants under "hepatic steatosis" and the Web site, clinicaltrials.gov, lists 128 studies related to this topic. Major objectives for studies on hepatic steatosis include understanding its causation, delineating its consequences, and defining its response to therapeutic intervention.

In summary, accurate and precise quantification of liver fat is important for diagnosis and treatment of patients with NAFLD and facilitates research on this condition.

Percutaneous Liver Biopsy

Nontargeted percutaneous liver biopsy with direct histologic visualization is the current gold standard for diagnosing hepatic steatosis, permitting comprehensive evaluation not only of liver fat content but also of other key histologic features, such as steatosis zonality, fat droplet size (macrovesicular vs microvesicular), iron overload, inflammation, cellular injury, and fibrosis. Evaluation of disease activity and staging of fibrosis is generally determined by the specific disease. For example, many centers use the grading/staging system proposed by Brunt and colleagues[34] for the evaluation of steatohepatitis (NASH). The Brunt scoring system is a semiquantitative score of necroinflammatory disease activity based on a combination of steatosis, inflammation, and ballooning degeneration as well as a staging score of fibrosis severity. More recently, Kleiner and colleagues[35] proposed a modified scoring system for NAFLD, the NAFLD activity score, to encompass a broader spectrum of NAFLD that includes isolated steatosis and not just steatohepatitis. The METAVIR scoring system is commonly used to provide semiquantitative disease activity in patients with hepatitis C.[36]

Steatosis is typically graded on a 0–3 scale based on the number of cells with intracellular vacuoles of fat[34]:

Grade 0 (normal) = up to 5% of cells affected
Grade 1 (mild) = 5% to 33% of cells affected
Grade 2 (moderate) = 34% to 66% of cells affected
Grade 3 (severe) = 67% or greater of cells affected

The percentage of cells affected with intracellular fat does not correspond directly to the MR imaging fat fraction (discussed later).

A major limitation of liver biopsy is lack of representation of the liver as a whole because most features of diffuse liver disease (steatosis, fibrosis, iron overload, and so forth) are inherently heterogeneous, and, therefore, biopsy suffers from sampling variability.[37-39] The underlying assumption that biopsy, which collects a tissue sample 1/50,000 the overall size of the liver, is representative of the entire organ is currently being challenged. A recent study by Ratziu and colleagues[37] in 51 patients undergoing two closely localized biopsies (30° to 45° apart) demonstrated a κ-reliability score of 0.64 for grading steatosis, which indicates poor agreement, inadequate for reliable grading. Other studies have shown significant sampling variability when more than one sample is analyzed.[40-46] Vuppalanchi and colleagues,[47] recently reported a dependence of diagnosis of NAFLD on the length and number of liver biopsy samples. The degree of sampling error depends not only on biopsy size but also on the stage of liver disease. Biopsy also carries significant risk of complications leading to hospitalization (1% to 3%) and death (1:10,000)[48] and necessitates several hours of postprocedure recovery. Thus, biopsy is impractical to diagnose or monitor the many tens of millions of Americans with or at risk for diffuse liver disease. Biopsy is also not feasible in many research studies, including epidemiologic and genetic studies.

Ultrasound

Ultrasound, the most common imaging modality used to evaluate hepatic steatosis,[49-51] infers the presence and severity of liver fat based on qualitative sonographic features, including liver echogenicity, echotexture, vessel visibility, and beam attenuation. Ultrasound is operator and machine dependent and suffers from poor repeatability and reproducibility. The positive predictive value of ultrasound for detection of steatosis is only 62% to 77%.[51,52] Moreover, ultrasound is particularly challenging in obese patients, the population at highest risk for the disease,[53] due to impaired beam penetration and limited liver visualization.

CT

CT, a widely available modality capable of rapid volumetric imaging, can provide objective assessment of hepatic X-ray attenuation, which is related to liver fat content.[51,54-56] The presence of iron, copper, glycogen, fibrosis, or edema confounds attenuation values, leading to errors in fat quantification[56] and CT has low sensitivity for mild to moderate steatosis. The use of some drugs, such as amiodarone or gold, is also well known to increase the attenuation of liver and confounds the ability of CT to quantify fat. Moreover, use of ionizing radiation by CT precludes its use for quantifying liver fat in children[57] or for repeated follow-up in adults.

Magnetic Resonance Spectroscopy

Magnetic resonance spectroscopy (MRS) noninvasively measures proton signals as a function of their resonance frequency. The signal intensity at frequencies corresponding to water or fat can be quantified, and the fat-signal fraction (FSF) can be calculated. When performed properly, MRS is sensitive to even trace amounts of liver fat, and MRS is accepted by many as the most accurate noninvasive method to quantify liver fat. MRS has important limitations, however, that preclude its widespread clinical and research implementations. It is restricted in spatial coverage. Sampling error is difficult to avoid, which is problematic for longitudinal monitoring. It is time consuming to perform, requires expertise to analyze, and is generally available only at academic centers. Imaging-based methods that evaluate the entire liver and that are simple to perform and analyze are preferable.

The acceptance of MRS as an accurate method derives primarily from landmark publications in the 1990s by Longo and colleagues,[58,59] Thomsen and colleagues,[60] and Szczepaniak and colleagues.[14,61] These investigators conducted seminal studies showing proof of concept that MRS quantitatively assesses liver fat content using independent tissue-based reference standards. Although groundbreaking, these investigations were small preclinical or clinical studies; multicenter validation studies in human subjects have not yet been performed. Thus, although MRS is used as the reference standard for most preliminary studies of emerging quantitative MR imaging methods (discussed later), more rigorous validation is needed. Such validation necessitates comparison with tissue triglyceride concentration as an independent tissue-based reference standard.

QUANTIFICATION OF FATTY ACCUMULATION IN THE LIVER WITH MR IMAGING
Conventional In-Phase and Opposed-Phase Imaging for Detection of Fat

Conventional MR imaging has been used to detect liver fat for more than 25 years.[62] As with MRS, MR imaging exploits the difference of the resonance frequencies between water and fat proton signals. By acquiring the images at echo times at which water and fat signals are approximately in-phase (W + F) and opposed-phase (W − F), volumetric liver fat detection is possible based on the relative signal loss on opposed-phase (also known as out-of-phase) images.[62]

Echo times for IOP imaging are based on the relative chemical shift between water and the methylene peak ($-CH_2-$) of fat. At 1.5T and at body temperature, this peak resonates approximately −217 Hz slower than water (−434 Hz at 3.0T). Thus, at 1.5T (3.0T) the main peak of fat is in-phase every 360° of phase between water and fat or every 4.6 ms (2.3 ms) (ie, 4.6 ms [2.3 ms], 9.2 ms [4.6 ms], 13.4 ms [6.9 ms], and so forth). Likewise, at 1.5T (3T), water and fat have opposed-phase at 2.3 ms (1.15 ms) and at every subsequent multiple of 4.6 ms (2.3 ms) (ie, 2.3 ms [1.15 ms], 6.9 ms [3.5 ms], 11.5 ms [5.8 ms], and so forth).

Fig. 1 shows several examples of patients with hepatic steatosis detected with in-phase and opposed-phase (IOP) imaging. A wide variety of patterns, including diffuse steatosis, lobar, geographic, perivascular, and even diffuse steatosis with mass-like sparing, among others, have been described.[63] IOP imaging is widely accepted as the gold standard noninvasive imaging method for qualitative detection and characterization of fat within the liver.

Several investigators have explored the extension of IOP imaging toward quantification of fat. Unlike CT where the pixel value directly reflects X-ray attenuation (in Hounsfield units), the signal intensity in MR images is arbitrary and depends on receiver gain and the sensitivity of receive radiofrequency coils (B_1 sensitivity). Therefore, normalization of the signal from MR images is a helpful way to remove the influence of coil sensitivity and, therefore, avoids errors introduced by inhomogeneous coil sensitivity when muscle or spleen is used as an internal calibration or normalization measurement. FSF (η) can be calculated as in Equation 1:

$$\eta = \frac{F}{W+F} \tag{1}$$

where W and F are the signal contributions from water and fat. The FSF only reflects the concentrations fat if the signals from W and F are corrected for confounding factors (discussed in detail later).

For IOP imaging, even though the water and fat signals are not separated, an FSF map can be calculated, noting that in phase, IP = W + F and opposed phase, OP = W−F (Equation 2):

$$\eta = \frac{IP - OP}{2IP} \tag{2}$$

Opposed-Phase   In-Phase

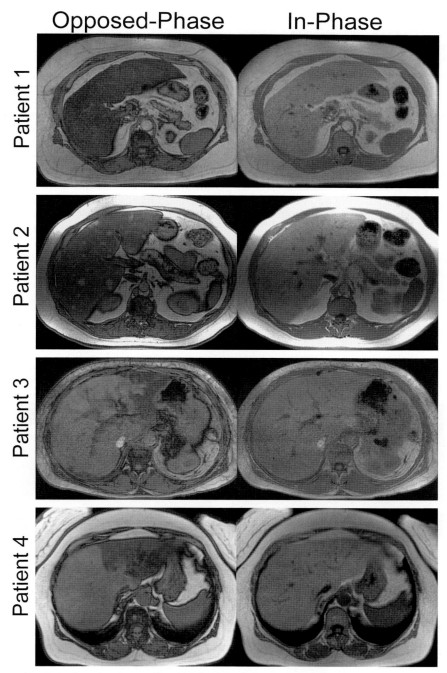

Fig. 1. Conventional IOP imaging is a well-established qualitative method for detection and characterizing fat within the liver. Examples of IOP imaging in patients with steatosis demonstrate a variety of patterns, including diffuse (*top row*), diffuse with mass-like sparing (*second row*), geographic steatosis (*third row*), and ever lobar (*bottom row*). Other patterns, including focal mass—like steatosis and perivascular distributions, have also been described.[63]

Fig. 2 illustrates how IOP imaging can be used to calculate an FSF image, or map, through combination of the in-phase (IP) and opposed-phase (OP) images.

Using this approach, it only possible to achieve a dynamic range of 0 to 50% FSF when magnitude images are used. This occurs because of a natural ambiguity with magnitude-only images with FSF greater than 50%. For example, the opposed-phase signal in a liver with 40% fat is the same as from a liver with 60% fat. This ambiguity can only be resolved with additional information, such as complex-phase information used with chemical shift–based water-fat separation methods[64–70] or through elegant methods that exploit differences in T_1 between water and fat.[71] These methods all require acquisition of additional images beyond IOP imaging. Fat fractions greater than 50% are uncommon in the liver.

As discussed later, however, there are multiple confounding factors that corrupt the ability of conventional IOP imaging to quantify fat, and this is particularly true at low fat fractions, where confounding factors have their largest impact and compromise the ability of IOP to quantify fat.[72–75]

Conventional Fat-Suppressed Imaging for Detection of Liver Fat

Another approach for the detection liver fat is to compare images acquired with and without fat suppression. Fat-suppression pulses have the effect of suppressing fat signal, decreasing the overall liver signal in a fat-containing liver. This is true for both T_1-weighted gradient-echo and T_2-weighted fast spin-echo (FSE) methods. Qayyum and colleagues[70] demonstrated better correlation between signal loss in fat-suppressed, T_2-weighted FSE imaging with biopsy steatosis grade than with IOP imaging. **Fig. 3** shows an example of a patient with severe steatosis seen on IOP imaging. The signal from the liver in the corresponding fat-suppressed, T_2-weighted FSE is dark compared with the spleen in contradistinction to the T_2-weighted, **s**ingle-**s**hot FSE image (without

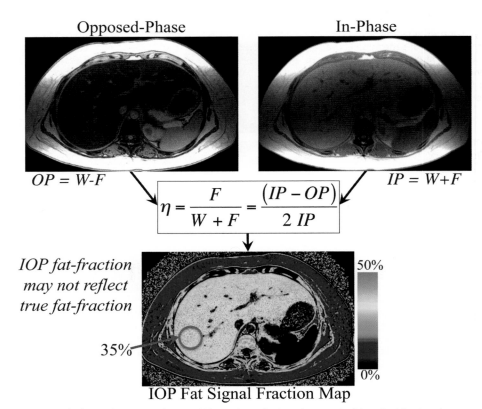

Fig. 2. FSF maps with dynamic range of 0 to 50% can be calculated on a pixel-by-pixel basis using conventional IOP imaging using Equation 2. Such IOP fat-signal maps do not accurately reflect the concentration of fat within the liver unless all confounding factors are addressed.

Opposed-Phase   In-Phase

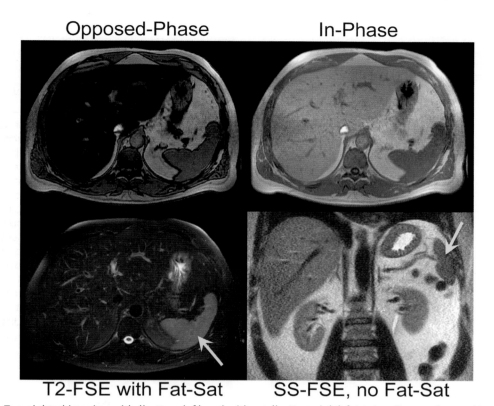

T2-FSE with Fat-Sat   SS-FSE, no Fat-Sat

Fig. 3. T$_2$-weighted imaging with (*bottom left*) and without (*bottom right*) fat saturation can be used to detect steatosis. When no fat saturation is used, the liver is bright compared with the spleen (*arrow*). When steatosis is present, the signal intensity of the liver drops because the fat-saturation pulse suppresses the signal from fat within the liver. Note the relative signal intensity of fat relative to the spleen in the fat-saturated image. IOP imaging (*top row*) demonstrates marked signal dropout on opposed-phase imaging, indicating the presence of steatosis.

fat suppression) where the liver appears relatively bright due to the presence of fat. **Fig. 4** shows a second example, in a patient with geographic fatty sparing seen on IOP imaging. The signal in the region of sparing is relatively bright on the T$_2$- weighted image compared with the surrounding liver. This occurs because the fat-suppression pulse suppresses the fat signal in the surrounding liver, leaving the region of sparing relatively unaffected.

In-Phase   Opposed-Phase   T2-FSE with Fat-Sat

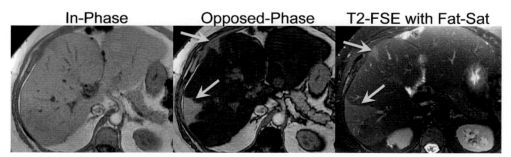

Fig. 4. IOP imaging demonstrates steatosis with regions of geographic sparing (*arrows*) in a patient with NAFLD. Fat-saturated T$_2$-weighted imaging shows diffuse decrease in signal in the liver in regions with fat accumulation. Regions of geographic sparing are unaffected by the fat-saturation pulse and, therefore, have higher relative signal intensity compared with regions of steatotic liver.

Complex Chemical Shift–Based Water-Fat Separation Methods can Measure 0 to 100% Fat

One approach to creating a proton density fat fraction (PDFF) map is to use a chemical shift–based water-fat separation method[68,74,76–78] that separates the signal from water and fat into water-only and fat-only images. Just as in-phase and opposed-phase images are coregistered, separated water and fat images are coregistered and can be recombined

into an FSF map. Fully separating water and fat signals (unlike in magnitude methods, such as IOP imaging), permits achievement of a full dynamic range of 0 to 100% FSF. **Fig. 5** contains a schematic overview of how the separated water and fat signals can be recombined into an FSF map. This particular example was generated using the chemical shift–based water-fat separation method described by Reeder and colleagues.[68,77,78] **Fig. 5** also illustrates how fat fraction maps can be displayed in gray scale or color scale.

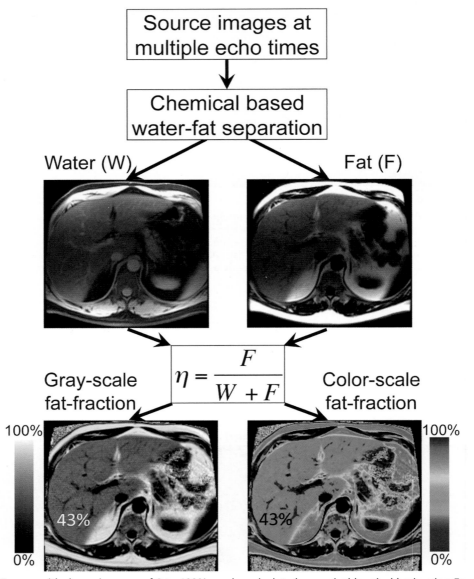

Fig. 5. FSF maps with dynamic range of 0 to 100% can be calculated on a pixel-by-pixel basis using Equation 1, when chemical shift–based water-fat separation methods are used to provide separate water-only and fat-only images. The FSF map does not accurately reflect the concentration of fat within the liver unless all confounding factors are addressed.

As with FSF maps generated with IOP imaging, FSF maps generated with chemical shift–based water-fat separation methods are independent of B_1 coil sensitivities that produce signal variation across an MR image. Just as IOP fat fraction maps do not directly measure the concentration of fat in the liver, neither does the FSF map generated with chemical shift–based water-fat separation methods. In order for the FSF map to reflect the concentration of fat, it must be corrected for confounding factors (discussed later).

Emerging MR Imaging Methods Measure Proton Density Fat Fraction

Technical development in recent years has transformed qualitative MR imaging techniques into rigorous quantitative methods. Accurate separation of the signal from mobile protons in fat from other mobile protons (ie, water) and correction for all factors that influence MR signal intensity permit calculation of PDFF. The authors define PDFF as the density of hydrogen protons attributable to fat, or the fraction of unconfounded proton signal from mobile fat, normalized by the total hydrogen proton density from all mobile proton species. This is equivalent to the ratio of the total unconfounded nuclear magnetic resonance (NMR) visible signal from fat protons, normalized by the total unconfounded NMR visible signal from fat and water protons. PDFF is a standardized, objective magnetic resonance–based measurement of an inherent tissue property. Accurate measurement of PDFF has the potential to provide a platform-independent biomarker unaffected by technical or biologic variability. To provide an accurate estimate of PDFF, the following five confounders must be addressed:

1. T_1 bias
2. T_2^* decay
3. Spectral complexity of fat
4. Noise bias
5. Eddy currents.

T_1 bias

T_1 bias occurs if the image acquisition is T_1 weighted and the two species (water and fat) have different values for T_1. T_1-weighted methods artificially amplify the relative signal of the shorter T_1 proton species (fat), referred to as T_1 bias. Methods to avoid T_1 weighting or correct for differences in T_1 are essential—otherwise, the apparent fat fraction is dependent on sequence parameters, such as repetition time, for example. Use of low flip angle gradient imaging to avoid T_1 weighting is the strategy generally adopted by most emerging

approaches that attempt to avoid T_1-related bias (**Fig. 6**).[71,77-84]

T_2^* decay

Nearly all MR imaging fat-quantification methods acquire images at different echo times, during which T_2^* decay occurs. Even in normal livers, T_2^* decay corrupts estimates of fat content. Bias from T_2^* decay is amplified in iron overload, which can coexist with fat in diffuse liver disease. The confounding effect of T_2^* can be removed by either incorporating T_2^* into the signal model used to separate water and fat, thereby correcting for T_2^* decay as part of the fitting,[78,81,85,86] or by measuring T_2^* separately and correcting for the effects of T_2^*.[71,80,87] **Fig. 7** demonstrates the importance of T_2^* correction in a patient with steatosis before and after the injection of superparamagnetic iron oxide (SPIO) particles that accumulate in the Kupffer cells in the liver, simulating hemosiderosis. Without the use of T_2^* correction, the PDFF is underestimated by the presence of liver iron.

Spectral complexity of fat

At clinical magnetic field strengths, fat has at least six distinct spectral peaks at different resonance frequencies. Accurate quantification should account for proton signal from all fat peaks. **Fig. 8** shows a spectrum of pure fat (vegetable oil) measured at 3.0T, demonstrating that a considerable fraction of signal from fat hydrogen protons is found at peaks remote from the main methylene ($-CH_2-$) fat peak (at -434 Hz). At least two of the fat peaks lie close to the water resonance and would not be suppressed with fat-saturation methods and would be incorrectly mapped to water signal in chemical shift–based fat-water imaging methods that (incorrectly) model fat as a single resonance peak. In **Fig. 8**, the chemical shifts of the fat peaks relative to water are shown in Hertz for 3.0T and in parts per million, based on the work of Hamilton and colleagues[88] In this work, Hamilton also determined the relative amplitudes of the fat peaks from human liver fat, which are relatively constant across large groups of patients. From this work, the relative amplitudes and frequencies (at 3.0T) of these peaks are approximately 4.7% (77 Hz), 3.9% (-64 Hz), 0.6% (-249 Hz), 12.0% (-332 Hz), 70.0% (-434 Hz), 8.8% (-485 Hz). The amplitudes are the same at 1.5T, although the resonance frequencies relative to water scale linearly with field strength.

Conventional IOP imaging and conventional chemical shift–based water-fat separation methods assume that fat has a single NMR peak, leading to inadvertent misidentification of some signal from fat as arising from water. This leads

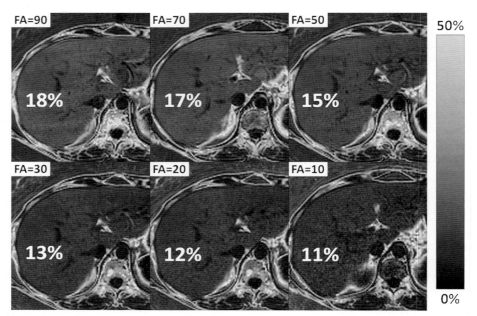

Fig. 6. Differences in T_1 between water and fat lead to bias if the image acquisition is T_1 weighted. Most MR imaging methods used to acquire fat raction images use gradient-echo methods, which are T_1 weighted using typical flip angles. Because the T_1 of fat is shorter than the water signal in the liver, the use of T_1-weighted imaging results in an apparent fat fraction greater than the true fat fraction. Reducing the flip angle can minimize T_1 bias, although at a cost of reduced SNR performance. It is important to avoid T_1 bias—otherwise, the apparent fat fraction depends on image parameters, such as repetition time and flip angle, and it is difficult to compare results using different protocols or different scanners. This example of MRI-M demonstrates how reducing the flip angle reduces the T_1 bias (true PDFF is approximately 11%), although it also degrades SNR performance.

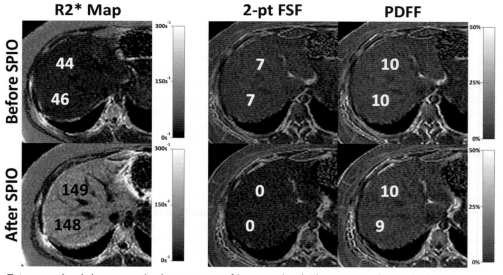

Fig. 7. T_2^* correction is important in the presence of iron overload. The top row shows the PDFF map measured using the MRI-M method (*right*) before (*top row*) and after (*bottom row*) the injection of intravenous SPIOs (Feridex, Bayer Healthcare Pharmaceuticals, Wayne, NJ, USA). SPIOs rapidly accumulate in the Kupffer cells within the liver and simulate iron overload from hemosiderosis and serve as an excellent model of iron overload in the liver. The R_2^* maps on the left demonstrate the increase in R_2^* from approximately 45 s^{-1} ($T_2^* = 22$ ms) to 148 s^{-1} ($T_2^* = 6.8$ ms) resulting from the SPIOs. No change in the PDFF is seen using the MRI-M method, which uses T_2^* correction, compared with the FSF measured with 2-point IOP imaging (see Equation 2). Large changes in the apparent fat fraction are seen with 2-point IOP imaging, even though the true fat concentration in the liver is identical, after the injection of SPIOs.

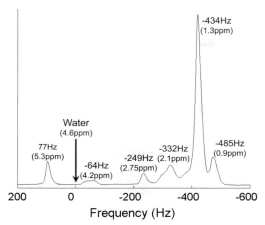

Fig. 8. Single-voxel MR spectrum of vegetable oil at 3.0T demonstrates the spectral complexity of fat. Triglycerides, such as those in human liver fat, have at least 6 identifiable peaks at clinical field strengths, similar to those shown in this figure. Methods, such as IOP imaging and chemical shift–based water-fat separation methods that model fat as a single NMR peak at −434 Hz (−217 Hz at 1.5T), inaccurately estimate the concentration of fat within tissue if all peaks are not included in signal measurements. The frequencies that are shown present the chemical shifts of the different peaks at 3.0T relative to water.

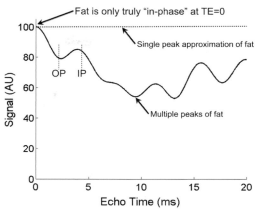

Fig. 9. Fat is only truly in-phase when TE = 0 or at a spin echo. This occurs because fat has multiple spectral peaks that interfere with one another in a complex pattern with increasing TE. This effect is shown in a simulation of the signal from pure fat, in the absence of T_2^* decay, and at 1.5T. Large drops in signal, up to 50%, occur (near TE = 10 ms) because of this interference. Therefore, methods that attempt to measure fat concentration must consider the spectral complexity of fat. In addition, methods that attempt to measure T_2^* decay in the presence of fat must also consider fat's spectral complexity. The interference of fat with itself leads to highly inaccurate measurements of T_2^*. As a result, the terminology, "in-phase" and "opposed-phase", loses its meaning because of the spectral complexity of fat. Conventional in-phase (IP) and opposed-phase (OP) echo times are shown for reference.

to significant quantification errors.[82,83] To account for the additional peaks of fat, spectral modeling of fat can easily be incorporated, if the frequency and relative amplitudes of the six fat peaks are known a priori. This strategy, referred to as spectral modeling, is based on the biochemical structure of human liver triglycerides and has been developed independently by Bydder and colleagues[81] and Yu and colleagues[78] based on an algorithm for chemical shift species separation for hyperpolarized ^{13}C imaging.[89]

Fig. 9 demonstrates the effects of multiple fat peaks with a simulation of the signal evolution that occurs in pure fat at 1.5T, ignoring T_2^* decay. A flat line would be expected in pure fat if it had a single NMR peak. In reality, the multiple peaks of fat destructively interfere with one another, attenuating the signal, even in pure fat. For this reason, except at TE = 0 or at a spin echo, fat is never in phase with itself. Considering the multiple peaks of fat, the terms, "in-phase" and "opposed-phase", lose their meaning, because these terms can only be used when referring to the relative phase of two NMR species (water and single-peak fat, for example). For historical reasons, this article uses this terminology in the context of the relative phase between water and the main methylene peak (−CH$_2$−) of fat at −217 Hz (−434 Hz) at 1.5T (3.0T).

Fig. 10 demonstrates the combined effects of T_2^* decay and spectral complexity of fat in a simulation for a fat-water mixture with 40% fat at 1.5T. The plot includes the expected signal behavior when (1) fat is approximated as a single NMR peak and no T_2^* decay, and when fat is modeled with multiple peaks with (2) no T_2^* decay; (3) $T_2^* =$ 25 ms (normal[90]); and (4) $T_2^* =$ 10 ms (simulating coexisting iron overload). Calculating the apparent fat fraction using the IOP fat fraction calculation (Equation 2) for these four cases demonstrates an apparent fat fraction of 40% (as expected), 35%, 33%, and 31%, respectively. This simulation demonstrates that spectral complexity of fat and T_2^* (even normal values of T_2^*) results in large discrepancies between the true fat fraction and the apparent fat fraction measured with conventional IOP imaging. When fat fractions are very low, the presence of T_2^* decay can even lead to apparent fat fractions that are negative, which have no physical meaning. The influence of T_2^* decay and spectral complexity of fat has been described in detail in phantom experiments reported recently by Hines and colleagues.[75] In summary, accurate quantification of fat is not

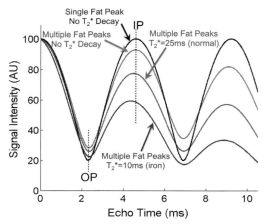

Fig. 10. $T_2{}^*$ decay and the spectral complexity of fat corrupt the ability of IOP imaging to quantify fat. Four simulations are shown for 40% fat at 1.5T, plotting: (1) "ideal" model of water and fat with single peak model and no $T_2{}^*$ decay (*black*); (2) complex spectrum of fat with no $T_2{}^*$ decay (*red*); (3) complex spectrum of fat with normal $T_2{}^*$ decay (= 25 ms)[90] (*green*); and (4) complex spectrum of fat with $T_2{}^* = 10$ ms (*blue*); to simulate iron overload. These plots indicate very large deviations from the expected signal pattern (*black curve*), demonstrating explicitly how $T_2{}^*$ decay and the spectral complexity of fat corrupt the ability of IOP imaging to quantify fat. Erroneous estimates of fat fraction occur without considering these important confounding factors.

possible with conventional IOP imaging unless $T_2{}^*$ decay and spectral complexity of fat are considered.

Noise bias
Recombination of separated water and fat images into a fat fraction image can cause bias at low fat fractions when using chemical shift–based water-fat separation methods. Noise bias occurs if magnitude water and fat images are recombined, because areas of low signal (eg, fat signal from a liver with no fat) have only positive noise after the magnitude operation. Noise bias is relevant to methods that fully separate water and fat signals before magnitude reconstruction and can be avoided using phase-constrained or magnitude discrimination methods developed by Liu and colleagues.[77] Methods that create fat fraction maps from IOP images (see Equation 2) are more immune to these effects except near fat fractions of 50% when the signal intensity of opposed-phase images approaches zero and noise bias has an impact on fat fraction calculations. Because low fat fractions (near zero) are more clinically relevant, noise bias effects are more important in chemical shift–based water-fat separation methods.

Eddy currents
Rapidly switching gradients lead to phase shifts on complex images acquired at different echo times. These phase shifts can corrupt estimates of fat fraction. Eddy currents affect methods that use phase information in images acquired at different echo times to quantify fat, such as chemical shift–based water-fat separation methods. Correction for eddy current can be performed using a hybrid complex–magnitude approach recently reported by Yu and colleagues[91] Magnitude-based methods, including conventional IOP imaging and other magnitude-based methods,[70,71,79–82,86,87,92–101] discard all phase information and should be immune to the effects of eddy currents.

Magnetic field strength is another potential confounding factor, because it is well known that T_1 and $T_2{}^*$ change with field strength and that the chemical shift of the fat peaks scales linearly with field strength. Therefore, if low flip angles are used to avoid T_1 bias and $T_2{}^*$ correction is performed with spectral modeling accounting for changes in field strength, then field strength is not expected to influence the measurement of fat fraction.

Quantitative Fat Fraction Imaging Methods

After correction for the five confounding factors, the FSF and PDFF are equivalent. In recent years, several research groups have proposed advanced MR imaging techniques that address one or more of these confounding factors (as shown in **Table 1**).[68,70,71,74,76–87,91–101] For simplification, the corrected fat quantification techniques may be separated into two categories: (1) magnitude based and (2) complex based.

Magnitude based
The magnitude-based technique is simpler to implement and uses two or more (6 echo times) IOP images or magnitude images (ie, discards phase information).[70,71,79–82,86,87,92–101] These methods provide estimates of fat fraction with a dynamic range of 0 to 50% fat signal, which is probably sufficient to estimate the range of liver fat concentrations encountered clinically, although it may not capture all individuals. Moreover, it does not measure fat in fat-dominant tissues, such as adipose tissue or marrow. Magnitude-based methods still require approaches that compensate or correct for T_1, $T_2{}^*$, and the spectral complexity of fat.

Complex based
The complex-based technique uses both magnitude and phase information from three or more images, acquired at echo times appropriate for

Table 1
Overview of gradient-echo–based MR imaging techniques to assess liver fat

	MR Imaging Technique	Confounders Addressed					Output	Refs
		T_1	T_2*	Fat Spectrum	Noise Bias	Eddy Currents		
Magnitude based	T_1w IOP (conventional MR imaging)	No	No	No	N/A	N/A	FSF	70,92–101
	Low-FA IOP	✓	No	No			T_1-independent FSF	79
	T_1w multiecho	No	✓	No			T_2*-corrected FSF	86,105
	Low-FA multiacquisition IOP	✓	✓	No			T_1-independent, T_2*-corrected FSF	71
		✓	✓	No				80
	Low-FA multiecho with T_2* correction and spectral modeling (MRI-M)	✓	✓	✓			PFDD	81,82
Complex based	T_1w triple echo	No	No	No	No	No	FSF	68,74,76
	Low-FA triple echo	✓	No	No	✓	No	T_1-independent, noise bias–corrected FSF	77
	Low-FA multiecho	✓	✓	No	✓	No	T_1-independent, T_2*-corrected FSF	85
	Low-FA triple echo with spectral modeling	✓	No	✓	✓	No	T_1-independent, noise bias–corrected, spectrally modeled FSF	83
	Low-FA multiecho with T_2* correction, spectral modeling, and eddy current correction (MRI-C)	✓	✓	✓	✓	✓	PFDD	78,84,91

Two methods, the MRI-M method, refined at UCSD, and the MRI-C method, refined at UW, correct for all confounding factors known to corrupt estimates of PDFF. MRI-M and MRI-C are the only methods, to the authors' knowledge, able to measure PDFF—these two methods that be validated in this proposal. Note that correction for eddy currents and noise bias are not required for magnitude-based methods.

Abbreviations: FA, flip angle; N/A, not applicable; T_1w, T_1-weighted; UCSD, University of California, San Diego; UW, University of Wisconsin.

more accurate separation of water and fat signals (based on the identification of three fat peaks rather than the commonly used single dominant fat peak to determine separation of water and fat signals).[68,74,76−78,83−85,91] These methods provide estimates of fat fraction with a dynamic range of 0 to 100%. Although a dynamic range of 0 to 100% is important for imaging adipose tissue,[102] it may be not necessary for quantifying the hepatic PDFF, which infrequently exceeds 50%. In addition to correction for T_1, T_2^*, and the spectral complexity of fat, complex-based MR imaging methods also require correction for noise bias and eddy currents.

As shown in **Table 1**, there are currently only two published methods that correct for all confounding factors; therefore, they are the only methods that can measure PDFF. These methods include a magnitude-based method, described by Bydder and colleagues,[81,82] and the complex-based techniques, described by Reeder and colleagues.[68,77,78,83−85,91] For convenience, this article refers to the magnitude-based method of Bydder and colleagues as MRI-M and the complex-based method of Reeder and colleagues as MRI-C. Most of the examples discussed in this article were acquired using MRI-C, MRI-M, or both, because these are the two methods used at the authors' institutions.

Of the two approaches, the magnitude-based approach may be simpler to implement but is not a comprehensive solution because it provides a limited dynamic range from 0 to 50%. Although a dynamic range of 0 to 50% captures the vast majority of individuals with liver fat, it may not capture all individuals. Moreover, it does not measure fat in fat-dominant tissues, such as adipose tissue or marrow. The complex-based approach is a general solution that holds the potential to quantify fat in all fat depots in the human body.

Fig. 11 shows a comparison of MRI-C and MRI-M at 3.0T, diagramming the source images needed for each method to reconstruct fat fraction images. **Figs. 12** and **13** show additional examples of MRI-C and MRI-M in the same patients. As shown, both MRI-M and MRI-C generate maps that display PDFF of every pixel on the image. The range of PDFF values for MRI-M is 0 to 50% and for MRI-C is 0 to 100%. These images were acquired using fundamentally different techniques, yet PDFF estimates in the liver are virtually identical. These figures also demonstrate the heterogeneity of fat distribution that can occur over the liver, underscoring the need for a biomarker that samples fat over the entire liver, unlike biopsy.

Magnetic field strength is another potential confounding factor that was not included in list of confounding factors discussed previously. If all other

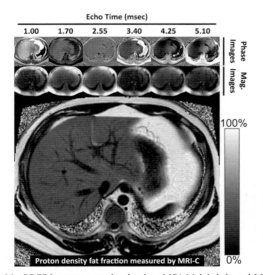

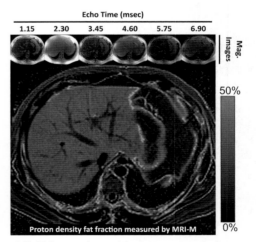

Fig. 11. PDFF images acquired using MRI-M (*right*) and MRI-C (*left*) in a patient with severe steatosis demonstrate excellent agreement both qualitatively and quantitatively for fat within the liver. Both methods generate PDFF images using fundamentally different approaches: MRI-M uses magnitude source images acquired at six different echo times to generate a PDFF image with dynamic range of 0 to 50%, which spans the relevant dynamic range of hepatic fat content encountered clinically. MRI-C uses complex (magnitude and phase) source images acquired at six echo times to generate a PDFF image with dynamic range of 0 to 100%. Source magnitude images for MRI-M and source complex images for MRI-C are shown along the top. Notice that adipose tissue outside the liver exceeds the 0 to 50% PDFF dynamic range of MRI-M and so appears dark on the corresponding PDFF map.

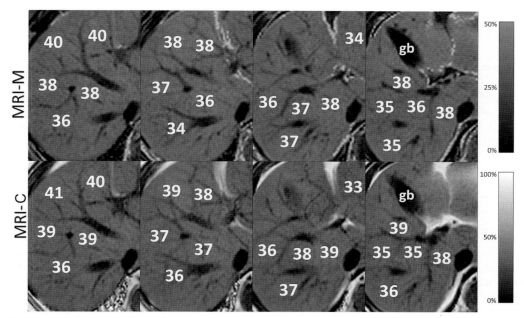

Fig. 12. Magnified MRI-M (*top row*) and MRI-C (*bottom row*) from four adjacent slices demonstrate excellent qualitative agreement in the appearance and quantitative agreement in PDFF measurements, in a patient with fatty liver. MRI-M and MRI-C images acquired in the same patient at 3T. gb, gall bladder.

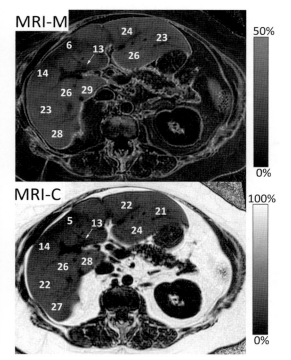

Fig. 13. MRI-M (*top*) and MRI-C (*bottom*) PDFF images acquired at 3T in a patient with heterogeneous liver fat show excellent qualitative agreement and quantitative agreement. A wide range of PDFF values from approximately 5% to 29% also underscores the advantages of volumetric imaging methods that assess the entire liver, unlike MRS or biopsy.

confounding factors (T_1, T_2*, and so forth) are addressed, however, PDFF measurements should be field strength independent. **Fig. 14** shows an example of MRI-C and MRI-M in the same patient at both 1.5T and 3.0T showing excellent agreement in the measurement of PDFF in all cases.

Performance and Usefulness of Emerging Fat Quantification Imaging Methods

The MRI-C and MRI-M methods have demonstrated excellent correlation and agreement with known fat fractions in phantom experiments,[75,81] animal experiments,[103] and clinical studies comparing these methods with single-voxel MRS. Yokoo and colleagues[82] reported excellent agreement between PDFF measured with MRI-M compared with MRS in 110 patients scanned at 1.5T, demonstrating excellent correlation (slope = 0.98; CI, 0.92, 1.04 and intercept = 0.91%; CI −0.18%, 1.99%). In addition, Meisamy and colleagues[84] had similar results in 54 patients scanned at 1.5T using MRI-C, also demonstrating excellent agreement (correlation of r^2 = 0.99, slope = 1.00 ± 0.01%, and intercept = 0.2% ± 0.1%). More recently Yokoo and colleagues[104] demonstrated similar results at 3.0T in a large patient cohort.

Methods such as these also hold great potential for the detection of steatosis using a predetermined fat fraction threshold to classify patients

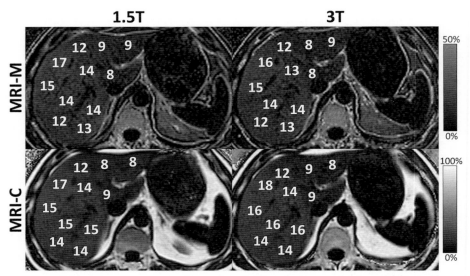

Fig. 14. Field strength is not an independent confounding factor for quantification of fat. Although T_1 and T_2^* change with field strength as well as the chemical shift, correction for these confounding factors shows no change in PDFF measured between 1.5T and 3T using either MRI-C or MRI-M. This demonstrates that field strength is not a factor that affects fat fraction, independently.

as having clinically significant steatosis. Although the exact threshold between normal and abnormal is not fully understood, a commonly used fat fraction threshold of 5.56% is commonly used to distinguish normal from abnormal. This threshold is based on a large MRS study performed by Szczepaniak and colleagues[14] in 2349 participants of the Dallas Heart Study. The 95th percentile

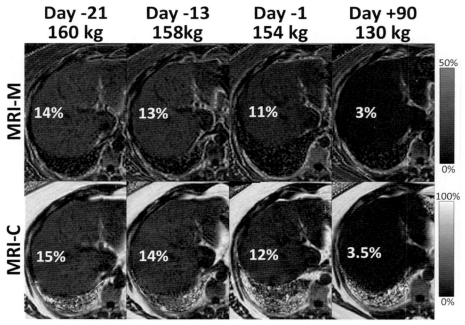

Fig. 15. Serial MR imaging examinations can be used to demonstrate meaningful changes in liver fat during weight loss in an obese patient who underwent LAGB. In this patient, MRI-M and MRI-C PDFF maps obtained 21 days, 13 days, and 1 day before LAGB and 90 days after LAGB are shown. A modest decrease in PDFF was seen during a very low calorie liquid diet, and near complete resolution of liver fat was seen 3 months after LAGB. In this patient, a 30-kg weight loss resulted in resolution of liver fat to normal levels.

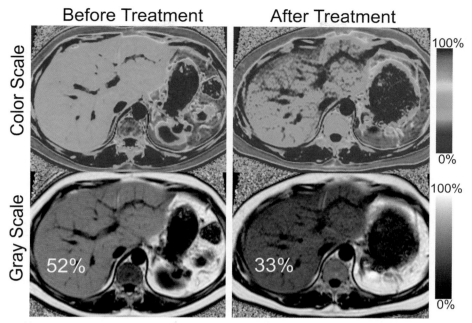

Fig. 16. Serial liver MR imaging examinations can be used to demonstrate changes in liver fat. Serial PDFF maps obtained with MRI-C were acquired in a 41-year-old man with insulin resistance and recalcitrant hypertriglyceridemia undergoing plasmapheresis and on multiple drugs to lower serum triglycerides. Follow-up MR imaging demonstrates a large decrease in the concentration of fat (from 52% to 33%) and marked decrease in the size of the liver. This example demonstrates that fat fractions greater than 50% occur and also compares the use of gray-scale and color-scale PDFF maps.

cutoff of 5.56% fat fraction was determined from a subset of 345 patients with no identifiable risk factors for steatosis. Using this threshold, both MRI-M and MRI-C have accuracies close to 100% for the detection of steatosis.[82,84]

Quantitative fat fraction measurements can also be used to track liver fat concentration during treatment monitoring. For example, **Fig. 15** shows MRI-C and MRI-M PDFF maps in an obese patient undergoing a very low calorie liquid diet for 2 weeks followed by LAGB (at day 0). A marked drop in PDFF from approximately 14% to 3% can be seen during the period of weight loss, demonstrating how quantitative MR imaging methods can monitor changes in liver fat concentration.

Quantitative fat measurements can also be performed during pharmacologic therapy. **Fig. 16** shows MRI-C fat fraction maps in a patient with recalcitrant hypertriglyceridemia, treated aggressively with lipid-lowering agents and plasmapheresis. A marked drop in fat fraction from 52% to 33% can be demonstrated after approximately 4 months of therapy. These findings correlate with a drop in triglycerides from 815 to 448 during this period. In addition, the size of the liver has also decreased, a feature that cannot be assessed

with biopsy. This figure also demonstrates that fat fractions greater than 50% can occur (albeit uncommon) and also compares the usefulness of display fat fraction maps in color scale or gray scale. Changes in fat fraction may be visually more apparent on the color-scale images.

SUMMARY

The use of MR imaging as a quantitative biomarker of intracellular liver fat has shown tremendous progress in recent years and holds great promise for providing cost-effective, accessible, and accurate evaluation of diffuse liver disease. The authors anticipate widespread clinical use of fat quantification methods within 1 to 3 years and perhaps 3 to 5 years for validated fat quantification methods. Given the rising epidemic of liver disease, especially NAFLD, and increasing recognition of their role in systemic diseases, the need for such methods is greater than ever. Despite the great promise these methods offer, continued technical development and validation are still required as these methods mature into well-accepted biomarkers of liver disease.

REFERENCES

1. Adams LA, Lymp JF, St Sauver J, et al. The natural history of nonalcoholic fatty liver disease: a population-based cohort study. Gastroenterology 2005; 129(1):113–21.
2. Adams LA, Waters OR, Knuiman MW, et al. NAFLD as a risk factor for the development of diabetes and the metabolic syndrome: an eleven-year follow-up study. Am J Gastroenterol 2009;104(4):861–7.
3. Dunn W, Xu R, Wingard DL, et al. Suspected nonalcoholic fatty liver disease and mortality risk in a population-based cohort study. Am J Gastroenterol 2008;103(9):2263–71.
4. Fabbrini E, deHaseth D, Deivanayagam S, et al. Alterations in fatty acid kinetics in obese adolescents with increased intrahepatic triglyceride content. Obesity (Silver Spring) 2009;17(1):25–9.
5. Korenblat KM, Fabbrini E, Mohammed BS, et al. Liver, muscle, and adipose tissue insulin action is directly related to intrahepatic triglyceride content in obese subjects. Gastroenterology 2008;134(5): 1369–75.
6. Lok AS, Everhart JE, Chung RT, et al. Evolution of hepatic steatosis in patients with advanced hepatitis C: results from the hepatitis C antiviral long-term treatment against cirrhosis (HALT-C) trial. Hepatology 2009;49(6):1828–37.
7. Lok AS, Everhart JE, Chung RT, et al. Hepatic steatosis in hepatitis C: comparison of diabetic and nondiabetic patients in the hepatitis C antiviral long-term treatment against cirrhosis trial. Clin Gastroenterol Hepatol 2007;5(2):245–54.
8. Matteoni CA, Younossi ZM, Gramlich T, et al. Nonalcoholic fatty liver disease: a spectrum of clinical and pathological severity. Gastroenterology 1999; 116(6):1413–9.
9. Rubinstein E, Lavine JE, Schwimmer JB. Hepatic, cardiovascular, and endocrine outcomes of the histological subphenotypes of nonalcoholic fatty liver disease. Semin Liver Dis 2008;28(4):380–5.
10. Sanyal AJ, Banas C, Sargeant C, et al. Similarities and differences in outcomes of cirrhosis due to nonalcoholic steatohepatitis and hepatitis C. Hepatology 2006;43(4):682–9.
11. Ekstedt M, Franzen LE, Mathiesen UL, et al. Long-term follow-up of patients with NAFLD and elevated liver enzymes. Hepatology 2006;44(4):865–73.
12. Clark JM, Diehl AM. Defining nonalcoholic fatty liver disease: implications for epidemiologic studies. Gastroenterology 2003;124(1):248–50.
13. Ioannou GN. Development and validation of a model predicting graft survival after liver transplantation. Liver Transpl 2006;12(11):1594–606.
14. Szczepaniak LS, Nurenberg P, Leonard D, et al. Magnetic resonance spectroscopy to measure hepatic triglyceride content: prevalence of hepatic steatosis in the general population. Am J Physiol Endocrinol Metab 2005;288(2):E462–8.
15. Ludwig J, Viggiano T, McGill DB, et al. Nonalcoholic steatohepatitis: Mayo Clinic experience with a hitherto unnamed disease. Mayo Clin Proc 1980;55:434–8.
16. Angulo P, Keach JC, Batts KP, et al. Independent predictors of liver fibrosis in patients with nonalcoholic steatohepatitis. Hepatology 1999;30(6): 1356–62.
17. Gramlich T, Kleiner DE, McCullough AJ, et al. Pathologic features associated with fibrosis in nonalcoholic fatty liver disease. Hum Pathol 2004;35(2): 196–9.
18. Angelico M. Donor liver steatosis and graft selection for liver transplantation: a short review. Eur Rev Med Pharmacol Sci 2005;9(5):295–7.
19. Ploeg RJ, D'Alessandro AM, Knechtle SJ, et al. Risk factors for primary dysfunction after liver transplantation—a multivariate analysis. Transplantation 1993;55(4):807–13.
20. Yoong KF, Gunson BK, Neil DA, et al. Impact of donor liver microvesicular steatosis on the outcome of liver retransplantation. Transplant Proc 1999; 31(1–2):550–1.
21. Guzman G, Brunt EM, Petrovic LM, et al. Does nonalcoholic fatty liver disease predispose patients to hepatocellular carcinoma in the absence of cirrhosis? Arch Pathol Lab Med 2008;132(11):1761–6.
22. Schindhelm RK, Diamant M, Heine RJ. Nonalcoholic fatty liver disease and cardiovascular disease risk. Curr Diab Rep 2007;7(3):181–7.
23. Targher G, Arcaro G. Non-alcoholic fatty liver disease and increased risk of cardiovascular disease. Atherosclerosis 2007;191(2):235–40.
24. Heath ML, Kow L, Slavotinek JP, et al. Abdominal adiposity and liver fat content 3 and 12 months after gastric banding surgery. Metabolism 2009; 58(6):753–8.
25. Phillips ML, Boase S, Wahlroos S, et al. Associates of change in liver fat content in the morbidly obese after laparoscopic gastric banding surgery. Diabetes Obes Metab 2008;10(8):661–7.
26. Lin HZ, Yang SQ, Chuckaree C, et al. Metformin reverses fatty liver disease in obese, leptin-deficient mice. Nat Med 2000;6(9):998–1003.
27. Bugianesi E, Gentilcore E, Manini R, et al. A randomized controlled trial of metformin versus vitamin E or prescriptive diet in nonalcoholic fatty liver disease. Am J Gastroenterol 2005;100(5): 1082–90.
28. Promrat K, Lutchman G, Uwaifo GI, et al. A pilot study of pioglitazone treatment for nonalcoholic steatohepatitis. Hepatology 2004;39(1):188–96.
29. Sanyal AJ, Mofrad PS, Contos MJ, et al. A pilot study of vitamin E versus vitamin E and pioglitazone for the treatment of nonalcoholic

steatohepatitis. Clin Gastroenterol Hepatol 2004; 2(12):1107–15.

30. Chalasani NP, Sanyal AJ, Kowdley KV, et al. Pioglitazone versus vitamin E versus placebo for the treatment of non-diabetic patients with non-alcoholic steatohepatitis: PIVENS trial design. Contemp Clin Trials 2009;30(1):88–96.

31. Lavine JE, Schwimmer JB, Molleston JP, et al. Treatment of nonalcoholic fatty liver disease in children: TONIC trial design. Contemp Clin Trials 2010; 31(1):62–70.

32. Busuttil RW, Tanaka K. The utility of marginal donors in liver transplantation. Liver Transpl 2003; 9(7):651–63.

33. Sanyal AJ. AGA technical review on nonalcoholic fatty liver disease. Gastroenterology 2002;123(5): 1705–25.

34. Brunt EM, Janney CG, Di Bisceglie AM, et al. Nonalcoholic steatohepatitis: a proposal for grading and staging the histological lesions. Am J Gastroenterol 1999;94(9):2467–74.

35. Kleiner DE, Brunt EM, Van Natta M, et al. Design and validation of a histological scoring system for nonalcoholic fatty liver disease. Hepatology 2005; 41(6):1313–21.

36. Bedossa P, Poynard T. An algorithm for the grading of activity in chronic hepatitis C. The METAVIR Cooperative Study Group. Hepatology 1996; 24(2):289–93.

37. Ratziu V, Charlotte F, Heurtier A, et al. Sampling variability of liver biopsy in nonalcoholic fatty liver disease. Gastroenterology 2005;128(7):1898–906.

38. Emond MJ, Bronner MP, Carlson TH, et al. Quantitative study of the variability of hepatic iron concentrations. Clin Chem 1999;45(3):340–6.

39. Villeneuve JP, Bilodeau M, Lepage R, et al. Variability in hepatic iron concentration measurement from needle-biopsy specimens. J Hepatol 1996; 25(2):172–7.

40. Abdi W, Millan JC, Mezey E. Sampling variability on percutaneous liver biopsy. Arch Intern Med 1979; 139(6):667–9.

41. Baunsgaard P, Sanchez GC, Lundborg CJ. The variation of pathological changes in the liver evaluated by double biopsies. Acta Pathol Microbiol Scand Am 1979;87(1):51–7.

42. Bedossa P, Dargere D, Paradis V. Sampling variability of liver fibrosis in chronic hepatitis C. Hepatology 2003;38(6):1449–57.

43. Labayle D, Chaput JC, Albuisson F, et al. [Comparison of the histological lesions in tissue specimens taken from the right and left lobe of the liver in alcoholic liver disease (author's transl)]. Gastroenterol Clin Biol 1979;3(3):235–40 [in French].

44. Maharaj B, Maharaj RJ, Leary WP, et al. Sampling variability and its influence on the diagnostic yield

of percutaneous needle biopsy of the liver. Lancet 1986;1(8480):523–5.

45. Olsson R, Hagerstrand I, Broome U, et al. Sampling variability of percutaneous liver biopsy in primary sclerosing cholangitis. J Clin Pathol 1995;48(10):933–5.

46. Regev A, Berho M, Jeffers LJ, et al. Sampling error and intraobserver variation in liver biopsy in patients with chronic HCV infection. Am J Gastroenterol 2002;97(10):2614–8.

47. Vuppalanchi R, Unalp A, Van Natta ML, et al. Effects of liver biopsy sample length and number of readings on sampling variability in nonalcoholic Fatty liver disease. Clin Gastroenterol Hepatol 2009;7(4):481–6.

48. Bravo A, Sheth S, Chopra S. Liver Biopsy. N Engl J Med 2001;344(7):495–500.

49. Charatcharoenwitthaya P, Lindor KD. Role of radiologic modalities in the management of non-alcoholic steatohepatitis. Clin Liver Dis 2007;11(1):37–54, viii.

50. Mishra P, Younossi ZM. Abdominal ultrasound for diagnosis of nonalcoholic fatty liver disease (NAFLD). Am J Gastroenterol 2007;102(12):2716–7.

51. Saadeh S, Younossi ZM, Remer EM, et al. The utility of radiological imaging in nonalcoholic fatty liver disease. Gastroenterology 2002;123(3): 745–50.

52. Graif M, Yanuka M, Baraz M, et al. Quantitative estimation of attenuation in ultrasound video images: correlation with histology in diffuse liver disease. Invest Radiol 2000;35(5):319–24.

53. Mottin CC, Moretto M, Padoin AV, et al. The role of ultrasound in the diagnosis of hepatic steatosis in morbidly obese patients. Obes Surg 2004;14(5): 635–7.

54. Kodama Y, Ng CS, Wu TT, et al. Comparison of CT methods for determining the fat content of the liver. AJR Am J Roentgenol 2007;188(5):1307–12.

55. Lee SW, Park SH, Kim KW, et al. Unenhanced CT for assessment of macrovesicular hepatic steatosis in living liver donors: comparison of visual grading with liver attenuation index. Radiology 2007;244(2): 479–85.

56. Limanond P, Raman SS, Lassman C, et al. Macrovesicular hepatic steatosis in living related liver donors: correlation between CT and histologic findings. Radiology 2004;230(1):276–80.

57. Fazel R, Krumholz HM, Wang Y, et al. Exposure to low-dose ionizing radiation from medical imaging procedures. N Engl J Med 2009;361(9): 849–57.

58. Longo R, Pollesello P, Ricci C, et al. Proton MR spectroscopy in quantitative in vivo determination of fat content in human liver steatosis. J Magn Reson Imaging 1995;5(3):281–5.

59. Longo R, Ricci C, Masutti F, et al. Fatty infiltration of the liver. Quantification by 1H localized magnetic resonance spectroscopy and comparison with

computed tomography. Invest Radiol 1993;28(4): 297–302.

60. Thomsen C, Becker U, Winkler K, et al. Quantification of liver fat using magnetic resonance spectroscopy. Magn Reson Imaging 1994;12(3):487–95.

61. Szczepaniak LS, Babcock EE, Schick F, et al. Measurement of intracellular triglyceride stores by H spectroscopy: validation in vivo. Am J Physiol 1999;276(5 Pt 1):E977–89.

62. Dixon WT. Simple proton spectroscopic imaging. Radiology 1984;153(1):189–94.

63. Hamer OW, Aguirre DA, Casola G, et al. Fatty liver: imaging patterns and pitfalls. Radiographics 2006; 26(6):1637–53.

64. Glover GH, Schneider E. Three-point Dixon technique for true water/fat decomposition with B0 inhomogeneity correction. Magn Reson Med 1991;18(2):371–83.

65. Xiang Q, An L. Water-fat imaging with direct phase encoding. J Magn Reson Imaging 1997;7:1002–15.

66. Ma J. Breath-hold water and fat imaging using a dual-echo two-point Dixon technique with an efficient and robust phase-correction algorithm. Magn Reson Med 2004;52(2):415–9.

67. Reeder SB, Pineda AR, Wen Z, et al. Iterative decomposition of water and fat with echo asymmetry and least-squares estimation (IDEAL): application with fast spin-echo imaging. Magn Reson Med 2005;54(3):636–44.

68. Reeder SB, McKenzie CA, Pineda AR, et al. Water-fat separation with IDEAL gradient-echo imaging. J Magn Reson Imaging 2007;25(3):644–52.

69. Hernando D, Haldar JP, Sutton BP, et al. Joint estimation of water/fat images and field inhomogeneity map. Magn Reson Med 2008;59(3): 571–80.

70. Qayyum A, Goh JS, Kakar S, et al. Accuracy of liver fat quantification at MR imaging: comparison of out-of-phase gradient-echo and fat-saturated fast spin-echo techniques—initial experience. Radiology 2005;237(2):507–11.

71. Hussain HK, Chenevert TL, Londy FJ, et al. Hepatic fat fraction: MR imaging for quantitative measurement and display—early experience. Radiology 2005;237(3):1048–55.

72. Martin J, Sentis M, Puig J, et al. Comparison of in-phase and opposed-phase GRE and conventional SE MR pulse sequences in T1-weighted imaging of liver lesions. J Comput Assist Tomogr 1996;20(6):890–7.

73. Siegelman ES, Rosen MA. Imaging of hepatic steatosis. Semin Liver Dis 2001;21(1):71–80.

74. Kim H, Taksali SE, Dufour S, et al. Comparative MR study of hepatic fat quantification using single-voxel proton spectroscopy, two-point dixon and three-point IDEAL. Magn Reson Med 2008;59(3): 521–7.

75. Hines CD, Yu H, Shimakawa A, et al. T1 independent, T2* corrected MRI with accurate spectral modeling for quantification of fat: validation in a fat-water-SPIO phantom. J Magn Reson Imaging 2009;30(5):1215–22.

76. Kovanlikaya A, Guclu C, Desai C, et al. Fat quantification using three-point dixon technique: in vitro validation. Acad Radiol 2005;12(5):636–9.

77. Liu CY, McKenzie CA, Yu H, et al. Fat quantification with IDEAL gradient echo imaging: correction of bias from T(1) and noise. Magn Reson Med 2007; 58(2):354–64.

78. Yu H, Shimakawa A, McKenzie CA, et al. Multiecho water-fat separation and simultaneous R2* estimation with multifrequency fat spectrum modeling. Magn Reson Med 2008;60(5):1122–34.

79. Fishbein MH, Gardner KG, Potter CJ, et al. Introduction of fast MR imaging in the assessment of hepatic steatosis. Magn Reson Imaging 1997; 15(3):287–93.

80. Guiu B, Petit JM, Loffroy R, et al. Quantification of liver fat content: comparison of triple-echo chemical shift gradient-echo imaging and in vivo proton MR spectroscopy. Radiology 2009;250(1): 95–102.

81. Bydder M, Yokoo T, Hamilton G, et al. Relaxation effects in the quantification of fat using gradient echo imaging. Magn Reson Imaging 2008;26(3): 347–59.

82. Yokoo T, Bydder M, Hamilton G, et al. Nonalcoholic fatty liver disease: diagnostic and fat-grading accuracy of low-flip-angle multiecho gradient-recalled-echo MR imaging at 1.5 T. Radiology 2009;251(1):67–76.

83. Reeder SB, Robson PM, Yu H, et al. Quantification of hepatic steatosis with MRI: the effects of accurate fat spectral modeling. J Magn Reson Imaging 2009;29(6):1332–9.

84. Meisamy S, Hines C, Hamilton G, et al. Validation of chemical shift based fat-fraction imaging with MR spectroscopy. Paper presented at: the International Society of Magnetic Resonance in Medicine 17th Meeting. Honolulu (HI), 2009.

85. Yu H, McKenzie CA, Shimakawa A, et al. Multiecho reconstruction for simultaneous water-fat decomposition and T2* estimation. J Magn Reson Imaging 2007;26(4):1153–61.

86. O'Regan DP, Callaghan MF, Wylezinska-Arridge M, et al. Liver fat content and T2*: simultaneous measurement by using breath-hold multiecho MR imaging at 3.0 T—feasibility. Radiology 2008; 247(2):550–7.

87. d'Assignies G, Ruel M, Khiat A, et al. Noninvasive quantitation of human liver steatosis using magnetic resonance and bioassay methods. Eur Radiol 2009;19(8):2033–40.

88. Hamilton G, Middleton M, Yokoo T, et al. In-vivo determination of the full 1H MR spectrum of liver fat; The International Society of magnetic resonance in medicine 18th Meeting. Honolulu (HI), 2009.

89. Reeder SB, Brittain JH, Grist TM, et al. Least-squares chemical shift separation for (13)C metabolic imaging. J Magn Reson Imaging 2007; 26(4):1145–52.

90. Schwenzer NF, Machann J, Haap MM, et al. T2* relaxometry in liver, pancreas, and spleen in a healthy cohort of one hundred twenty-nine subjects-correlation with age, gender, and serum ferritin. Invest Radiol 2008;43(12):854–60.

91. Yu H, Shimakawa A, Reeder S, et al. Magnitude fitting following phase sensitive water-fat separation to remove effects of phase errors. Paper presented at: The International Society of Magnetic Resonance in Medicine 17th Meeting. Honolulu (HI), 2009.

92. Mitchell DG, Kim I, Chang TS, et al. Fatty liver. Chemical shift phase-difference and suppression magnetic resonance imaging techniques in animals, phantoms, and humans. Invest Radiol 1991;26(12):1041–52.

93. Levenson H, Greensite F, Hoefs J, et al. Fatty infiltration of the liver: quantification with phase-contrast MR imaging at 1.5 T vs biopsy. AJR Am J Roentgenol 1991;156(2):307–12.

94. Kawamitsu H, Kaji Y, Ohara T, et al. Feasibility of quantitative intrahepatic lipid imaging applied to the magnetic resonance dual gradient echo sequence. Magn Reson Med Sci 2003;2(1):47–50.

95. Rinella ME, McCarthy R, Thakrar K, et al. Dual-echo, chemical shift gradient-echo magnetic resonance imaging to quantify hepatic steatosis: Implications for living liver donation. Liver Transpl 2003;9(8):851–6.

96. Pacifico L, Celestre M, Anania C, et al. MRI and ultrasound for hepatic fat quantification:relationships to clinical and metabolic characteristics of pediatric nonalcoholic fatty liver disease. Acta Paediatr 2007;96(4):542–7.

97. Schuchmann S, Weigel C, Albrecht L, et al. Non-invasive quantification of hepatic fat fraction by fast 1.0, 1.5 and 3.0 T MR imaging. Eur J Radiol 2007;62(3):416–22.

98. Yoshimitsu K, Kuroda Y, Nakamuta M, et al. Noninvasive estimation of hepatic steatosis using plain CT vs. chemical-shift MR imaging: significance for living donors. J Magn Reson Imaging 2008; 28(3):678–84.

99. Cowin GJ, Jonsson JR, Bauer JD, et al. Magnetic resonance imaging and spectroscopy for monitoring liver steatosis. J Magn Reson Imaging 2008;28(4):937–45.

100. Borra RJ, Salo S, Dean K, et al. Nonalcoholic fatty liver disease: rapid evaluation of liver fat content with in-phase and out-of-phase MR imaging. Radiology 2009;250(1):130–6.

101. McPherson S, Jonsson JR, Cowin GJ, et al. Magnetic resonance imaging and spectroscopy accurately estimate the severity of steatosis provided the stage of fibrosis is considered. J Hepatol 2009;51(2):389–97.

102. Bornert P, Keupp J, Eggers H, et al. Whole-body 3D water/fat resolved continuously moving table imaging. J Magn Reson Imaging 2007; 25(3):660–5.

103. Hines CD, Yu H, Shimakawa A, et al. Quantification of hepatic steatosis with 3-T MR imaging: validation in ob/ob mice. Radiology 2010;254(1):119–28.

104. Yokoo T, Shiehmorteza M, Bydder M, et al. Spectrally-modeled hepatic fat quantification by multi-echo gradient-recalled-echo magnetic resonance imaging at 3.0T 2009; the International Society of magnetic resonance in medicine 17th Meeting. Honolulu (HI), 2009.

105. He T, Gatehouse PD, Kirk P, et al. Myocardial T-2* measurement in iron-overloaded thalassemia: an ex vivo study to investigate optimal methods of quantification. Magn Reson Med 2008;60(2): 350–6.

Magnetic Resonance Imaging Quantification of Liver Iron

Claude B. Sirlin, MD[a],*, Scott B. Reeder, MD, PhD[b,c,d,e]

KEYWORDS

- Iron quantification • Magnetic resonance imaging
- Hepatic iron overload • Quantitative biomarkers

This article reviews emerging magnetic resonance imaging (MR imaging) techniques that attempt to quantify liver iron noninvasively. The content is divided into the following sections:

- Overview of iron deposition and diseases where liver iron overload is clinically relevant.
- Review why quantitative noninvasive biomarkers of liver iron would be beneficial.
- Describe current state-of-the-art methods for quantifying iron with MR imaging, including remaining challenges and unsolved problems.
- Explore the challenge and new approaches for quantifying iron overload when both iron and fat are present in the liver.

After reading this content, the reader should understand the scope of diffuse liver disease with regard to iron deposition and the limitations of biopsy, and be familiar with emerging quantitative MR imaging methods for measuring liver iron.

IRON METABOLISM AND OVERLOAD

Hepatic iron overload is the abnormal and excessive intracellular accumulation of iron in hepatocytes, Kupffer cells, or both hepatocytes and Kupffer cells, primarily as ferritin particles and hemosiderin aggregates.[1,2] Iron overload may occur selectively in the liver but more commonly iron overload is a systemic condition that affects extrahepatic organs as well as liver. In this section, we briefly review normal iron metabolism and the pathogenesis and clinical relevance of iron overload.

Normal Iron Metabolism

An essential nutrient, iron is required by every human cell.[1,3] Under physiologic conditions, about 10% of dietary iron (1 to 2 mg/d) is absorbed daily, while a similar amount of iron is lost via sloughing of cells from the skin and mucosal surfaces.[4–6] An additional 2 mg/d is lost in premenopausal women because of menstruation.[4] The intestinal absorption of iron adjusts to physiologic needs and is carefully regulated to balance losses.[3] As a result, iron concentration is normally maintained in a narrow homeostatic range, about 40 mg Fe/kg body weight in women and 50 mg Fe/kg in men.[1,3] About 80% of body iron is functional, located in hemoglobin in red blood cells, myoglobin in muscle, and in iron-containing

[a] Liver Imaging Group, Department of Radiology, University of California San Diego, 408 Dickinson Street, San Diego, CA 92103-8226, USA
[b] Liver Imaging Research Program, Department of Radiology, University of Wisconsin, E1/374 CSC, 600 Highland Avenue, Madison, WI 53792-3252, USA
[c] Department of Medical Physics, University of Wisconsin, E1/374 CSC, 600 Highland Avenue, Madison, WI 53792, USA
[d] Department of Biomedical Engineering, University of Wisconsin, E1/374 CSC, 600 Highland Avenue, Madison, WI 53792, USA
[e] Department of Medicine, University of Wisconsin, E1/374 CSC, 600 Highland Avenue, Madison, WI 53792, USA
* Corresponding author.
E-mail address: csirlin@ucsd.edu

Magn Reson Imaging Clin N Am 18 (2010) 359–381
doi:10.1016/j.mric.2010.08.014
1064-9689/10/$ — see front matter © 2010 Elsevier Inc. All rights reserved.

enzymes.[7,8] A small fraction of iron is bound to transferrin, an intravascular transport protein that delivers iron to the liver, bone marrow, and other tissues.[7,9] About 20% of body iron is in storage form and contained within the storage protein, ferritin, a hollow apoprotein shell with a central cavity, (7–8 nm in diameter, filled with iron oxyhydroxide nanocrystals).[8,10] In normal mammalian liver tissues, ferritin is found mainly in the cytoplasm of hepatic Kupffer cells as well as spleen and in bone marrow macrophages.

Hepatic Iron Overload

Although the body is capable of regulating intestinal absorption of iron, the body has no mechanism for regulating iron elimination. Thus, increased supply of iron leads to systemic iron overload. If sustained, the overload eventually overwhelms the capacity of ferritin to sequester the excess iron. When ferritin storage capacity is exceeded, free iron accumulates in the cells of the affected organ or organs. Additionally, ferritin molecules cluster in the cystoplasm and inside lysosomes of affected cells. Some of the ferritin denatures to form insoluble aggregates of hemosiderin,[8,10] nanoscale particles with a relatively broad range of size and shape.[10] Thus, in normal conditions, iron is stored mainly as ferritin molecules in the cytoplasm, but in iron overload states, iron is stored not only as cytoplasmic ferritin molecules but also as cytoplasmic ferritin clusters, lysosomal ferritin clusters, and insoluble hemosiderin aggregates. The functional iron pool is unaffected.

The free intracellular iron reacts with hydrogen and lipid peroxides and generates toxic hydroxyl and lipid radicals that attack cell membranes, cellular proteins, and nucleic acids.[11,12] The damage, if sustained, leads to progressive fibrosis and organ dysfunction. Clinical manifestations depend on the pattern and severity of organ involvement, which in turn depend on the route and cause of the iron overload.

Iron overload may result from excess intestinal absorption, repeated intravenous blood transfusions, or a combination of the two:

Excess intestinal absorption leads initially to accumulation of iron in periportal hepatocytes and later to hepatocytes throughout the liver lobule.[13] With further progression, iron accumulates in Kupffer cells and biliary epithelium. Eventually, there is spillage of iron into the circulation, where it binds to transferrin.[7] The transferrin delivers the excess iron to organs with high transferrin-receptor density (pancreas, myocardium, thyroids, gonads, hypophysis, skin), leading to iron overload at these sites. Extrahepatic reticuloendothelial organs (spleen, marrow, and lymph nodes) are relatively spared.

Intravenous blood transfusions lead to preferential involvement of the reticuloendothelial system. Red blood cell transfusions provide 200 to 250 mg iron per unit, and the iron contained in the transfused red blood cells accumulates in the reticuloendothelial cells of liver, spleen, bone marrow, and lymph nodes, where it is safely sequestered as ferritin until the storage capacity of the reticuloendothelial system (10 g of iron, or the amount of iron delivered by 40 to 50 transfusions) is saturated.[7] After saturation, the iron accumulates in hepatocytes and in parenchymal cells of the pancreas, myocardium, and endocrine glands.[7]

Conditions associated with hepatic iron overload include hereditary hemochromatosis (HH), thalassemia, sickle cell disease (SCD), sideroblastic anemia, chronic hemolytic anemias, transfusional and parenteral iron overload, dietary iron overload, myelodysplasia, and chronic hepatopathies.[14] In the following sections, we briefly discuss iron overload in HH, thalassemia, SCD, and chronic hepatopathy. In the first 3 conditions, excess iron deposits in an otherwise normal liver and may cause liver disease; in the latter condition, iron deposits in an already abnormal liver and may accelerate disease progression.

Hereditary hemochromatosis

HH is a genetic disorder associated with mutations in genes regulating iron metabolism,[6] the most common of which are in the HFE gene.[15,16] These gene mutations result in dysregulated constitutive intestinal iron uptake. Affected patients absorb iron at 5 to 10 times the normal rate (up to 10 mg/d),[6] which may lead to total-body iron overload and accumulation of excess iron in liver, heart, and other organs, as discussed previously.[3] Liver iron stores are often more than 10 times that of normal liver.[17] HH is the most common genetic disorder in populations of Northern European ancestry. In the United States, about 6% of persons have a mutation in one of the causative genes.[6,10] The penetrance of disease is lower,[6] and the prevalence of clinically relevant disease is about 1 in 300 to 400 in Caucasian populations and lower in other racial groups.[10] Complications of HH include liver fibrosis, cirrhosis (5% of patients), arthritis, diabetes, and assorted cardiac disturbances owing to iron deposition in the liver, joints, pancreas, and heart, respectively.[1,3,6,18] These complications are more common in and occur at a younger age in men than women,[3] in whom menstruation helps to check the progression of iron overload.[4] Patients with cirrhosis may develop hepatocellular carcinoma, which is a leading cause of death in these patients.[14,18] In patients with HH, the severity of hepatic iron overload is an important prognostic biomarker for development of both hepatic and extrahepatic complications.

Thalassemias

These are genetic disorders in hemoglobin synthesis that prevent the body from producing sufficient hemoglobin and red blood cells. Thalassemias are prevalent in people of Mediterranean origin. The prevalence is low in Northern Europe. Chronic blood transfusion is life saving, but the repeated transfusions cause progressive accumulation of iron in the reticuloendothelial system. Patients with thalassemia major and other transfusion-dependent anemias receive roughly 0.4 mg/kg/d of heme iron, 10 to 50 times the physiologic rate of iron absorption.[19] This transfusional overload is exacerbated by increased intestinal iron absorption stimulated by tissue hypoxia, apoptosis of defective erythroid precursors generated by ineffective erythropoiesis, as well as hemolysis of native and transfused red blood cells.[20] Because of the additive iron-loading mechanisms, systemic iron overload becomes severe in infancy or early childhood. Without aggressive iron chelation therapy, affected patients die from endocrine and cardiac dysfunction in the second decade of life.[21–23] Liver disease caused by hepatic iron overload may cause morbidity and contribute to poor quality of life but, in the absence of concomitant viral hepatitis,[24] death attributable to cirrhosis is rare.[20] The relative rarity of end-stage liver disease in these patients can be attributed in part to premature death from cardiac and endocrine disease and in part to preferential accumulation of iron in Kupffer cells rather than hepatocytes as part of the hepatic involvement.

Sickle cell disease

SCD is a common, genetic blood disorder with high prevalence in African Americans. Although sickle cell disease is associated with anemia, erythropoiesis is virtually normal and so there is no significant increase in intestinal iron absorption. Thus, nontransfused patients with SCD do not spontaneously load iron.[7] Patients with SCD, however, may receive blood transfusions to alleviate symptoms that occur during a sickle crisis and consequently develop transfusional iron overload.[25] SCD also is associated with intravascular (extrasplenic) hemolysis. Free hemoglobin is released from destroyed red blood cells into the blood and filtered by the kidneys; some of the filtered hemoglobin is excreted in the urine but some is reabsorbed by the proximal convoluted tubules and deposits in the renal cortex as ferritin and hemosiderin.[7]

Chronic hepatopathy

Chronic liver diseases (hepatitis B and C virus infection, alcohol-induced liver disease, nonalcoholic fatty liver disease, and porphyria cutanea tarda) are sometimes associated with hepatic iron overload[3,14]; this has been attributed to diminished functional hepatocyte mass, aberrant hepatic signaling with excess intestinal iron absorption,[26] and reduced mobilization of storage iron from the liver. In these diseases, the primary liver condition is the paramount abnormality and the secondary iron overload is less important. Emerging evidence suggests, however, that hepatic iron accumulation in patients with preexisting liver disease plays a synergistic role in the development of hepatic fibrosis and cirrhosis, reduces response to antiviral interferon therapy, and contributes to the development of hepatocellular carcinoma (HCC).[24,27,28]

TREATMENT OF IRON OVERLOAD

The treatment of iron overload is based on its cause, severity, and organ involvement. The primary treatment for patients with HH is lifelong therapeutic phlebotomy (regular extractions of about 500 mL of blood), which aims to remove excess iron and prevent iron-mediated tissue damage.[3,14,26] Phlebotomy is initially performed weekly, with longer intervals between sessions once hemoglobin levels decrease or an acceptable liver iron concentration (LIC) is achieved. Liver fibrosis may regress in response to therapy,[29] and life expectancy may return to that of a healthy person.[18]

Iron overload in patients with transfusion-dependent anemias cannot be treated by phlebotomy. Instead, these patients are treated with chelation therapy.[3,30,31] Currently, 3 chelating agents are available: deferasirox, deferiprone, and deferoxamine.[21,32,33] The aim of therapy is to maintain total body iron at a level sufficiently low to prevent or even reverse iron toxicity while simultaneously minimizing treatment side effects. Close monitoring of iron levels is necessary.[1,32]

In patients with viral hepatitis and hepatic iron overload, iron-chelating therapy is under investigation.

QUANTIFICATION OF LIVER IRON IS IMPORTANT

Liver iron quantification is important. In HH, measuring the liver iron content permits identification of individuals suitable for phlebotomy therapy and helps exclude clinical disease in individuals at risk for HH based on genetic studies.[1] Liver iron content also provides important prognostic information regarding the risk for developing hepatic complications such as hepatic fibrosis and cirrhosis.[14,34,35]

In thalassemia and other iron-loading anemias, liver iron content serves as an indirect marker of total body iron.[26] The liver contains about 70% of total body iron and is the main iron storage site in the body.[1,36] It correlates closely with total body iron and accounts for 98% of the variation in total iron stores.[26] Thus, measuring liver iron provides a reliable marker of total body iron to guide, monitor, and titrate therapy.[1] Liver iron also serves as prognostic biomarker for endocrine and cardiovascular complications in patients with thalassemia. It should be emphasized, however, that whereas liver iron content correlates with total body iron, it is not a perfect marker.[1,33] In iron-loading anemias, most iron-mediated toxicities occur in extrahepatic organs that account for only a fraction of total body iron.[19] Moreover, iron loading and clearance rates in these conditions are organ dependent; thus, liver iron content may not reflect iron content in iron-sensitive target organs such as heart, pituitary, and pancreas.[1,20] Although high liver iron levels convey prognostic risk, low liver iron values do not exclude iron overload in the myocardium or other specific target tissues.[19] Finally, the relationship of liver iron to total body iron depends on the etiology and route of iron overload: iron preferentially accumulates in the liver in patients with HH, especially early in the course of iron loading, whereas it accumulates throughout the reticuloendothelial system in iron-loading anemias and other conditions in which recurrent blood transfusions are a major source of iron.

With the recognition that mild iron overload may be a cofactor in the progression of hepatic disorders,[27] evaluation of liver iron content is now considered relevant in the management of chronic liver diseases such as viral hepatitis, alcoholic liver disease, nonalcoholic fatty liver disease (NAFLD), and porphyria cutanea tarda.[28]

COEXISTENCE OF FATTY LIVER AND IRON OVERLOAD

Intracellular hepatic fat and iron overload may occur together. In fact, abnormally elevated intrahepatic stores of iron are considered by some as a potential cofactor in the development of inflammation and fibrosis in the aggressive form of NAFLD, nonalcoholic steatohepatitis (NASH).[37–39] Despite this, the role of role of iron in NAFLD remains unknown. In some studies, up to 40% of patients with NAFLD have concomitant iron overload,[39,40] with a strong association between iron and aggressive histology. In our experience, combined steatosis and iron overload occur occasionally. In patients with HH, accumulation of iron within hepatocytes creates oxidative stress that can lead to end-stage cirrhosis, liver failure, and the development of hepatocellular carcinoma,[41] which is a major cause of death in patients with hemochromatosis.[41] Moreover, in patients with iron overload from HH, coexisting steatosis can accelerate disease progression.[42] Thus, iron and steatosis are important and common features of diffuse liver disease whose coexistence is common and important because of probable synergistic injury mechanisms to the liver. Importantly, as we discuss later, the coexistence of fat and iron has important technical implications for quantification of these disease features with MR imaging.

CURRENT METHODS FOR QUANTIFYING HEPATIC IRON—BIOPSY, IMAGING, SPECTROSCOPY, AND SUSCEPTOMETRY
Percutaneous Liver Biopsy

Nontargeted percutaneous liver biopsy with direct histologic visualization is the current gold standard to diagnose diffuse liver disease, including iron overload. Iron deposition is typically evaluated on a semiquantitative scale based on Prussian Blue staining of iron granules. The most commonly used method is the scoring system of Rowe and colleagues,[43] based on detection of iron granules and the magnifications at which discrete granules are resolved. This method uses a 5-point grading scale: grade 0 = granules absent/barely discernible at ×400 power, grade 1+ = iron granules barely discernible (×250); grade 2+ = discrete iron granules resolved (×100); grade 3+ = discrete granules resolved (×25); grade 4+ = masses visible (×10 or grossly visible). This is the most reproducible method and has been shown to correlate with liver iron concentration (LIC), a more precise measure of iron. Direct measurement of LIC requires the use of atomic absorption spectrophotometry, which is often performed when the specific diagnosis of iron overload is suspected or to monitor therapy. Normal LIC ranges from 0.2 mg Fe/g dry weight (3.6 μmol Fe/kg dry weight) to 2 mg Fe/g dry weight (36 μmol Fe/kg dry weight). Iron overload is defined as iron that exceeds the upper limit of normal. In HH, the LIC may range up to 10 times the upper limit of normal (20 mg Fe/g dry weight or, equivalently, 360 μL Fe/dry weight). In iron overload associated with transfusion-dependent anemias, the LIC may exceed 20 times the upper limit of normal

(40 mg Fe/g dry weight or 720 μL Fe/g dry weight). Unfortunately, atomic absorption spectrophotometry for LIC quantification[44] is available only at specialized centers. It is a destructive technique and the specimen submitted for chemical analysis cannot also be evaluated histologically.

Owing to nonuniformity in the distribution of liver iron, measurement of LIC from biopsy specimens is subject to sampling error. In one study, the average coefficient of variation (CV) of LIC values in multiple needle biopsies was 19% in nondiseased livers and 40% in cirrhotic livers. Biopsy also carries significant risk of complications leading to hospitalization (1%–3%) and death (1:10,000),[45] and is also not feasible in many research studies, including epidemiologic and genetic studies. In summary, because of the invasiveness, discomfort, risk, and sampling variability of biopsy, there is an urgent need for accurate, precise, and noninvasive methods to assess liver fat and iron.

Quantitative Phlebotomy

In quantitative phlebotomy, the amount of iron in the removed blood is measured. This method can assess total body iron stores,[26] but cannot be used in transfusion-dependent patients with iron overload and is generally acceptable only if the procedure provides therapeutic benefit.[1]

Ultrasound

Iron deposition is not detectable at ultrasound, and ultrasound has no clinical role in the evaluation of the iron-overloaded liver, other than assessing the sequela of liver injury, such as cirrhosis and portal hypertension.

Computed Tomography

Iron overload in the liver is well known to increase the overall attenuation of liver through increased absorption of x-rays by iron, and CT has been described for the qualitative detection of iron overload from genetic hemochromatosis and hemosiderosis.[46,47] Unfortunately, just as with fat quantification, many confounding factors, including steatosis, may alter hepatic attenuation and CT is not a reliable method for detection and quantification of hepatic iron overload.[3,48]

Magnetic Resonance Spectroscopy

Magnetic resonance spectroscopy (MRS) also can be used to assess liver iron. Wang and colleagues[49] developed a multi-echo MRS sequence. Single-voxel spectra were acquired at multiple echo times in human subjects with varying degrees of hepatic iron overload. The T_2 relaxation value of the liver water peak was measured from the multi-echo spectra. T_2 relaxation values showed high correlation with corresponding LIC values measured from synchronous liver biopsies, showing proof of concept that MRS could be used to estimate LIC values in human subjects. Although the method is promising, the use of MRS for assessment of liver iron has the same limitations as MRS for liver fat, as discussed in the article by Reeder and Sirlin elsewhere in this edition of *Magnetic Resonance Imaging Clinics of North America*.

Susceptometry

Liver iron susceptometry using a superconducting quantum interference device (SQUID) is generally regarded as the most accurate noninvasive method to quantify liver iron.[11] This susceptometric technique, first proposed more than 40 years ago,[50,51] is based on the concept that iron is the only nontrace element with high susceptibility. Thus, normal tissue is diamagnetic and has susceptibility close to that of the water; in the presence of iron, the susceptibility of the liver is modified. The instrument measures the magnetic field variation produced outside the body adjacent to the liver in response to an external magnetic field. The magnetic field variation is proportional to the amount of tissue iron.[52] Other paramagnetic materials (oxygen, deoxyhemoglobin, some trace metals) make negligible contributions to the hepatic magnetic susceptibility and their effects can be ignored. Hence, magnetic measurements are highly specific for iron concentration. The SQUID has been validated by experiments showing excellent correlation with chemical assay–determined LIC. Although the SQUID has been calibrated, validated, and used for clinical studies, its complexity, high cost, and limited availability (only 4 instruments in the whole world) have precluded widespread implementation.[3,11] Another limitation is that the SQUID assesses liver iron only[11]; because iron loading and clearance rates are organ specific, a method that measures iron at other body sites, if comparable in accuracy, would be preferable.

QUANTIFICATION OF IRON ACCUMULATION IN THE LIVER WITH MR IMAGING
Conventional MR Imaging for Detection of Iron

Similar to its use in detection of liver fat, conventional MR imaging has been used to detect liver iron for more than 25 years.[53,54] MR imaging does not image the iron directly but instead detects the effect of iron on water protons in the tissue of interest. The basis of using MR imaging for iron detection is that iron accelerates T_2 relaxation and T_2^* signal decay, thereby causing signal loss on T_2-weighted spin-echo/fast spin-echo and T_2^*w gradient-echo MR images.

Iron also accelerates T_1 relaxation and may cause signal augmentation on T_1-weighted images[53,55]; the T_1-shortening effect may be difficult to observe on clinical MR images because, and unless the echo time (TE) is very short, signal loss from T_2 or T_2^* shortening typically dominates signal augmentation from T_1 shortening. In clinical practice, therefore, T_1-weighted imaging is not used to detect iron.

The detailed mechanisms that underlie T_2 and T_2^* shortening are not well understood, but the following concepts are accepted by many investigators. On a cellular scale, iron is distributed as ferritin particles and hemosiderin aggregates in a nonuniform fashion.[10,13] The nonuniformly distributed iron depots act like tiny bar magnets that create microscopic focal magnetic field inhomogeneities. These inhomogeneities cause protons within the voxel to precess at different precessional frequencies. The resulting frequency spread generates phase differences through the voxel between excitation and readout, causing accumulation of static dephasing and signal decay.[10,19] Static dephasing and the resulting signal decay are reversible using spin-echo methods and therefore contribute to T_2^* signal decay but not to T_2 relaxation.

To explain T_2 relaxation, investigators have proposed "outer sphere" and "inner sphere" theories. According to the outer sphere theory, water protons diffusing through the field inhomogeneities experience different magnetic field inhomogeneities and accrue different phase shifts depending on their specific path of diffusion.[8,19] This leads to diffusion-dependent dephasing and signal decay. Unlike static dephasing and signal decay, diffusion-dependent dephasing and signal decay are not reversible with spin-echo methods and hence contribute to T_2 as well as T_2^* relaxation. The degree of diffusion-dependent dephasing and signal decay depend on several factors, including the number, size, shape, and distribution of iron-containing depots; the diffusivity of the water molecules; and the echo spacing.[10,17] According to the inner sphere theory, iron electrons enhance the relaxation of protons of water molecules bound to iron-containing proteins. Through chemical exchange, enhanced relaxation of bound water protons is then transferred to the bulk water protons.[8,56]

Regardless of the mechanism, the T_2 and T_2^* shortening caused by iron can be detected by conventional MR imaging using T_2-weighted or T_2^*-weighted images. On such images, iron overload can be inferred if the liver (or other tissue of interest) has lower signal intensity than normal. For example, on T_2-weighted and T_2^*-weighted images, the normal liver has slightly lower signal intensity than spleen and kidneys. Moderate or marked hypointensity of liver relative to spleen or kidneys is abnormal and suggests iron overload. The degree of signal loss depends on the amount of iron and the echo time; in general, the greater the echo time, the greater the signal loss (**Fig. 1**).

Importantly, iron-induced T_2^* shortening exceeds iron-induced T_2 shortening. Hence, T_2^*-weighted images have greater sensitivity for detecting iron[10] and are superior for delineating its distribution, as illustrated in **Fig. 2**.

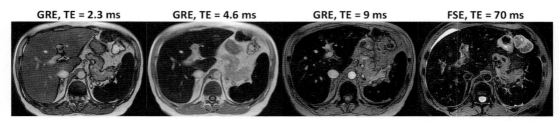

GRE, TE = 2.3 ms   GRE, TE = 4.6 ms   GRE, TE = 9 ms   FSE, TE = 70 ms

Fig. 1. Conventional T_2^*-weighted GRE and T2-weighted imaging is a well-established qualitative method for detecting iron overload within the liver and assessing involvement of other organs. Shown are breath-held GRE images with TEs of 2.3, 4.6, and 9 ms and a respiratory-triggered fat-saturated fast spin echo image with TE of 70 ms at 1.5T through the same slice of the liver in a male patient with transfusional iron overload. Notice abnormally low signal intensity of liver, spleen, and marrow on all images, indicating iron overload in these reticuloendothelial tissues. The pancreas, which has normal signal intensity, is spared. The pattern of organ involvement is typical for transfusional overload. The liver is mildly hypointense at 2.3 but then shows progressive signal loss with increasing TE on the gradient echo images, indicating fast T_2^* decay. The spleen is markedly hypointense at 2.3 ms, indicating even faster T_2^* decay. As its signal intensity at 2.3 ms is already very low, the spleen does not appreciably lose additional signal with increasing TE.

Baseline   **4 Months**   **8 Months**

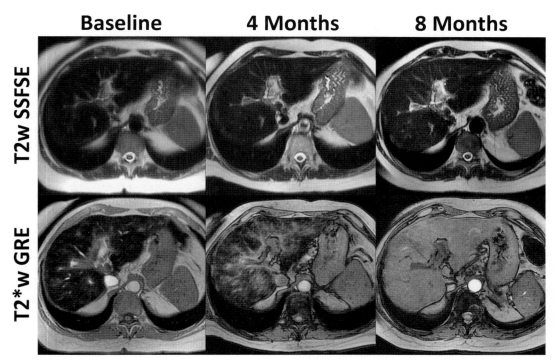

Fig. 2. T_2*-weighted GRE sequences are more sensitive to the presence and distribution of hepatic iron overload than T_2-weighted single shot fast spin echo (SSFSE) sequences. Shown are co-localized SSFSE (*top row*) and GRE (*bottom row*) images in a woman with transfusional iron overload at baseline and at 4 and 8 months after chelation therapy. The T_2-weighted SSFSE images look similar at all 3 time points, but the T_2*-weighted GRE images show diffuse iron overload at baseline, partial regression of iron overload at 4 months, and near complete regression at 8 months. Notice that at 4 months, the GRE image shows normal signal intensity in a branching periportal pattern with persistent hypointensity in intervening parenchyma and along the periphery, suggesting that different parts of the liver may clear excess iron at different rates.

The distribution of iron overload is usually diffuse and homogeneous but it may be heterogeneous with a lobar/segmental, heterogeneous, or patchy pattern (see **Fig. 2**). In patients with cirrhosis, the accumulation also may be focal, reflecting selective accumulation of iron in siderotic nodules[7]; these nodules may be distributed in a patchy or diffuse fashion (**Fig. 3**). As expected, the pattern of organ involvement reflects the etiology. In patients with HH, there is preferential involvement of the liver, pancreas, and heart, with sparing of extrahepatic reticuloendothelial organs (spleen, bone marrow, lymph nodes).[7,57] By comparison, in thalassemia and other transfusion-dependent anemias, preferential involvement of the reticuloendothelial system (liver, spleen, marrow, nodes) is characteristic (**Fig. 4**).[58] Involvement of the pancreas, heart, and other nonreticuloendothelial system organs suggests the storage capacity of the RE system has been exceeded.[7] As opposed to patients with transfusion-dependent anemias, patients with transfusion-independent anemias may exhibit an HH-type pattern, presumably

because of upregulated intestinal absorption of iron. In SCD, the renal cortex may show iron accumulation related to intravascular hemolysis (**Fig. 5**).[7] The liver in patients with SCD is usually spared in the absence of transfusion therapy; involvement of the liver in nontransfused patients with SCD suggests a coexisting cause for hepatic iron overload such as HH.[7]

Historically, T_2*-weighted images were obtained as single-echo gradient echo (GRE) sequences with long echo times (eg, 10–15 ms) to impart T_2* weighting. Although opposed-phase and in-phase (OP and IP) imaging were developed for liver fat detection, it also permits iron detection because the second echo has a longer echo time than the first echo and is therefore more T_2* weighted (see **Figs. 1** and **5**). Most commercial 1.5T scanners implement the dual-echo sequence using an OP-IP sequence design: the first echo has a TE of about 2.3 ms (OP at 1.5T) and the second echo has a TE of about 4.6 ms (IP at 1.5T). On such sequences, appreciable signal loss between the first echo (OP) and the

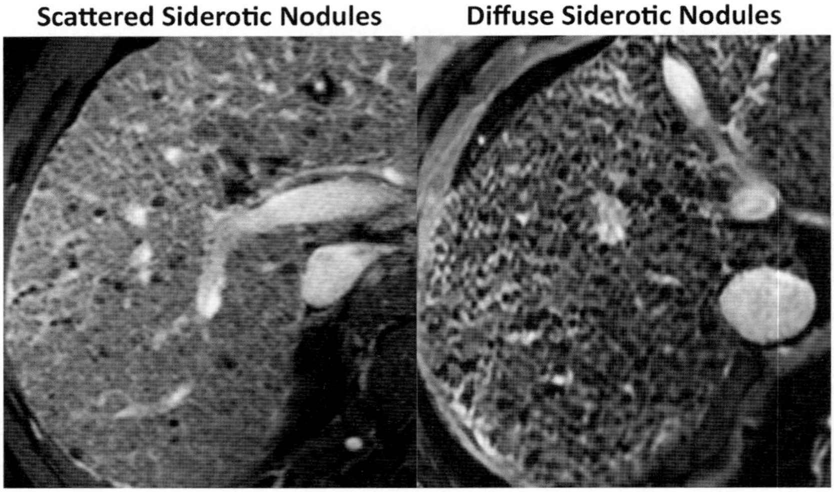

Scattered Siderotic Nodules   Diffuse Siderotic Nodules

Fig. 3. In patients with preexisting cirrhosis, iron may accumulate in regenerating nodules. Iron-laden regenerating nodules are known as siderotic nodules. Shown are T_2*-weighted GRE images after administration of a gadolinium-based contrast agent in 2 patients with cirrhosis secondary to hepatitis C viral infection. Siderotic nodules are hypointense because of T_2* shortening effects of iron. In the patient on the left, scattered siderotic nodules are evident in a patchy distribution, whereas in the patient on the right they are diffusely distributed. Hyperintense reticulations in the liver in both patients represent gadolinium-enhanced fibrotic bands. These are more conspicuous in the patient on the right because of greater contrast between the hyperintense fibrotic bands and the diffusely distributed hypointense siderotic nodules.

second echo (IP) indicates short T_2* decay and suggests the presence of parenchymal iron. The normal liver has a long T_2* relaxation time (greater than 20 ms) and loses only minimal signal intensity across closely spaced gradient echoes; iron accumulation, however, shortens the transverse relaxation and increases the amount of signal intensity loss. Concomitant liver steatosis may confound the interpretation, however, because signal loss owing to fat-water signal cancellation on the first echo (OP) may mask or even dominate T_2* signal decay on the second echo (IP).

Many commercial 3T scanners implement the dual-echo sequence using an IP-OP sequence design: the first echo has a TE of 2.3 ms (IP at 3T) and the second echo has a TE of about 5.8 ms (OP at 3T) (see **Fig. 4**). On IP-OP design sequences, signal loss on the second echo is nonspecific, as it could be attributable to steatosis with fat-water signal cancellation, iron overload

TE 2.3 ms   TE 5.8 ms

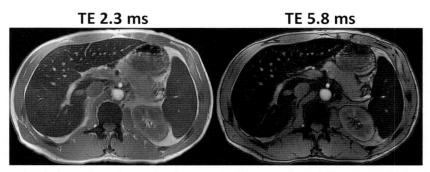

Fig. 4. Patients with thalassemia and secondary iron overload have preferential involvement of reticuloendothelial tissues. Shown are dual-echo GRE images obtained at 3T with TEs of 2.3 and 5.8 ms. Notice low signal of liver and spleen at 2.3 ms and incremental signal loss at 5.8 msec because of iron-mediated T_2* shortening. In principle, the signal loss of the liver at 5.8 ms (nominally out of phase at 3T) could be attributed to steatosis rather than iron overload, which is a limitation of the IP-OP sequence design commonly implemented at 3T. In this case, a fat quantification sequence (not shown) excluded the presence of concomitant fat. The pancreas and kidney are spared, suggesting the storage capacity of the reticuloendothelial system has not been exceeded.

OP (TE = 2.3 ms) **IP (TE = 4.6 ms)**

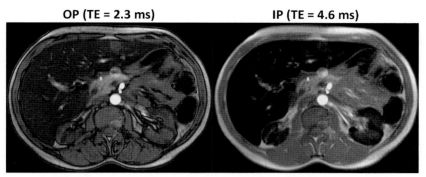

Fig. 5. Patients with SCD and secondary iron overload may have iron accumulation in the renal cortex. In this patient with SCD and history of transfusion therapy, notice low signal in the renal cortex and liver on T1-weighted dual-echo GRE images acquired at 1.5T with echo times as shown. The low signal is more pronounced on the second echo (TE = 4.6 ms). As illustrated in this case, dual-echo T_1-weighted imaging can be used to detect iron overload in tissue. Signal loss on the second echo compared with the first echo indicates short T_2* decay and suggests the presence of iron. As discussed in the text, hepatic iron overload does not occur in patients with SCD in the absence of transfusion therapy.

with short T_2*, or coexisting steatosis and iron overload with both fat-water signal cancellation and short T_2*. Thus, caution should be exercised in the interpretation of any T_2*-weighted GRE image if the TE is nominally OP because tissue hypointensity could be attributed to fat-water signal cancellation, T_2* shortening, or both. If the IP-OP dual-echo sequence shows signal loss on the second echo, obtaining a non–fat-saturated T_2-weighted sequence may help: moderate to marked hypointensity of the liver on the T_2-weighted image suggests iron overload whereas higher-than-normal signal intensity of the liver suggests fat.

Advanced MR Imaging for Quantification of Liver Iron

Although detection of liver iron using qualitative MR imaging is possible, qualitative MR imaging methods do not reliably assess the degree of iron overload and hence do not reliably guide treatment initiation or therapy monitoring. This requires quantitative methods that can predict the exact LIC based on MR imaging data. An ideal technique would measure LIC accurately over its entire clinical range from 2 mg Fe/g dry weight (36 μmol Fe/kg) to more than 40 mg Fe/g dry weight (720 μL Fe/g dry weight)[59] in a manner that is reproducible across most clinical MR imaging platforms. Two general MR imaging-based strategies for measuring LIC are

- Signal intensity ratios (SIRs) based on T_2-weighted or T_2*-weighted imaging
- Relaxometry based on T_2 or T_2* relaxation times (or R_2 or R_2* relaxation rates).

Although the methods differ in their details, as discussed later, they fundamentally have the same approach. For each method, MR images are obtained and MR imaging measurements (SIRs or relaxation times) are made. The MR imaging measurements are compared cross-sectionally to chemically determined LIC values from liver biopsies in human[13] subjects to generate empirical calibration curves.[10,60] An empirical approach is required, because there is not yet sufficient understanding of the underlying relaxation mechanisms to derive the curves based on first principles. Owing to the sampling variability of LIC values derived from biopsy samples, large numbers of subjects are required to generate reliable calibration curves that may be suitable for eventual implementation into clinical practice.

In the subsections that follow, we discuss the 2 strategies (SIR and relaxometry), review the leading specific methods for each strategy, and discuss their relative advantages and disadvantages. We conclude the section on iron quantification with a discussion on current limitations and unsolved problems.

Signal intensity ratio

In SIR methods, the signal intensity of the liver on spin-echo or GRE sequences is divided by the signal intensity of a reference tissue that does not accumulate iron (eg, fat, skeletal muscle) or noise.[38,61–66] To reduce depth-dependent signal intensity drop off, images are acquired using a body coil.[62] Large regions-of-interest (ROIs) are placed in the liver and the reference object on the same image, while avoiding artifacts, vessels, and boundaries. The mean signal intensity of the liver ROIs is then divided by the mean signal intensity of the reference ROIs. Comparison with a reference is necessary because the absolute signal intensity measured by MR imaging is arbitrary and depends on acquisition parameters and instrumentation. The most commonly used reference is skeletal muscle. One advantage of using skeletal muscle is that liver usually has higher signal intensity than muscle, so visual comparison can corroborate a slight decline in relative liver signal intensity. Moreover, acquisition parameters such as voxel size or bandwidth only minimally impact the liver-to-muscle ratio, whereas these parameters may alter the liver-to-noise ratio considerably. The use of adipose tissue as a reference is problematic because the signal intensity of fat varies strongly with echo time and measurements of fat signal may be difficult in children and thin adults.

Although many SIR methods have been proposed, the leading such method is the one described by Gandon and colleagues.[62] In this method, 5 breath-hold GRE sequences are obtained while adjusting the flip angle or TE (as listed in **Table 1**) to modulate the weighting and generate nominally T_1-weighted, proton density–weighted, or mildly, moderately, or heavily T_2*-weighted images. On each sequence, the liver signal intensity is measured in 3 operator-defined ROIs in the peripheral aspect of the right lobe, while muscle signal intensity is measured in 2 regions of interest on right and left paraspinous muscles (**Fig. 6**). The mean liver signal intensity is then divided by the mean muscle signal intensity to yield a liver/muscle ratio. The investigators evaluated

this technique in 149 patients with LIC values ranging from 36 to 709 µmol Fe/g. By combining the signal intensity ratio data from the 5 sequences, they designed a computer-based algorithm (Available at: http://www.radio.univ-rennes1.fr) that[62] estimates the LIC with high accuracy (mean difference of 0.8 µmol/g, 95% confidence interval [CI] 6.3 to 7.9) over a range of LIC values from 3 to 375 µmol Fe/g dry weight (0.2 to 20.9 mg iron/g dry weight).

Although promising, the Gandon method has limitations. In principle, the liver-to-muscle ratio is affected by numerous variables including choice of sequence (spin echo or GRE), scan parameters (field strength, repetition time, echo time, flip angle), and type of coil (surface or body) used. Thus, standardization of parameters is necessary. Even with standardization of parameters, however, LIC estimates made by the Gandon method depend on the scanner type,[67] suggesting that results may not be reproducible across platforms or sites. Also, the liver-to-muscle ratio derived from each sequence has a different empirical correlation with chemically determined LIC values as well as a different dynamic range. Initially, the curves are linear and show decline of the liver-muscle ratio with increasing LIC, but all sequences eventually saturate (ie, the liver-muscle ratio has reached the noise floor and cannot decline further with increasing LIC values).[62] Consequently, the method cannot quantify LIC values greater than 375 µmol/kg (20.9 mg/kg) and hence does not capture the entire relevant range of values.[59] Another limitation is that biologic factors (eg, hepatic steatosis and fat with muscle fascial

Table 1
Acquisition techniques of Gandon and colleagues,[62] St Pierre and colleagues,[76] and Wood and colleagues[77]

Author	Method Type	Sequence Type	Number of Acquisitions	Acquisition Parameters	Total Scan Duration
Gandon[62]	SIR	Single-echo GRE	5 breath-held acquisitions	TR 120 ms FA 90° — TE 4 ms FA 20° — TE 4 ms FA 20° — TE 9 ms FA 20° — TE 14 ms FA 20° — TE 21 ms	10 minutes
St Pierre[76]	R_2	Single-echo spin echo	7 free-breathing acquisitions	TR 2500 ms TE 6, 7, 8, 9, 12, 15, 18 ms	20+ minutes
Wood[77]	R_2*	Single-echo GRE	17 during a single breath hold	TR 25 ms FA° 20 TE 0.8–4.8 ms at 0.25 ms intervals	One breath hold

Abbreviations: FA, flip angle; GRE, gradient echo; SIR, signal intensity ratio; TE, echo time; TR, repetition time.

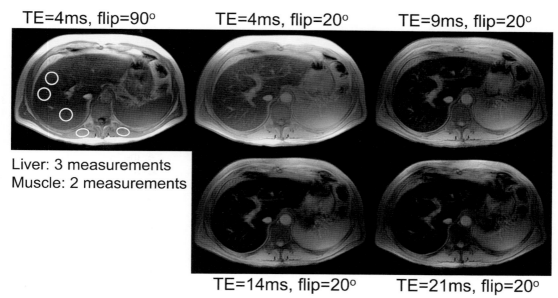

TE=4ms, flip=90° **TE=4ms, flip=20°** **TE=9ms, flip=20°**

Liver: 3 measurements
Muscle: 2 measurements

TE=14ms, flip=20° **TE=21ms, flip=20°**

Fig. 6. Quantification of iron can be performed using multiple GRE images acquired with T_1 weighting (TE = 4 ms, flip = 90°), and increasing amounts of T_2*-weighting (TE = 4, 9, 14, and 21 ms, with flip = 20°) according to Gandon and colleagues.[62] At least 3 ROIs are placed in the liver, and 2 in the muscle to provide normalization for B1 sensitivity and provide signal ratios. ROIs are propagated to all 5 images and values entered in the Web site available online at: http://www.radio.univ-rennes1.fr/Sources/EN/HemoCalc15.html. Based on the signal intensities entered, an estimated LIC is provided automatically.

planes) may confound the interpretation, as these factors are known to affect the signal intensity of the liver and muscle, respectively. Chemical fat saturation can be applied to reduce the confounding effects of fat, but this requires homogeneous fat saturation of both the liver and the reference tissue. Also, body habitus may affect the homogeneity of the signal intensity across the image and complicate the analysis of SIRs. Finally, the technique requires several breath holds and total acquisition time, including inter-breath hold intervals, is about 10 minutes.[65]

Relaxometry

Overview Compared with SIR methods, relaxometry is a theoretically more robust approach for estimating LIC. In relaxometry, a series of images is acquired with increasing echo times, the signal intensity of the tissue of interest (eg, liver) is modeled as a function of echo time, and signal decay constants (eg, T_2 or T_2*) are calculated.[68] As opposed to SIR methods, in which the signal intensity of 2 tissues (eg, liver and reference tissue) is compared at a given TE, relaxometry models the signal intensity of a single tissue (eg, liver) across multiple TEs. Because the tissue of interest is measured at a co-localized location at each TE, depth-dependent signal intensity changes in the image do not confound the results. Thus, use of

surface coils to acquire the data is acceptable. Depending on whether a spin-echo or GRE-based sequence is performed, T_2 or T_2* values can be calculated. Some investigators report rates of signal decay, R_2 or R_2*, instead of the time constants T_2 or T_2*. These rates are simply the reciprocals of T_2 and T_2*, ie, $R_2 = 1000/T_2$ and R_2* = $1000/T_2$*. Typically, T_2 and T_2* are expressed in ms, while R_2 and R_2* are expressed in s^{-1}. The observed T_2 or T_2* value is inversely related to the iron concentration: the lower the T_2 or T_2*, the greater the iron concentration. By comparison, the observed R_2 or R_2* value is directly related to the iron concentration: the greater the R_2 or R_2*, the greater the iron concentration. The time (T_2 or T_2*) or rate (R_2 or R_2*) calculations can be repeated pixel by pixel from the coregistered images to generate parametric maps (**Fig. 7**). These maps demonstrate the quantity and distribution (see **Figs. 7–9**) of the measured parameter. By placing ROIs on the maps, representative parameter (T_2, T_2*, R_2, R_2*) values can be recorded. The R_2 or R_2* values can be used for diagnosis or treatment monitoring (**Fig. 10**).

Technical issues Key technical issues in performing relaxometry are (1) field strength, (2) parameter of interest (R_2, R_2*), (3) pulse sequence design, (4)

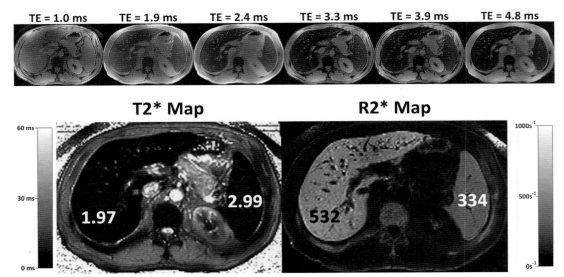

Fig. 7. R_2* mapping can be performed in a single breath hold using rapid GRE methods that acquire multiple images at increased echo times, within the same TR. Results are typically displayed as an R_2* map (*bottom right*), where areas of high iron concentration appear bright. Alternatively, results can also be displayed as a T_2* map (*bottom left*), which may be more intuitive because regions of elevated iron appear dark, corresponding to the appearance of iron overloaded tissue in heavily T_2*-weighted images. Both approaches are equally valid.

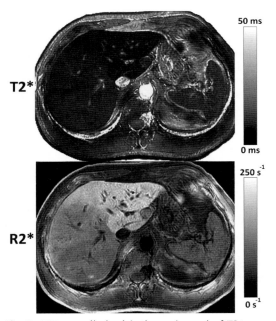

Fig. 8. R2* map (*below*) is the reciprocal of T2* map (*above*). Both maps depict the distribution of iron in the liver. In this patient, the left lobe has greater iron content than the right lobe, and it appears darker than the right lobe on the T2* map and brighter on the R2* map. As illustrated in this case, R2* maps may depict heterogeneity in iron distribution to better advantage than T2* maps because of their wider gray-level dynamic range.

choice of TEs, and (5) model for data fitting. These are discussed in the following sections.

Field strength Relaxation rates R_2 and R_2* increase with field strength.[8,10,69] Because of the dependency of relaxation rates on field strength, calibration curves obtained at one field strength (eg, 1.5T) cannot be transferred directly to another field strength (eg, 3T). Thus, calibration curves at different field strengths should be derived and validated. Also, whereas 3T imaging provides higher signal to noise than 1.5T, it has theoretical disadvantages for LIC estimation. For example, susceptibility artifacts are worse than at 1.5T, which may degrade GRE image quality.[19] More importantly, owing to faster signal decay at 3T, the maximum quantification limit may be lower than at 1.5T,[19] potentially lowering the utility of 3T scanners for iron quantification.

Parameter of interest (R_2 or R_2)* R_2 and R_2* methods have different theoretical advantages and disadvantages. R_2 measurements are less sensitive than R_2* measurements to confounding factors unrelated to iron content; these include technical factors (scanner, voxel size and shape, receive bandwidth), external magnetic inhomogeneities, and artifacts caused by metal clips, gas–soft tissue interfaces, and other sources of susceptibility.[2,70] By comparison, R_2* measurements are less sensitive than R_2 measurements to variations in the size and distribution of iron

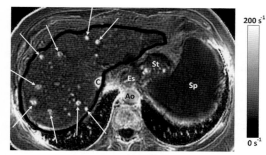

Fig. 9. R2* map shows scattered siderotic nodules (*arrows*) in a patient with alcoholic cirrhosis. C, cava; Ao, aorta; St, stomach; Sp, spleen. The liver margins have been highlighted in black to improve demarcation of the liver.

particles[71] and hence are less confounded by factors (eg, etiology and severity of iron overload, presence and severity of cirrhosis) that affect these features.[57] Another advantage of R_2* techniques is that they can be performed in a single breath hold,[55,57,72–75] whereas R_2 techniques take 5 to 20 minutes (depending on methodology).[23,70,76]

Although there is not yet consensus regarding the optimal relaxation rate parameter (R_2 or R_2*) for LIC estimation, R_2 and R_2* values generated comparable noninvasive estimates of LIC in a recent study.[77] Given the much shorter acquisition time required for R_2* techniques, the use of R_2 techniques may be difficult to justify if additional studies confirm equivalent accuracy.

Pulse sequence design R_2 can be measured using a series of single spin echoes, each acquired after a separate excitation,[23,25] or a train of spin echoes, each acquired after a single excitation (ie, a Carr-Purcell-Meiboom-Gill, or CPMG, sequence).[20,25,68,78] Compared with those made with a series of single spin echoes, R_2 measurements made with a train of spin echoes will be lower (because of more frequent application of refocusing pulses) and will vary with the echo spacing.[2,79] R_2* is usually measured using a breath-hold multi-echo GRE technique,[72,80] as most modern scanners now permit acquisition of multiple coregistered GRE images across a range of echo times after a single excitation. In general, R_2* measurements made with a multi-echo GRE technique are less affected by echo spacing than R_2 measurements made with an echo-train spin-echo (CPMG) technique.

Choice of TE To reliably measure relaxation parameters, it is important that the TEs span the range of expected clinically relevant T_2 (2.5 to 60 ms) or T_2* (0.5 to 30 ms) values.[70] Optimally, the first echo time should be as short as possible: 5 ms or less for spin-echo (T_2 measurements) and 1 ms or less for GRE (T_2* measurements) sequences.[70] The last echo time should be as long as reasonable without degradation by motion and other artifacts. Practically, this usually corresponds to a TE of 15 to 30 ms for spin-echo (T_2 measurements) and 10 to 15 ms for GRE (T_2* measurements) sequences.[70]

The optimal number of echoes has not been determined. Two reasonable approaches would

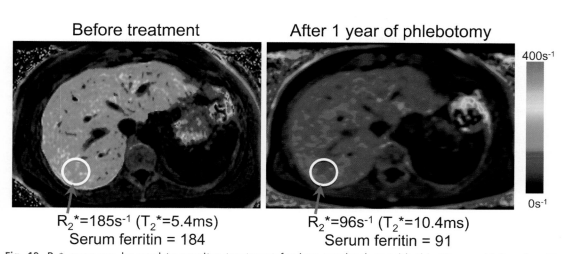

Before treatment

After 1 year of phlebotomy

$R_2*=185s^{-1}$ ($T_2*=5.4ms$)
Serum ferritin = 184

$R_2*=96s^{-1}$ ($T_2*=10.4ms$)
Serum ferritin = 91

Fig. 10. R_2* maps can be used to monitor treatment for iron overload, as with this 52-year-old female with known genetic hemochromatosis. R_2* maps acquired 1 year after treatment with phlebotomy demonstrate a marked decrease in R_2* from 185 s^{-1} to 96 s^{-1}, with a corresponding decrease in the serum ferritin, which is an indirect marker of iron overload. These particular R_2* maps were acquired with the Yu method, which automatically produces an R_2* map as part of the correction needed for fat quantification.

be to acquire as many echoes as possible between the first and last echoes or to space the echoes logarithmically. To achieve the appropriate echo spacing, it may be necessary to use a small frequency matrix (192 or 224), fractional echo sampling, and high receive bandwidth (>100 kHz).

Liver fat alters the signal decay observed in hepatic tissue and may confound the T_2^* measurements. To suppress the potentially confounding signals from fat, one option is to collect echoes only at in-phase echo times, but this approach is problematic in heavily iron-overloaded livers. In such livers, considerable signal decay may occur by the first in-phase echo time (2.3 ms at 3T, 4.6 ms at 1.5T), and sampling of the decay curve may be inadequate for reliable R_2^* estimation. The use of quantitative MR imaging techniques in patients with coexisting steatosis and iron overload is discussed further in a subsequent section.

Model for data fitting The simplest model for data fitting is a *monoexponential* model given by,

$$S(TE) = Ae^{-TE \times R_2^*} \qquad (1)$$

Where, S is measured signal intensity and A is the signal intensity expected at TE = 0. An important limitation is that the model assumes uniform iron concentration within each tissue voxel. This assumption is incorrect,[60] as voxels may contain both iron-dense (iron-loaded hepatocytes and/or Kupffer cells) and iron-sparse components (bile, blood, interstitial fluid).[70] The iron-dense component generates rapidly decaying signal, whereas the iron-sparse component generates slowly decaying signal. The monoexponential model assumes, as a simplification, that a single exponential describes the contributions of both components; although a monoexponential model describes the early part of the composite signal decay curve reasonably well (ie, over early echo times), it may not describe the tail end of the composite signal decay curve (ie, over late echo times). Also, the model neglects the confounding effect of image noise. Transverse relaxation measurements are usually derived from magnitude MR images. Such images have non- zero baseline signal intensity owing to the presence of additive noise (noise in the real and imaginary components of the complex MR signal has a Gaussian distribution with zero mean, but noise in the displayed magnitude image has a Rician distribution with non-zero mean). The additive noise produces a signal level offset in the magnitude images, prevents the observed signal intensity from decaying to zero,[25] and prolongs the apparent decay curve.[81] Ignoring the long-T_2^* contribution of the iron-sparse component and the confounding effect of Rician noise in magnitude images introduces estimation errors: the time constants T_2 and T_2^* are overestimated, whereas the rate constants R_2 and R_2^* are underestimated.[70]

Numerous data-fitting models have been proposed to address the limitations of the mono-exponential model,[23,25,33,55,60,81,82] including those listed as follows.

1. Monoexponential with truncation (echoes with low signal intensity are excluded until a good fit to mono-exponential decay is achieved).
2. Monoexponential model with weighting (signal decay is assumed to be exponential but progressively less weight is given to echoes with decreasing signal intensity).
3. Monoexponential model with offset (a constant offset is added to account for noise and long T_2^* components. The model is given by,

$$S(TE) = Ae^{-TE\ R_2^*} + C \qquad (2)$$

4. Monoexponential model with baseline subtraction (measured image noise is subtracted directly from the tissue signal intensity at each echo time; the corrected signal intensity of the tissue is then entered into a monoexponential model).
5. Bi-exponential model (2 components are modeled: an iron-dense, short-T_2^* component and an iron-sparse, long-T_2^* component). The model is given by,

$$S(TE) = Ae^{-TER_2^*|_A} + Be^{-TER_2^*|_B} \qquad (3)$$

Where, A and B are the iron-dense, short-T_2^* and iron-sparse, long-T_2^* components, respectively).

Each of the 5 models has advantages and disadvantages, and consensus has not yet been reached regarding which model is optimal. For example, although the bi-exponential model provides a more complete description of the multicomponent nature of liver tissue, it has 4 degrees of statistical freedom.[70] This makes the fitting process unstable unless mathematical constraints are imposed. Further research is needed to identify the most accurate model.

Specific relaxometry methods Numerous specific methods to measure R_2 and R_2^* for LIC estimation have been published. The most rigorously validated methods are those of St Pierre and colleagues[2,59,76] (R_2 mapping) and Wood and colleagues[77] (R_2^* mapping), and are discussed in the following sections.

St Pierre method (FerriScan) The St Pierre method[59,76] was approved by the Food and Drug Administration (FDA) and is marketed as FerriScan (www.ferriscan.com/). The method uses 7 T_2-weighted single spin-echo free-breathing sequences under fixed gain control with constant repetition time (TR) and increasing TE spaced at 1- to 3-ms intervals.[76] Images are acquired in half-Fourier mode to reduce acquisition time. An external calibration phantom with very long T_2 is placed within the field of view to permit correction for instrumental drift across sequences. Image analysis is centralized and requires several post-processing steps including gain drift correction,[60] respiratory motion correction, background noise subtraction,[60] estimation of effective initial signal intensity at zero TE, and bi-exponential modeling pixel by pixel to generate liver R_2 parametric maps.[2,60] (The model assumes a dual-compartment system with slow-R_2 and fast-R_2 components. The R_2 values of the slow and fast components are computed from the model. The composite R_2 is calculated as the average of the R_2 values of the individual components weighted by their relative population densities in each voxel.) The largest slice is then selected and the mean composite R_2 value across the slice is calculated.

The investigators evaluated this technique in more than 100 patients with LIC values ranging from 0.3 to 42.7 mg Fe/g dry weight (5 to 747 μmol Fe/g). Liver R_2 demonstrated a curvilinear relationship with LIC over the entire LIC range with a correlation coefficient of 0.98.[76] The iron concentration could be predicted from the measured liver R_2 as:

$$[Fe] = \left(29.75 - \sqrt{900.7 - 2.283\,R_2}\right)^{1.424} \qquad (4)$$

with prediction errors comparable to those expected from the variability in liver biopsy.

The curvilinear relationship between R_2 and LIC indicates that R_2 values plateau at high LIC values. The plateau has been attributed to clustering of iron into large aggregates in patients with severe iron overload.[76,77] These aggregates are thought to cause magnetic inhomogeneities greater than the diffusion-dependent movement of water molecules. In the presence of such large inhomogeneities, diffusing water molecules experience a relatively constant magnetic field between excitation and refocusing pulses and hence there is relatively little diffusion-dependent dephasing and signal decay.

Although FDA approved, the St Pierre method has limitations.[76] The data analysis is centralized and cannot be completed directly by the radiologist. An external calibration phantom is required.

Acquisition time is long (~20 minutes) because of the multiple free-breathing sequences. Finally, as the relationship between R_2 and LIC is curvilinear, the method is relatively insensitive to longitudinal changes in LIC in patients with extreme iron overload, which may limit the suitability of the technique for monitoring such patients.

Wood method The Wood method uses 17 T_2^*-weighted single-echo GRE sequences in a single-breath hold with constant TR, constant flip angle, and increasing TE spaced at equal 0.25-ms intervals (as listed in **Table 1**).[83] Dummy scans are performed to achieve longitudinal steady-state before data acquisition. R_2^* is measured by fitting the observed data to a mono-exponential model with offset (data-fitting model 3 listed previously) pixel by pixel to generate a parametric map. The mean R_2^* value from all liver pixels on a single midhepatic slice is the calculated, excluding major vessels and areas of susceptibility artifact such as lung-liver interfaces.

The investigators evaluated this technique in more than 20 patients with LIC values ranging from 1.3 to 32.9 mg iron/g dry weight (23 to 590 μmol iron/g dry weight). Liver R_2^* demonstrated a linear relationship with LIC with a correlation coefficient of 0.97. The iron concentration could be predicted from the measured liver R_2^* as:

$$[Fe] = -0.63 + 0.0267R_2^* \qquad (5)$$

with prediction errors comparable to those of the St Pierre method. In an independent confirmatory study, Hankins and colleagues[80] derived a similar calibration curve using a single-breath-hold R2* technique in a separate patient population.

Importantly, the linear relationship between R_2^* and LIC indicates that R_2^* values do not plateau at high LIC values, presumably because R_2^* values are relatively unaffected by iron particle size and distribution. A limitation of the Wood method is that quantification linearity has been shown only up to a LIC of 32.9 mg iron/g dry weight. Further study is needed to determine if the Wood method maintains linearity through the upper end of LIC values encountered clinically. It is possible that linearity is not maintained: in the investigators' study, a single patient had a LIC of 57.8 mg iron/g dry weight; this patient's R2* value underestimated the chemically determined LIC and the patient was excluded from analysis.[77] A possible reason for LIC underestimation by the Wood method in patients with extreme iron overload is that the first echo time of 0.8 msec may be too long to reliably measure ultrafast signal decay. For such measurements, it may be necessary to use sequences with ultrashort first echo times.[83]

CURRENT LIMITATIONS OF MR IMAGING—BASED IRON QUANTIFICATION METHODS

Although published SIR and relaxometry methods have shown high accuracy for predicting LIC values, limitations remain. Most importantly, all current MR imaging methods are based on a "black box" approach in which MR measurements are correlated with chemically determined LIC values to derive empirical calibration curves.[13,82] This is in contradistinction to proton density fat-fraction (PDFF), the biomarker for liver fat accumulation, which is based on first principles. A consequence of the black box approach for MR imaging—based iron quantification is that recalibration in patients is necessary for any pulse sequence modifications, even minor changes such as TR—a tedious, time-consuming, and expensive process.[13] Furthermore, an empirical approach is not suitable for extrahepatic organs that may accumulate iron such as heart, brain, pituitary, and pancreas. Finally, empirical approaches implicitly assume that iron is the only variable that affects the MR imaging parameter being measured, even though many biologic and technical factors may confound the MR imaging measurement—LIC calibration,[8] as described briefly in the following sections.

Iron Particle Size, Distribution, and Other Features

Iron deposits in the iron-overloaded liver show heterogeneity in size and distribution over spatial scales spanning 3 orders of magnitude[13]:

- Intracellular (variable number and size of iron particles within different parts of individual cells; spatial scale in microns)
- Intercellular (variable amount of iron in adjacent cells; spatial scale tens of microns)
- Zonal (variable amount of iron between aggregates of cells in different zones of the hepatic lobule; spatial scale hundreds of microns).

The loading factor of ferritin varies widely from 2500 to more than 4500 iron atoms per molecule.[10] MR imaging particles may have round, cylindrical, or irregular shapes.[84] These features (particle size, distribution, loading factor, and shape) may vary between individual patients, between patient groups, or in response to different chelating agents.[11,85] They are thought to affect the relationship between LIC and R_2 relaxation values[10,11,71,84,86,87] and, because they cannot be determined noninvasively, introduce unavoidable error in R_2-based LIC estimation. Finally,

the biochemical form of the iron (hemosiderin vs ferritin) is known to affect relaxivity measurements in vitro, and possibly affect signal relaxation in vivo.

Technical Factors

Numerous technical factors may confound the MR imaging measurement—LIC calibration curve. These include field strength,[8,69] type of sequence (spin-echo, CPMG, fast spin-echo, GRE),[13] echo spacing,[13,60,84,87] voxel size and shape, receive bandwidth, type of coil (surface or body), and data-fitting model.[13,60,81] The effect of many of these factors on MR imaging—based LIC estimation has not been well studied.

Normal Variability

The range of liver T_2 and T_2^* values in individuals without iron overload is wide. For example, Schwenzer and colleagues[74] found that normal T_2^* values ranged from 14 to 46 ms at 1.5T (mean 28 ms, standard deviation 7 ms). The wide range of T_2 and T_2^* values in individuals without iron overload is in contradistinction to PDFF, the liver steatosis biomarker, which varies narrowly in individuals without excess liver fat. The wide T_2 and T_2^* range makes relaxometry methods inherently inaccurate for quantifying mild iron overload; the reason is that depending on an individual's baseline T_2 or T_2^* value, the amount of iron in mild overload states may fail to drive the T_2 or T_2^* into the abnormal range. Thus, while relaxometry methods may be accurate for quantifying iron in subjects with moderate to severe iron overload (eg, patients with thalassemia or HH), they may not be accurate for quantifying iron in subjects with mild iron overload (eg, patients' chronic hepatopathy and secondary iron overload).

Concomitant Fibrosis, Inflammation, and Fat

Hepatic fibrosis and inflammation may confound the MR imaging measurement—LIC relationship because they prolong T_2 relaxation and so may partially offset the T_2-shortening effect of iron.[9] Also, both inflammation and fibrosis are associated with restricted diffusion of water molecules in the liver parenchyma.[88,89] As the effects of diffusion contribute strongly to iron-mediated relaxation mechanisms,[13,17,84] diffusion restriction may reduce the sensitivity of relaxation parameters to the presence of iron. Moreover, fibrosis alters the spatial distribution of iron,[2] which may affect R_2 as discussed previously. The confounding effect of fat is discussed in the next section.

QUANTIFICATION OF IRON AND FAT WHEN BOTH ARE PRESENT

Does the presence of fat corrupt our ability to quantify iron? Some investigators have described the use of T_2^*-weighted imaging[63] and multi-echo R_2^* map measurements by only acquired "in-phase" echoes.[77] If fat had a single discrete nuclear magnetic resonance (NMR) peak, this would be an excellent approach to avoid the effects of fat when quantifying R_2^*. However, fat signal is never truly "in-phase" except at TE = 0. The interference of the multiple resonance peaks of fat leads to destructive interference that accelerates signal decay, shortening the apparent T_2^* ($T_2^*{}_{app}$). **Fig. 11** contains a simulation that illustrates the signal behavior of tissue containing 0%, 20%, and 40% fat with a true T_2^* of 25 ms, all at 1.5T. When signal is acquired at 3 "in-phase" echo times (4.6 ms, 9.2 ms, 13.8 ms) and the apparent T_2^* is estimated, considerable error results owing to the accelerated signal decay from the interference caused by the multiple peaks

of fat, with apparent T_2^* of 25 ms (as expected), 21 ms, and 18 ms for 0% fat, 20% fat, and 40% fat, respectively. **Fig. 12** further illustrates this point by demonstrating that the estimated T_2^* is highly dependent on the *number* of "in-phase" echoes, contrary to the concept that exponential signal decay time constants are, by definition, independent of the echo times.

The ability to measure iron through T_2^* decay (R_2^* mapping) is, therefore, heavily influenced by the presence of fat. Thus, it is not possible to measure fat-fraction and R_2^* without measuring the two simultaneously. Fortunately, 3 groups have described methods that simultaneously estimate water and fat signals, along with T_2^* decay.[90–93] Although these methods were all developed primarily in the context of measuring fat-fraction, they also offer new opportunities to quantify R_2^* by correcting for the presence of fat. Importantly, as demonstrated in **Figs. 11** and **12**, the multiple peaks of fat are the primary reason why the presence of fat creates bias in the measurement of R_2^*. Therefore, measurement of R_2^* in the presence of fat should incorporate spectral modeling of fat into their T_2^* correction methods.[90–92] To date, only the methods of Bydder and colleagues[91] and Yu and colleagues[90,92] incorporate both the effects of T_2^* decay and spectral modeling.

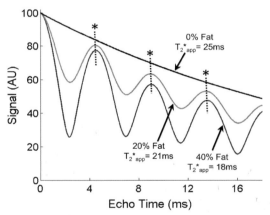

Fig. 11. Fat corrupts the ability of gradient echo methods to quantify T_2^* using conventional multi-echo imaging methods. In the simulation shown in this figure, the signal from a water-fat mixture with increasing amounts of fat at 0% (*black*), 20% (*red*), and 40% (*blue*) are shown for a true $T_2^* = 25$ ms at 1.5T. Even when images are acquired "in-phase" (*asterisks*), the fitted values of T_2^* are inaccurate when fat is present. This occurs because the spectral complexity of fat causes fat to interfere with itself and accelerates the effective signal decay. To measure T_2^* accurately, simultaneous measurement of fat and T_2^* is necessary, including spectral modeling of fat, such as performed by the methods of Bydder and colleagues[91] and Yu and colleagues.[90,92] Without simultaneous measurement of fat and T_2^* with spectral modeling, it is not possible to measure fat concentration and iron concentration (indirectly through T_2^*), when both iron and fat are present.

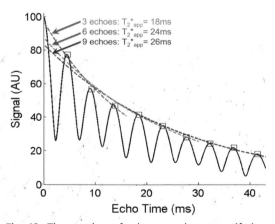

Fig. 12. The number of echoes used to quantify iron (indirectly, through measurement of T_2^*) also affects the ability of MR imaging to measure T_2^*, when fat is present. The presence of fat creates a complicated signal pattern because of the interference of multiple fat peaks, leading to signal decay that is no longer monoexponential. Without simultaneous measurement of fat and T_2^*, including spectral modeling, the ability of MR imaging to measure T_2^* accurately is corrupted, even when images are acquired at "in-phase" echo times (*squares*). In this simulation, the true $T_2^* = 25$ ms, and the fat-fraction is 40%.

Figs. 13–16 show examples of patients with co-existing steatosis and iron overload imaged using the methods of Bydder and colleagues[91] and Yu and colleagues[90,92] that both provide a simultaneous PDFF map and an R_2^* map. Interestingly, in **Fig. 14**, the conventional in-and-opposed-phase images demonstrated nearly *identical* signal intensity between the in-phase and opposed-phase images, indicating that the effects of iron and fat exactly balanced one another in this case. The complex method of Yu and colleagues[92] measured 13.5% fat and $T_2^* = 9.6$ ms, both of which are abnormal and clinically important. **Fig. 15** shows a different patient with severe steatosis (36.5% PDFF) and coexisting iron overload ($T_2^* = 9.4$ ms). **Fig. 16** shows an example of diffuse steatosis with nodular areas of focal fat, with superimposed iron overload imaged with 2-point IOP and the method of Bydder and colleagues[91] that illustrates the importance of T_2^* correction and spectral modeling when both fat and iron are present.

An important assumption made by these methods is that the T_2^* decay of water and fat are either the same[90] or closely dependent on one another.[91] Differences in T_2^* decay between water and fat will lead to an averaging effect if a common T_2^* decay parameter is assumed in the signal model. Very recently, Chebrolu and colleagues[94] described a reconstruction approach that allows independent estimation of T_2^* of water and fat, including the effects of spectral fat modeling. This method was shown to improve quantification of fat and iron in a water-fat-superparamagnetic iron oxides phantom. O'Regan and colleagues[93] have described a magnitude-based method that allows independent estimation of T_2^* for water and fat, although they did not incorporate spectral modeling of fat. This work measured the T_2^* of water and fat to be 21.8 ± 6.7 ms and 4.6 ± 1.8 ms, respectively, in 5 healthy volunteers. By comparison, Schwenzer and colleagues[74] measured the average T_2^* in 129 healthy volunteers, measuring an average of 25.4 ± 6.0 ms. These results suggest that the method of O'Regan and colleagues[93] underestimates the T_2^* of fat, and possible water, possibly because of the interference of the multiple fat peaks that causes apparent accelerated signal decay.

The effects of fat on iron estimation methods that acquire T_2-weighted imaging or R_2 maps using spin-echo techniques deserve a mention. Images acquired with these methods acquire signal at spin echoes where the phase of water and all fat peaks are in-phase. Thus, the destructive interference effects of fat that occur with R_2^* methods will not be a factor with R_2 methods. However, there is a dilutional effect of fat that may affect both R_2^* and R_2 methods. Iron

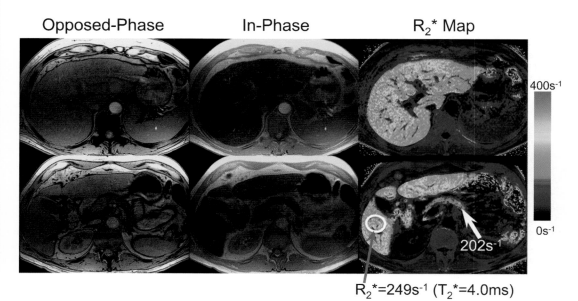

Opposed-Phase   In-Phase R_2^* Map

400s⁻¹

202s⁻¹

0s⁻¹

$R_2^*=249s^{-1} (T_2^*=4.0ms)$

Fig. 13. IOP imaging in a 60-year-old male with known genetic hemochromatosis shows paradoxic decrease in signal on the in-phase images (*middle column*) because these images are more heavily T_2^* weighted (TE = 4.6 ms, compared with 2.3 ms for opposed-phase images). R_2^* maps measured using the method of Yu and colleagues[90,92] demonstrate dramatically shortened T_2^* in the liver (4.0 ms) as well as the pancreas (*arrow*, $T_2^* = 5.0$ ms). Note that whereas the liver and pancreas are affected, the spleen is spared, typical of genetic hemochromatosis.

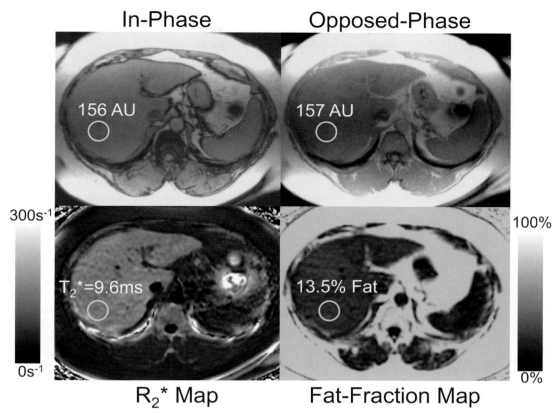

Fig. 14. Fat and iron corrupt the ability to detect and quantify the other using IOP imaging. In this obese patient with hemosiderosis, the signal intensity of the in-phase and opposed-phase images are essentially equal, suggesting that the liver is normal. However, quantitative imaging with the complex method of Yu and colleagues[92] shows markedly decreased T_2* (9.6 ms) and abnormally high fat concentration (13.5%) demonstrating how the presence of iron and fat corrupt the ability to measure the other, unless both are measured simultaneously. Also, note the shortened T_2* in the spleen, consistent with hemosiderosis. (*Courtesy of* S. Vasanawala, MD, PhD, Stanford University, Stanford, CA, and Huanzhou Yu, PhD, MR Global Applied Science Lab, GE Healthcare, Menlo Park, CA.)

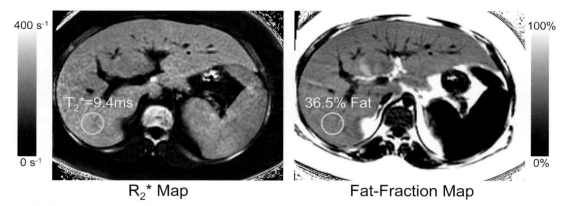

Fig. 15. High fat concentrations and elevated iron can coexist, necessitating the use of methods such as those by Bydder and colleagues[91] and Yu and colleagues[92] that can simultaneously estimate PDFF and T_2*. In this obese patient with hemosiderosis, the PDFF measured with the complex method of Yu and colleagues[92] was 36.5%, and the T_2* was 9.4 ms, both highly abnormal. (*Courtesy of* S. Vasanawala, MD, PhD, Stanford University, Stanford, CA, and Huanzhou Yu, PhD, MR Global Applied Science Lab, GE Healthcare, Menlo Park, CA.)

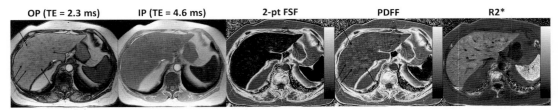

OP (TE = 2.3 ms)   IP (TE = 4.6 ms)   2-pt FSF   PDFF   R2*

Fig. 16. Simultaneous measurement of fat-fraction and R_2^* using the method of Bydder and colleagues.[91] Multiple unusual hypodense lesions were identified at CT (not shown), concerning for metastatic disease. Conventional in-and-opposed imaging reveals multiple hypointense nodules, best seen on OP images (*left*) corresponding to the hypodense nodules seen on CT. Fat signal fraction (FSF) calculated with 2-point IOP imaging (as explained in the article by Reeder and Sirlin elsewhere in this issue) shows no evidence of liver fat, because of T_2^* shortening. PDFF and R_2^* maps measured with the method of Bydder and colleagues[91] show diffuse fatty liver with nodular areas of focal fat, as well as elevated R_2^* (shortened T_2^*) in both the liver and spleen suggestive of hemosiderosis.

deposits in the liver exist in the form of iron oxide crystal within the cytoplasm of cells. Thus, they may have a differentially greater magnetic field perturbation on water signal, compared with fat signal. This could lead to bioexponential decay of water and fat signals owing to a mixing or dilutional effect from fat. The overall impact and importance of this effect remains to be determined, but should be considered in future studies in patients with concomitant iron overload and steatosis.

SUMMARY

Despite incomplete understanding of the underlying relaxation mechanisms, clinical studies have empirically established calibration curves that accurately predict chemically determined LIC values from MR imaging measurements (SIR, R_2, R_2^*). The leading methods are the ones published by Gandon and colleagues[62] (SIR), St Pierre and colleagues(R_2),[76] and Wood and colleagues (R_2^*).[77] The St Pierre method is FDA approved and commercially available (with a service charge), but is time consuming to perform. Preliminary studies suggest the Wood method may be of comparable accuracy but requires a single breath hold. A limitation of all SIR, R_2, and R_2^* methods is that they are based on empirical approaches. Many factors may confound the results but are not yet well understood.

New biomarkers of iron have the potential of benefiting a large number of patients with liver disease, because of increasing availability of MR technology and decreasing cost of MR examinations over the past decade. Today, estimated 10,000 to 15,000 MR imaging scanners are operational in the United States, which translates to approximately 30 to 45 MR imaging scanners per million (personal communication, Jason Polzin, PhD, GE Healthcare, 2009). MR imaging scanners

are now commonly found in both urban and rural communities and considered as accessible as CT and US. Moreover, it is generally agreed that MR imaging is more accessible than liver biopsy. The use of MR imaging as a quantitative biomarker of intracellular liver iron overload has shown tremendous progress in recent years and holds great promise to provide accessible and accurate evaluation of diffuse liver disease.

REFERENCES

1. Brittenham GM, Cohen AR, McLaren CE, et al. Hepatic iron stores and plasma ferritin concentration in patients with sickle cell anemia and thalassemia major. Am J Hematol 1993;42(1):81–5.
2. St Pierre TG, Clark PR, Chua-Anusorn W. Single spin-echo proton transverse relaxometry of iron-loaded liver. NMR Biomed 2004;17(7):446–58.
3. Alustiza JM, Castiella A, De Juan MD, et al. Iron overload in the liver diagnostic and quantification. Eur J Radiol 2007;61(3):499–506.
4. Bothwell TH, Charlton RW. A general approach to the problems of iron deficiency and iron overload in the population at large. Semin Hematol 1982; 19(1):54–67.
5. Cook JD, Skikne BS, Lynch SR, et al. Estimates of iron sufficiency in the US population. Blood 1986; 68(3):726–31.
6. Pietrangelo A. Hereditary hemochromatosis—a new look at an old disease. N Engl J Med 2004;350(23): 2383–97.
7. Siegelman ES, Mitchell DG, Semelka RC. Abdominal iron deposition: metabolism, MR findings, and clinical importance. Radiology 1996;199(1):13–22.
8. Gossuin Y, Muller RN, Gillis P. Relaxation induced by ferritin: a better understanding for an improved MRI iron quantification. NMR Biomed 2004;17(7):427–32.
9. Carneiro AA, Fernandes JP, de Araujo DB, et al. Liver iron concentration evaluated by two magnetic

methods: magnetic resonance imaging and magnetic susceptometry. Magn Reson Med 2005; 54(1):122–8.

10. Li TQ, Aisen AM, Hindmarsh T. Assessment of hepatic iron content using magnetic resonance imaging. Acta Radiol 2004;45(2):119–29.

11. Brittenham GM, Badman DG. Noninvasive measurement of iron: report of an NIDDK workshop. Blood 2003;101(1):15–9.

12. Andrews NC. Disorders of iron metabolism. N Engl J Med 1999;341(26):1986–95.

13. Ghugre NR, Coates TD, Nelson MD, et al. Mechanisms of tissue-iron relaxivity: nuclear magnetic resonance studies of human liver biopsy specimens. Magn Reson Med 2005;54(5):1185–93.

14. Adams P, Brissot P, Powell LW. EASL international consensus conference on haemochromatosis. J Hepatol 2000;33(3):485–504.

15. Feder JN, Gnirke A, Thomas W, et al. A novel MHC class I-like gene is mutated in patients with hereditary haemochromatosis. Nat Genet 1996;13(4): 399–408.

16. Beutler E, Gelbart T, West C, et al. Mutation analysis in hereditary hemochromatosis. Blood Cells Mol Dis 1996;22(2):187–94 [discussion: 194a–b].

17. Jensen JH, Chandra R. Theory of nonexponential NMR signal decay in liver with iron overload or superparamagnetic iron oxide particles. Magn Reson Med 2002;47(6):1131–8.

18. Niederau C, Fischer R, Sonnenberg A, et al. Survival and causes of death in cirrhotic and in noncirrhotic patients with primary hemochromatosis. N Engl J Med 1985;313(20):1256–62.

19. Wood JC. Magnetic resonance imaging measurement of iron overload. Curr Opin Hematol 2007; 14(3):183–90.

20. Papakonstantinou O, Alexopoulou E, Economopoulos N, et al. Assessment of iron distribution between liver, spleen, pancreas, bone marrow, and myocardium by means of R2 relaxometry with MRI in patients with beta-thalassemia major. J Magn Reson Imaging 2009;29(4):853–9.

21. Anderson LJ, Wonke B, Prescott E, et al. Comparison of effects of oral deferiprone and subcutaneous desferrioxamine on myocardial iron concentrations and ventricular function in beta-thalassaemia. Lancet 2002;360(9332):516–20.

22. Ehlers KH, Levin AR, Markenson AL, et al. Longitudinal study of cardiac function in thalassemia major. Ann N Y Acad Sci 1980;344:397–404.

23. Beaumont M, Odame I, Babyn PS, et al. Accurate liver T-2* measurement of iron overload: a simulations investigation and in vivo study. J Magn Reson Imaging 2009;30(2):313–20.

24. Angelucci E, Muretto P, Nicolucci A, et al. Effects of iron overload and hepatitis C virus positivity in determining progression of liver fibrosis in thalassemia following bone marrow transplantation. Blood 2002; 100(1):17–21.

25. Bonny JM, Zanca M, Boire JY, et al. T-2 maximum likelihood estimation from multiple spin-echo magnitude images. Magn Reson Med 1996;36(2):287–93.

26. Angelucci E, Brittenham GM, McLaren CE, et al. Hepatic iron concentration and total body iron stores in thalassemia major. N Engl J Med 2000;343(5): 327–31.

27. Fujita N, Sugimoto R, Urawa N, et al. Hepatic iron accumulation is associated with disease progression and resistance to interferon/ribavirin combination therapy in chronic hepatitis C. J Gastroenterol Hepatol 2007;22(11):1886–93.

28. Pietrangelo A. Non-invasive assessment of hepatic iron overload: are we finally there? J Hepatol 2005; 42(1):153–4.

29. O'Neil J, Powell L. Clinical aspects of hemochromatosis. Semin Liver Dis 2005;25(4):381–91.

30. Brittenham GM, Griffith PM, Nienhuis AW, et al. Efficacy of deferoxamine in preventing complications of iron overload in patients with thalassemia major. N Engl J Med 1994;331(9):567–73.

31. Borgna-Pignatti C, Castriota-Scanderbeg A. Methods for evaluating iron stores and efficacy of chelation in transfusional hemosiderosis. Haematologica 1991;76(5):409–13.

32. Drakonaki EE, Maris TG, Maragaki S, et al. Deferoxamine versus combined therapy for chelating liver, spleen and bone marrow iron in beta-thalassemic patients: a quantitative magnetic resonance imaging study. Hemoglobin 2010;34(1):95–106.

33. Positano V, Salani B, Pepe A, et al. Improved T2* assessment in liver iron overload by magnetic resonance imaging. Magn Reson Imaging 2009;27(2): 188–97.

34. Bassett ML, Halliday JW, Powell LW. Value of hepatic iron measurements in early hemochromatosis and determination of the critical iron level associated with fibrosis. Hepatology 1986;6(1):24–9.

35. Adams PC, Deugnier Y, Moirand R, et al. The relationship between iron overload, clinical symptoms, and age in 410 patients with genetic hemochromatosis. Hepatology 1997;25(1):162–6.

36. Carneiro AAO, Fernandes JP, Zago MA, et al. An alternating current superconductor susceptometric system to evaluate liver iron overload. Rev Sci Instrum 2003;74(6):3098–103.

37. Bonkovsky HL, Jawaid Q, Tortorelli K, et al. Non-alcoholic steatohepatitis and iron: increased prevalence of mutations of the HFE gene in non-alcoholic steatohepatitis. J Hepatol 1999;31(3): 421–9.

38. Bonkovsky HL, Rubin RB, Cable EE, et al. Hepatic iron concentration: noninvasive estimation by means of MR imaging techniques. Radiology 1999;212(1): 227–34.

39. George DK, Goldwurm S, MacDonald GA, et al. Increased hepatic iron concentration in nonalcoholic steatohepatitis is associated with increased fibrosis. Gastroenterology 1998;114(2):311–8.

40. Moirand R, Mortaji AM, Loreal O, et al. A new syndrome of liver iron overload with normal transferrin saturation. Lancet 1997;349(9045):95–7.

41. Harrison SA, Bacon BR. Relation of hemochromatosis with hepatocellular carcinoma: epidemiology, natural history, pathophysiology, screening, treatment, and prevention. Med Clin North Am 2005;89(2):391–409.

42. Powell EE, Ali A, Clouston AD, et al. Steatosis is a cofactor in liver injury in hemochromatosis. Gastroenterology 2005;129(6):1937–43.

43. Rowe JW, Wands JR, Mezey E, et al. Familial hemochromatosis: characteristics of the precirrhotic stage in a large kindred. Medicine (Baltimore) 1977;56(3):197–211.

44. Barry M, Sherlock S. Measurement of liver-iron concentration in needle-biopsy specimens. Lancet 1971;1(7690):100–3.

45. Bravo A, Sheth S, Chopra S. Liver biopsy. N Engl J Med 2001;344(7):495–500.

46. Rofsky NM, Fleishaker H. CT and MRI of diffuse liver disease. Semin Ultrasound CT MR 1995;16(1):16–33.

47. Mortele KJ, Ros PR. Imaging of diffuse liver disease. Semin Liver Dis 2001;21(2):195–212.

48. Guyader D, Gandon Y, Deugnier Y, et al. Evaluation of computed tomography in the assessment of liver iron overload. A study of 46 cases of idiopathic hemochromatosis. Gastroenterology 1989;97(3):737–43.

49. Wang ZJ, Haselgrove JC, Martin MB, et al. Evaluation of iron overload by single voxel MRS measurement of liver T2. J Magn Reson Imaging 2002;15(4):395–400.

50. Bauman JH, Hoffman RW. Magnetic susceptibility meter for in vivo estimation of hepatic iron stores. IEEE Trans Biomed Eng 1967;14(4):239–43.

51. Bauman JH, Harris JW. Estimation of hepatic iron stores by vivo measurement of magnetic susceptibility. J Lab Clin Med 1967;70(2):246–57.

52. Carneiro AAO, Baffa O, Fernandes JP, et al. Theoretical evaluation of the susceptometric measurement of iron in human liver by four different susceptometers. Physiol Meas 2002;23(4):683–93.

53. Stark DD, Bass NM, Moss AA, et al. Nuclear magnetic resonance imaging of experimentally induced liver disease. Radiology 1983;148(3):743–51.

54. Stark DD, Goldberg HI, Moss AA, et al. Chronic liver disease: evaluation by magnetic resonance. Radiology 1984;150(1):149–51.

55. Maris TG, Papakonstantinou O, Chatzimanoli V, et al. Myocardial and liver iron status using a fast T*2 quantitative MRI (T*2qMRI) technique. Magn Reson Med 2007;57(4):742–53.

56. Brooks RA, Moiny F, Gillis P. On T2-shortening by weakly magnetized particles: the chemical exchange model. Magn Reson Med 2001;45(6):1014–20.

57. Brewer CJ, Coates TD, Wood JC. Spleen R2 and R2* in iron-overloaded patients with sickle cell disease and thalassemia major. J Magn Reson Imaging 2009;29(2):357–64.

58. Siegelman ES, Mitchell DG, Rubin R, et al. Parenchymal versus reticuloendothelial iron overload in the liver: distinction with MR imaging. Radiology 1991;179(2):361–6.

59. St Pierre TG, Clark PR, Chua-Anusorn W. Measurement and mapping of liver iron concentrations using magnetic resonance imaging. Ann N Y Acad Sci 2005;1054:379–85.

60. Clark PR, Chua-anusorn W, St Pierre TG. Bi-exponential proton transverse relaxation rate (R2) image analysis using RF field intensity-weighted spin density projection: potential for R2 measurement of iron-loaded liver. Magn Reson Imaging 2003;21(5):519–30.

61. Ernst O, Sergent G, Bonvarlet P, et al. Hepatic iron overload: Diagnosis and quantification with MR imaging. Am J Roentgenol 1997;168(5):1205–8.

62. Gandon Y, Olivie D, Guyader D, et al. Non-invasive assessment of hepatic iron stores by MRI. Lancet 2004;363(9406):357–62.

63. Gandon Y, Guyader D, Heautot JF, et al. Hemochromatosis: diagnosis and quantification of liver iron with gradient-echo MR imaging. Radiology 1994;193(2):533–8.

64. Kreeftenberg HG, Mooyaart EL, Huizenga JR, et al. Quantification of liver iron concentration with magnetic resonance imaging by combining T1-, T2-weighted spin echo sequences and a gradient echo sequence. Neth J Med 2000;56(4):133–7.

65. Olthof AW, Sijens PE, Kreeftenberg HG, et al. Non-invasive liver iron concentration measurement by MRI: comparison of two validated protocols. Eur J Radiol 2009;71(1):116–21.

66. Rose C, Vandevenne P, Bourgeois E, et al. Liver iron content assessment by routine and simple magnetic resonance imaging procedure in highly transfused patients. Eur J Haematol 2006;77(2):145–9.

67. Virtanen JM, Komu ME, Parkkola RK. Quantitative liver iron measurement by magnetic resonance imaging: in vitro and in vivo assessment of the liver to muscle signal intensity and the R2* methods. Magn Reson Imaging 2008;26(8):1175–82.

68. Alexopoulou E, Stripeli F, Baras P, et al. R2 relaxometry with MRI for the quantification of tissue iron overload in beta-thalassemic patients. J Magn Reson Imaging 2006;23(2):163–70.

69. Bulte JW, Miller GF, Vymazal J, et al. Hepatic hemo-siderosis in non-human primates: quantification of liver iron using different field strengths. Magn Reson Med 1997;37(4):530–6.

70. Wood JC, Ghugre N. Magnetic resonance imaging assessment of excess iron in thalassemia, sickle cell disease and other iron overload diseases. Hemoglobin 2008;32(1–2):85–96.

71. Gossuin Y, Muller RN, Gillis P, et al. Relaxivities of human liver and spleen ferritin. Magn Reson Imaging 2005;23(10):1001–4.

72. Chandarana H, Lim RP, Jensen JH, et al. Hepatic iron deposition in patients with liver disease: prelim-inary experience with breath-hold multiecho T2*-weighted sequence. AJR Am J Roentgenol 2009; 193(5):1261–7.

73. McCarville MB, Hillenbrand CM, Loeffler RB, et al. Comparison of whole liver and small region-of-interest measurements of MRI liver R2* in children with iron overload. Pediatr Radiol 2010;40(8): 1360–7.

74. Schwenzer NF, Machann J, Haap MM, et al. T2* relaxometry in liver, pancreas, and spleen in a healthy cohort of one hundred twenty-nine sub-jects—correlation with age, gender, and serum ferritin. Invest Radiol 2008;43(12):854–60.

75. Westwood M, Anderson LJ, Firmin DN, et al. A single breath-hold multiecho T2* cardiovascular magnetic resonance technique for diagnosis of myocardial iron overload. J Magn Reson Imaging 2003;18(1): 33–9.

76. St Pierre TG, Clark PR, Chua-anusorn W, et al. Noninvasive measurement and imaging of liver iron concentrations using proton magnetic resonance. Blood 2005;105(2):855–61.

77. Wood JC, Enriquez C, Ghugre N, et al. MRI R2 and R2* mapping accurately estimates hepatic iron concentration in transfusion-dependent thalassemia and sickle cell disease patients. Blood 2005;106(4): 1460–5.

78. Voskaridou E, Douskou M, Terpos E, et al. Magnetic resonance imaging in the evaluation of iron overload in patients with beta thalassaemia and sickle cell disease. Br J Haematol 2004;126(5):736–42.

79. Wright GA, Hu BS, Macovski A. 1991 I.I. Rabi Award. Estimating oxygen saturation of blood in vivo with MR imaging at 1.5 T. J Magn Reson Imaging 1991;1(3):275–83.

80. Hankins JS, McCarville MB, Loeffler RB, et al. R2* magnetic resonance imaging of the liver in patients with iron overload. Blood 2009;113(20):4853–5.

81. He T, Gatehouse PD, Kirk P, et al. Myocardial T-2* measurement in iron-overloaded thalassemia: an ex vivo study to investigate optimal methods of quantification. Magn Reson Med 2008;60(2):350–6.

82. Christoforidis A, Perifanis V, Spanos G, et al. MRI assessment of liver iron content in thalassemic patients with three different protocols: comparisons and correlations. Eur J Haematol 2009;82(5): 388–92.

83. Chappell KE, Patel N, Gatehouse PD, et al. Magnetic resonance imaging of the liver with ultra-short TE (UTE) pulse sequences. J Magn Reson Imaging 2003;18(6):709–13.

84. Yablonskiy DA, Haacke EM. Theory of NMR signal behavior in magnetically inhomogeneous tis-sues—the static dephasing regime. Magn Reson Med 1994;32(6):749–63.

85. Wood JC, Aguilar M, Otto-Duessel M, et al. Influence of iron chelation on R1 and R2 calibration curves in gerbil liver and heart. Magn Reson Med 2008; 60(1):82–9.

86. Gutierrez L, Lazaro FJ, Abadia AR, et al. Bioinor-ganic transformations of liver iron deposits observed by tissue magnetic characterisation in a rat model. J Inorg Biochem 2006;100(11):1790–9.

87. Muller RN, Gillis P, Moiny F, et al. Transverse relaxiv-ity of particulate MRI contrast media: from theories to experiments. Magn Reson Med 1991;22(2): 178–82 [discussion: 195–6].

88. Taouli B, Chouli M, Martin AJ, et al. Chronic hepatitis: role of diffusion-weighted imaging and diffusion tensor imaging for the diagnosis of liver fibrosis and inflammation. J Magn Reson Imaging 2008; 28(1):89–95.

89. Taouli B, Tolia AJ, Losada M, et al. Diffusion-weighted MRI for quantification of liver fibrosis: preliminary experience. AJR Am J Roentgenol 2007;189(4):799–806.

90. Yu H, McKenzie CA, Shimakawa A, et al. Multiecho reconstruction for simultaneous water-fat decompo-sition and T2* estimation. J Magn Reson Imaging 2007;26(4):1153–61.

91. Bydder M, Yokoo T, Hamilton G, et al. Relaxation effects in the quantification of fat using gradient echo imaging. Magn Reson Imaging 2008;26(3): 347–59.

92. Yu H, Shimakawa A, McKenzie CA, et al. Multiecho water-fat separation and simultaneous R2* estima-tion with multifrequency fat spectrum modeling. Magn Reson Med 2008;60(5):1122–34.

93. O'Regan DP, Callaghan MF, Wylezinska-Arridge M, et al. Liver fat content and T2*: simultaneous measurement by using breath-hold multiecho MR imaging at 3.0 T—feasibility. Radiology 2008; 247(2):550–7.

94. Chebrolu VV, Hines CD, Yu H, et al. Independent estimation of T*2 for water and fat for improved accuracy of fat quantification. Magn Reson Med 2010;63(4):849–57.

Chronic Hepatitis and Cirrhosis on MR Imaging

Tatsuyuki Tonan, MD[a], Kiminori Fujimoto, MD, PhD[a,b],
Aliya Qayyum, MD, MRCP, FRCR[c,*]

KEYWORDS

- Liver cirrhosis • Hepatitis
- Liver-specific MR contrast agent • Fibrosis
- Regenerative nodule • Dysplastic nodule
- Well-differentiated hepatocellular carcinoma

Chronic liver diseases represent a major cause of morbidity and mortality worldwide. The major origins of chronic liver disease and also leading causes of cirrhosis and hepatocellular carcinoma (HCC) are chronic infection with hepatitis B virus (HBV) and hepatitis C virus (HCV), and alcoholic and nonalcoholic fatty liver disease. Magnetic resonance (MR) imaging has been increasingly used to evaluate diffuse parenchymal abnormalities of the liver. Morphologic changes and signal intensity effects not only facilitate the diagnosis of chronic liver disease with MR imaging, but may help to distinguish between differing etiology and assist in staging severity. Moreover, recent advances in the development of MR systems and liver-specific MR contrast agents such as superparamagnetic iron oxide (SPIO) and gadoxetic acid (Gd-EOB-DTPA) have expanded the potential utility of MR imaging in the accurate depiction of specific disorders and cirrhosis-associated hepatocellular nodules.

In this article, the authors focus on the current role of MR imaging in the detection and characterization of chronic hepatitis and cirrhosis. In particular, the characteristic MR imaging features of morphologic changes and focal manifestations of chronic liver disease are highlighted.

DEFINITION, ETIOLOGY, AND PREVALENCE

Chronic hepatitis is defined as a continuous or recurrent inflammation of the liver for more than 6 months, with histologic changes of chronic liver damage. Pathologically it is characterized by lymphocytic infiltration, liver cell injury, necrosis, and fibrosis.[1] Chronic hepatitis progresses from mild inflammation, to more severe inflammation and fibrosis, and eventually to cirrhosis. Cirrhosis is characterized by the replacement of liver tissue by fibrosis, scar tissue, and regenerative nodules, leading to the deterioration of liver function.[2]

The most common causes of cirrhosis in the United States[3] are HBV and HCV infection, either singly or combined, and alcohol abuse. Other causes of cirrhosis include nonalcoholic fatty liver disease, hemochromatosis, autoimmune disease, Wilson disease, primary sclerosing cholangitis, and primary biliary cirrhosis.

The clinical importance of chronic liver disease is reflected in the large numbers of affected patients and the frequency of the associated serious complications. Approximately 400 million people are chronically infected with HBV worldwide,[4] of whom 25% to 40% die of cirrhosis and its end-stage complications. Chronic hepatitis C further affects approximately 200 million people

[a] Department of Radiology, Kurume University School of Medicine, 67 Asahi-machi, Kurume 830-0011, Japan
[b] Department of Radiology, Center for Diagnostic Imaging, Kurume University Hospital, 67 Asahi-machi, Kurume 830-0011, Japan
[c] Department of Radiology and Biomedical Imaging, University of California San Francisco, 505 Parnassus Avenue, Room L-307, Box 0628, San Francisco, CA 94143, USA
* Corresponding author.
E-mail address: aliya.qayyum@radiology.ucsf.edu

Magn Reson Imaging Clin N Am 18 (2010) 383–402
doi:10.1016/j.mric.2010.08.011

with a greater prevalence in Western countries.[5] The development of cirrhosis is common in chronic HCV, and the risk of HCC is 3% to 4% per year.[6] Once chronic HCV infection is established, cirrhosis develops within 10 to 20 years in approximately 20% of patients.[7] An estimated 10,000 deaths annually have been attributed to HCV-related diseases, and it is suggested that HCV may be responsible for nearly half of all HCC cases.

Alcoholic liver disease is among the most important causes of morbidity and mortality in the United States, accounting for up to 12,000 deaths each year, and representing more than 50% of liver disease–related deaths.[8,9] Nonalcoholic fatty liver disease (NAFLD) is now recognized as an important clinical entity, affecting approximately 20% to 30% of the adult population in the Western world.[10] NAFLD represents a disease spectrum ranging from isolated steatosis to more advanced disease with necroinflammatory change and fibrosis (nonalcoholic steatohepatitis or NASH), to cirrhosis in its most severe form. The prevalence of obesity and NAFLD in the United States translates into a substantial clinical problem, with more than 19% of obese individuals and 2% to 3% of the general population presenting with NASH.[10]

MR IMAGING FEATURES
Morphologic and Signal Intensity Changes

Hepatitis is associated with infiltration of inflammatory cells in to the liver, which results in liver cell injury and edema. Such liver changes may be visualized as periportal edema, which is characterized by high signal intensity bands paralleling the portal vessels on T2-weighted images (**Fig. 1**).

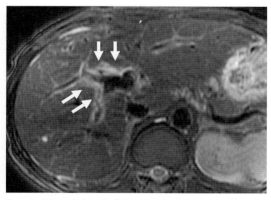

Fig. 1. T2-weighted fat-saturated turbo spin-echo (TSE) image (repetition time/echo time [TR/TE] = 4600/99 ms) in a patient with chronic hepatitis due to autoimmune hepatitis shows regions of high signal intensity bands paralleling the portal vessels (*arrow*).

Periportal edema is a common but nonspecific imaging finding in patients with severe acute hepatitis[11] and is also described in chronic viral hepatitis.[1] A similar appearance may also be seen in patients with malignant lymphadenopathy in the porta hepatis, biliary obstruction, cirrhosis, hepatic trauma, or transplant rejection.[12]

As cirrhosis progresses from early to advanced or end stage, it gives rise to several intra- and extrahepatic changes, including regional morphologic changes in the liver, nodularity of the liver surface, splenomegaly, regenerative nodules, iron and fat deposition, and ascites, and the development of varices and collaterals.[13] Although the classically described findings of cirrhosis are common in advanced cirrhosis, they are seen less frequently in the early stage of the disease, at which time the liver may appear normal on cross-sectional imaging, occasionally hampering imaging-based diagnosis.[14]

Enlargement of the hilar periportal space[14] (**Fig. 2**) on MR imaging has been shown to be a useful sign in the diagnosis of early cirrhosis. It has been reported that this sign is visible in 98% of patients with early cirrhosis who do not have conventional signs (ie, splenomegaly, portosystemic collateral vessels, ascites, or surface nodularity), whereas this sign is seen in only 11% of patients with normal livers.[15] Often, expansion of the major interlobar fissure[16] (see **Fig. 2**) is seen in these patients with early cirrhosis. These findings are attributed to atrophy of the medial segment of the left hepatic lobe, suggesting that medial segment atrophy may be an initial morphologic change in early cirrhosis.[17]

Hepatic morphologic changes typically seen in advanced cirrhosis include hypertrophy of the caudate lobe and lateral segments of the left lobe, and atrophy of both posterior segments of the right lobe and the medial segment of the left lobe.[17] Other morphologic changes with high specificity for a diagnosis of cirrhosis include the expanded gallbladder fossa sign (**Fig. 3**),[18] which is defined as enlargement of the pericholecystic space (ie, gallbladder fossa), and the right posterior hepatic notch sign (see **Fig. 3**),[19] which is defined as a sharp indentation in the right medial posterior surface of the liver (**Table 1**).

The patterns of hepatic morphologic and signal intensity changes overlap among the different causes of cirrhosis. However, certain imaging features may suggest particular etiological factors, such as enlargement of the lateral segment accompanied by shrinkage of both the right lobe and left medial segment, which reportedly frequently occurs in patients with viral-induced cirrhosis. Conversely, previous study showed

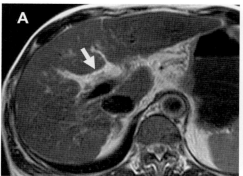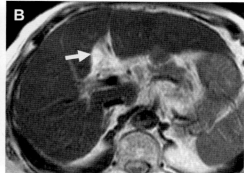

Fig. 2. T2-weighted TSE image in early cirrhosis shows enlargement of the hilar periportal space between the left medial segment and the right portal vein (*A*) (*arrow*) and expansion of the major interlobar fissure (*B*) (*arrow*) between the left medial and lateral segments.

that the mean values of the volume index of the caudate lobe were significantly greater in patients with alcoholic cirrhosis than in patients with viral cirrhosis.[20] Marked caudate lobe enlargement is typically associated with alcoholic cirrhosis.[20]

Primary sclerosing cholangitis (PSC) and primary biliary cirrhosis (PBC) have several distinctive features that may help to differentiate them from other types of cirrhosis (**Table 2**). PSC is reportedly associated with hypertrophy of the caudate lobe and atrophy of the other areas (medial segment, lateral segment, and right hepatic lobe, either individually or in combination)

(**Fig. 4**).[21] Previous study showed that these findings were observed in 68% (ie, hypertrophy of the caudate lobe) and 55% (ie, atrophy of the other areas) of patients with PSC, respectively.[21] Other etiologies, such as Budd-Chiari syndrome also demonstrate hypertrophy of the caudate lobe and variable atrophy/hypertrophy of the remaining portions of the liver.[22] In addition, irregular intra- and/or extrahepatic bile duct dilatation and stenosis are also observed. The arterial or delayed phase of contrast-enhanced dynamic MR imaging demonstrates increased enhancement of the hepatic parenchyma surrounding the dilated

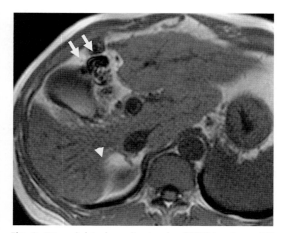

Fig. 3. T1-weighted gradient-echo (GRE) in-phase (TE, 4.7 ms) image in advanced cirrhosis shows enlargement of the pericholecystic space, presenting the expanded gallbladder fossa sign (*arrows*), and sharp indentation in the right medial posterior surface, presenting the right posterior hepatic notch sign (*arrowhead*).

Table 1
Typical morphologic changes of liver cirrhosis

Early Cirrhosis	Advanced Cirrhosis
Enlargement of the hilar periportal space	Hypertrophy of caudate lobe and/or lateral segments
Expansion of the major interlobar fissure	Atrophy of medial and/or posterior segments Enlargement of the pericholecystic space (expanded gallbladder fossa sign) Hepatic sharp indentation in the posterior surface (right posterior hepatic notch sign)

Data from Refs.[12–16]

Table 2
Distinctive morphologic changes and appearance of PSC and PBC at MR imaging

	Morphologic Changes	Appearance on MR Imaging
PSC	Hypertrophy of caudate lobe Atrophy of medial segment, lateral segment, right hepatic lobe (or all of 3 segments) Dilatation and stenosis of intra- and/or extrahepatic bile duct	Dynamic MR imaging[a] Increased enhancement of local hepatic parenchyma SPIO[b] Decreased enhancement of local hepatic parenchyma Gd-EOB-DTPA[c] Decreased enhancement of local hepatic parenchyma
PBC	Nonspecific	Periportal hyperintensity (hyperintense on T2WI) MR imaging periportal halo sign (hypointense on T1WI and T2WI)

Abbreviations: PBC, primary biliary cirrhosis; PSC, primary sclerosing cholangitis; WI, weighted imaging.
[a] T1-weighted GRE image on arterial- and portal phase after administration of gadolinium-based contrast agents.
[b] T2-weighted GRE image after administration of superparamagnetic iron oxide (SPIO).
[c] T1-weighted GRE image on hepatocyte-selective phase after administration of gadoxetic acid (Gd-EOB-DTPA).
Data from Refs.[17–19]

intrahepatic bile duct (**Fig. 5**), which is considered to represent fibrotic changes and hepatocyte damage.[21] In the authors' experience, the periductal parenchyma in PSC does not show uptake of SPIO, a liver-specific MR contrast agent normally taken up by hepatic Kupffer cells (**Fig. 6**). A reduced uptake of hepatobiliary-specific contrast agents (ie, Gd-EOB-DTPA, discussed later) is also observed (see **Fig. 6**).

MR findings that have been shown to be helpful in the diagnosis of PBC include periportal hyperintensity on T2-weighted images and the periportal halo sign (**Fig. 7**). Periportal hyperintensity on T2-weighted MR images has been attributed to

periportal inflammation.[23] One study reported that periportal hyperintensity (see **Fig. 7**) was observed in 100% of patients with PBC with histologic stage I or II disease, 75% of patients with stage III disease, and 33% of patients with stage IV disease.[24] Forty-three percent of patients with PBC are reported to demonstrate the periportal halo sign (see **Fig. 7**), which is depicted as periportal signal hypointensity on T1- and T2-weighted

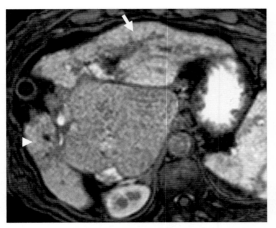

Fig. 5. Arterial-phase contrast-enhanced dynamic MR imaging shows slight increased enhancement of liver parenchyma in the lateral segment (*arrowhead*) and right hepatic lobe (*arrow*), which corresponds to the distribution of intrahepatic bile duct dilatation in comparison with that in caudate lobe. (Same patient as in **Fig. 4**.)

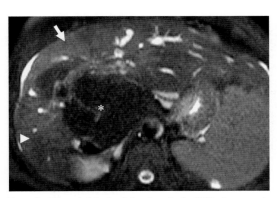

Fig. 4. T2-weighted fat-saturated TSE image in a patient with primary sclerosing cholangitis (PSC) shows hypertrophy of the caudate lobe (*asterisk*), and atrophy of the medial segment (*arrow*) and right hepatic lobe (*arrowhead*).

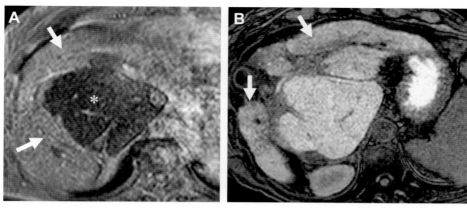

Fig. 6. T2-weighted GRE image (TE, 9.5 ms) within 10 minutes after administration of SPIO (*A*) demonstrates a high-intensity area in which SPIO particles are not taken up, presenting fibrotic change and hepatocyte damage (*arrows*). Conversely, uptake of SPIO particles is observed in the caudate lobe (*asterisk*). T1-weighted fat-saturated 3-dimensional (3D) gradient-echo (GRE) images (TR/TE = 3.6/1.7 ms, flip angle = 15°) in hepatocyte-selective phase (*B*) shows also decrease of uptake of Gd-EOB-DTPA (*arrows*). (Same patient as in **Fig. 4**.)

MR images.[23] It has been suggested that the MR imaging periportal halo sign may represent stellate, periportal, hepatocellular parenchymal extinction encircled by a rosette of large regenerating nodules.[23]

Portal Hypertension

In the cirrhotic liver, progressive hepatic fibrosis leads to increased vascular resistance at the level of the hepatic sinusoids, which results in a reduced portal contribution to liver perfusion.[25] The subsequent development of portal hypertension gives rise to complications such as ascites and the

development of collateral vessels at the lower end of the esophagus (**Fig. 8**).[26] Portosystemic shunts also form through reopened paraumbilical veins (see **Fig. 8**) and the left gastric vein, which both normally drain into the portal vein.

The decreased portal venous supply that occurs as a result of liver fibrosis is partially compensated by an increase in arterial blood supply.[27] Such an increase in arterial perfusion may be demonstrated by pronounced liver enhancement in the first seconds after administration of intravenous contrast media in cirrhotic patients. Early patchy enhancement of liver parenchyma on MR imaging is a feature of portal hypertension, and is

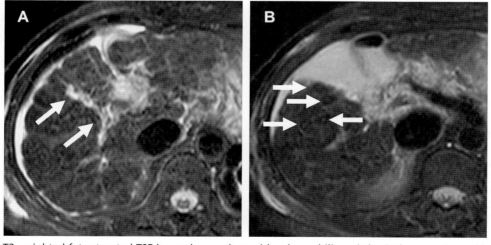

Fig. 7. T2-weighted fat-saturated TSE image in a patient with primary biliary cirrhosis shows periportal hyperintensity (*A*) (*arrows*) around portal tracts and around areas of low-intensity signal (*B*) (*arrows*) encircling the portal veins, presenting the periportal halo sign.

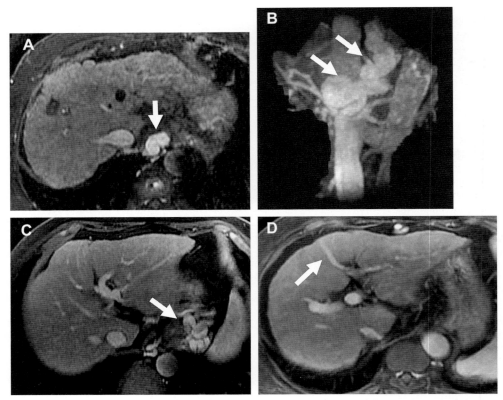

Fig. 8. Axial T1-weighted fat-saturated 3D GRE images (TR/TE = 3.3/1.5 ms, flip angle = 12°) (*A, C, D*) and maximum-intensity projection image (*B*) in portal phase after administration of Gd-EOB-DTPA at 3-T units shows examples of collateral vessel development in end-stage cirrhosis; dilated and tortuous esophageal varices (*A, B*) (*arrows*), gastric varices (*C*) (*arrow*), and recanalized paraumbilical veins (*D*) (*arrow*).

reportedly associated with the presence of numerous infiltrating macrophages, necrosis, tissue collapse, and increased steatosis (**Fig. 9**).[28]

Fibrosis

Pathologic characteristics and MR imaging features of liver fibrosis

Fibrosis is an inherent component of cirrhosis, and has MR imaging characteristics. In viral hepatitis, liver fibrosis begins and manifests as fibrous expansion of the portal triads (**Fig. 10**). Fibrous septa then grow from the expanded portal triad into the surrounding hepatic parenchyma. Subsequently, the fibrous septa lengthen and thicken to eventually form fibrous bridges that link adjacent portal triads and central veins (see **Fig. 10**). As the liver injury continues, the bridges continue to enlarge and coalesce and eventually divide the liver into rounded islands of hepatic parenchyma (regenerative nodules) surrounded by fibrosis tissue (see **Fig. 10**).[29] The pattern of early fibrosis

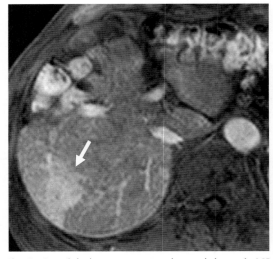

Fig. 9. Arterial-phase contrast-enhanced dynamic MR image shows increased enhancement of liver parenchyma (*arrow*), presenting early patchy enhancement.

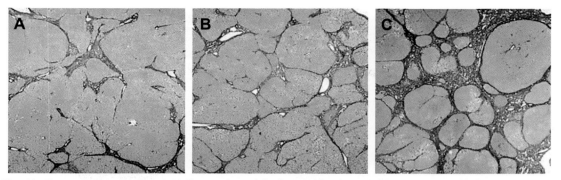

Fig. 10. Photomicrographs (Azan-Mallory stain, original magnification ×20) in a patient with hepatitis C virus infection (HCV) shows chronic hepatitis (*A*), early cirrhosis (*B*), and advanced cirrhosis (*C*). *A* shows moderate fibrosis without lobular distortion, and *B* shows advanced fibrosis having a tendency of lobular distortion. *C* shows multiple regenerative nodules and wider fibrous septa surrounding these nodules. (*Courtesy of* Osamu Nakashima, MD, Department of Pathology, Kurume University School of Medicine, Japan.)

differs in alcoholic hepatitis and nonalcoholic fatty liver disease because early fibrosis first develops adjacent to the central veins rather than in the portal triads, but progressive fibrosis eventually shows the same pathologic findings as cirrhosis caused by viral hepatitis.[29,30]

The current reference examination in the assessment of liver fibrosis is liver biopsy. However, this procedure is invasive with recognized morbidity and mortality, and repeated biopsy for the monitoring of disease progression is accordingly suboptimal. In addition, the accuracy of biopsy remains controversial because of sampling variability caused by the small size of hepatic samples and the heterogeneity of liver fibrosis.[31] These limitations have stimulated the search for noninvasive approaches to the assessment of liver fibrosis.

Conventional MR imaging techniques and fibrosis

The MR imaging appearance of the fibrotic septa and bridges comprises reticulations surrounding regenerative nodules giving rise to the so-called lacelike pattern. The fibrous septa appear hypointense on T1-weighted images and hyperintense on T2-weighted images (**Fig. 11**),[16] which in part is attributed to large water content.[22]

Most gadolinium-based contrast agent formulations freely equilibrate with extracellular volumes, such as liver fibrosis, and thereby improve the visibility of fibrosis on MR imaging.[32] MR images obtained at the equilibrium and delayed phase after gadolinium administration show fibrotic septa and bridges as linear and reticulation enhancement patterns.[28] These findings are more prominent in the periphery of the liver.

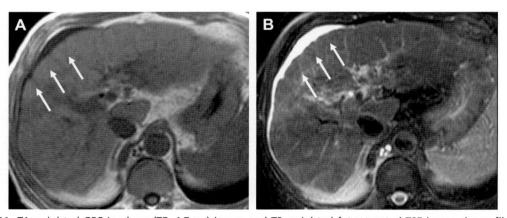

Fig. 11. T1-weighted GRE in-phase (TE, 4.7 ms) image and T2-weighted fat-saturated TSE image shows fibrotic septa and bridges as reticulations. The reticulations (*arrows*) are observed as hypointense on T1-weighted images (*A*) and as hyperintense on T2-weighted images (*B*).

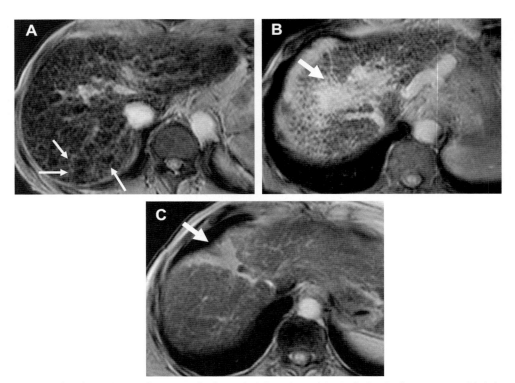

Fig. 12. T2-weighted GRE image (TE, 9.5 ms) after administration of SPIO distinctly demonstrates high-intensity reticulations (*A*) (*arrows*) and confluent fibrosis (*B* = wedge shape, *C* = geographic shape) (*arrow*), which do not take up SPIO particles in cirrhotic liver with HCV.

In end-stage liver cirrhosis, focal confluent fibrosis, which typically has a wedge shape or geographic shape with straight or concave borders, is occasionally observed in the subcapsular region.[22,29] The signal intensity and enhancement features of confluent fibrosis following administration of extracellular contrast agents are similar to those of fibrotic septa and bridges.

Liver-specific contrast agents and fibrosis
SPIO-enhanced MR imaging has been shown to be helpful in the detection of macroscopic fibrous bands and diffuse liver fibrosis. On T2-weighted turbo spin-echo and T2-weighted GRE images after administration of SPIO, the areas of fibrosis within the liver, which have reduced Kupffer cell density, accumulate less iron oxide

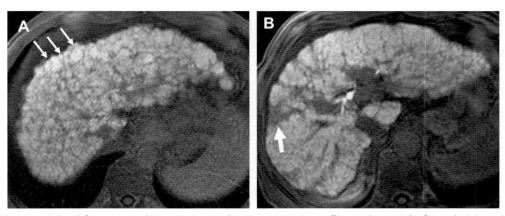

Fig. 13. T1-weighted fat-saturated 3D GRE image (TR/TE = 3.6/1.7 ms, flip angle = 15°) after administration of Gd-EOB-DTPA at hepatocyte-selective phases also clearly demonstrates fibrotic reticulations (*A*) and confluent fibrosis (*B* = wedge shape) (*arrows*).

Table 3
Macroscopic architectures and typical appearance of liver fibrosis at MR imaging

Macroscopic Findings	MR Imaging Form	Signal Intensity	Dynamic MR Imaging[a]	SPIO[b]	Gd-EOB-DTPA[c]
Fibrotic septa and bridge	Reticulation (lacelike pattern)	Hypointense (T1WI)	Increased enhancement	Hyperintense[d]	Hypointense[d]
Confluent fibrosis	Wedge shape or geographic shape	Hyperintense (T2WI)			

Abbreviations: Gd-EOB-DTPA, gadoxetic acid; SPIO, superparamagnetic iron oxide.
[a] T1-weighted GRE image on delayed phase after administration of gadolinium-based contrast agents.
[b] T2-weighted GRE image after administration of SPIO.
[c] T1-weighted GRE image on hepatocyte-selective phase after administration of Gd-EOB-DTPA.
[d] Appearance is described in comparison with the surrounding hepatic parenchyma.
Data from Refs.[13,23,24,26–28,30,31]

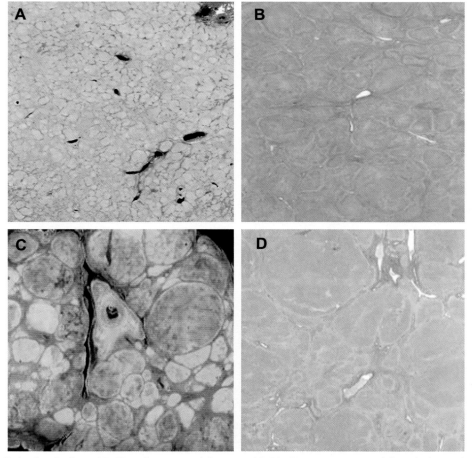

Fig. 14. Cirrhosis of micro- (*A, B*) and macronodular type (*C, D*). Gross appearance (*A*) and photomicrographs (Azan-Mallory stain, original magnification ×20) (*B*) show regenerative nodules (2–3 mm in size) with irregular shape in a case of cirrhotic liver with HCV. Gross appearance (*C*) and photomicrographs (Azan-Mallory stain, original magnification ×20) (*D*) show regenerative nodules (1–2 cm in size) with regular shape in a case of cirrhotic liver with HBV. (*Courtesy of* Osamu Nakashima, MD, Department of Pathology, Kurume University School of Medicine, Japan.)

and appear as hyperintense reticulations or areas (ie, confluent fibrosis)[33] compared with the surrounding hepatic parenchyma (**Fig. 12**). A recent study has shown the usefulness of double-contrast–enhanced MR imaging (sequential administration of SPIO and a gadolinium-based contrast agent) in the detection of liver fibrosis architecture. The investigators noted that the combination of these contrast agents was synergistic, and demonstrated liver fibrosis with greater clarity than could be achieved with either agent alone.[34]

Hepatobiliary-specific contrast agents such as mangafodipir trisodium (Mn-DPDP), gadobenate dimeglumine (Gd-BOPTA), and Gd-EOB-DTPA are taken up by functioning hepatocytes and excreted in the bile. The paramagnetic properties of these agents cause shortening of the longitudinal relaxation time (T1) of the liver and biliary tree. In visual analysis of images enhanced by Mn-DPDP, lower or heterogeneous enhancement areas are observed in cirrhotic liver, and it is considered that these areas contain the fibrous zone, indicating reticulation, confluent, and hepatocyte necrosis.[35,36] In the authors' experience, images enhanced by Gd-EOB-DTPA frequently show similar findings in cirrhotic liver, and this agent may also distinctly demonstrate liver fibrosis, such as fibrous septa, bridges (**Fig. 13**), and confluent fibrosis (see **Fig. 13**) (**Table 3**).

Emerging functional MR imaging techniques for fibrosis

Recently, several novel techniques for the assessment of liver fibrosis have been proposed, including MR elastography, diffusion-weighted MR imaging, and MR spectroscopy. MR elastography is a phase contrast-based MR imaging technique for direct visualization and quantitative measurement of propagating mechanical shear waves in biologic tissue.[37] Recent studies in patients with a spectrum of liver disease types have shown that liver stiffness as measured with MR elastography increases as the stage of fibrosis advances. The difference in stiffness between patients with early stages of fibrosis (F0 vs F1 vs F2) are small, with overlap between groups, but those between groups at higher stages (F2 vs F3 vs F4) are large, with little overlap.[38] Evaluation of the reproducibility and validity of MR

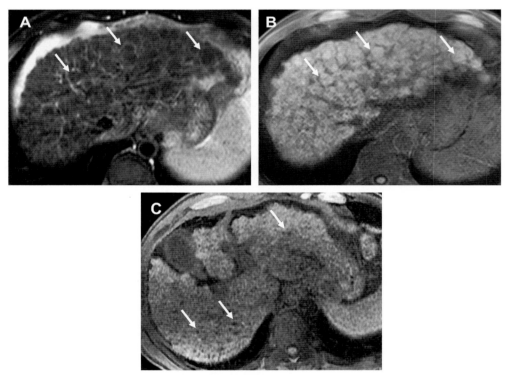

Fig. 15. Innumerable regenerative nodules have varying signal intensity, appearing isointense to hypointense on a T2-weighted fat-saturated TSE image (*A*) (*arrows*) and isointense to hyperintense on a T1-weighted fat-saturated 3D GRE image (TR/TE = 3.6/1.7 ms, flip angle = 15°) (*B*) (*arrows*). Hemosiderin deposition is common in regenerative nodules (siderotic nodules), producing such specific imaging features as hypointensity on T1-weighted fat-saturated 3D GRE image (*C*) (*arrows*).

Table 4
Characteristics and typical appearance of cirrhotic nodules at MR imaging

	Signal Intensity		Dynamic MR Imaging[a]	Kupffer Cell Density	SPIO[b]	Hepatocellular Function	Gd-EOB-DTPA[c]
	T1WI	T2WI					
RNs	Iso–Hyper (siderotic nodules; T1/T2WI, hypo)	Iso–Hypo	Iso–Hyper	Similar[d]	Iso[d]	Similar[d]	Iso[d]
DNs							
Low grade	Hypo–Hyper	Hypo	Iso–Hyper	Various[d]	Hypo–Hyper[d]	Various[d]	Hypo–Hyper[d]
High grade		Hypo–Slightly hyper					

Abbreviations: DNs, dysplastic nodules; Gd-EOB-DTPA, gadoxetic acid; Hypo, hypointense; Hyper, hyperintense; Iso, isointense; RNs, regenerative nodules; SPIO, superparamagnetic iron oxide.

[a] T1-weighted GRE image on delayed phase after administration of gadolinium-based contrast agents.
[b] T2-weighted GRE image after administration of SPIO.
[c] T1-weighted GRE image on hepatocyte-selective phase after administration of Gd-EOB-DTPA.
[d] Appearance is described in comparison with the surrounding hepatic parenchyma.
Data from Refs.[47–55,59–61]

elastography in an independent population of 35 healthy individuals and 48 patients with varying degrees of chronic liver disease showed a sensitivity of 86% and specificity of 85% for the detection of stages 2 to 4 fibrosis compared with liver histology from biopsy. A high negative predictive value (97%) for excluding the presence of fibrosis was also noted, suggesting that MR elastography might have a role in improving the ability to risk-stratify patients for liver biopsy to exclude occult advanced fibrosis.[39] MR elastography therefore appears to shows promise for the noninvasive staging of liver fibrosis, particularly in patients with advanced fibrosis.

Diffusion-weighted magnetic resonance imaging is a technique that assesses the freedom of diffusion of water protons within tissue by applying motion-sensitizing gradients that cause diffusing protons to lose signal. Recent advances in MR imaging technology have facilitated the performance of diffusion-weighted MR imaging of the liver, and it has also been used to detect liver fibrosis. Prior studies have reported that apparent diffusion coefficient (ADC) values acquired from b values of 500 (seconds/mm^2) and greater correlated significantly with liver fibrosis stage, and that ADC values with a combination of b value of 0 and 1000 (seconds/mm^2) showed the highest correlation (r = -0.654, $P<.001$).[40] On the other hand, several studies noted that there was no significant correlation between fibrosis stage and the ADC value using low b values (b values, 50 to 400 seconds/mm^2), because diffusion-weighted imaging with a low b value was influenced by perfusion contamination.[40,41] Luciani and colleagues,[42] reported that ADC calculated from low b values was significantly reduced in cirrhosis. Thus, the fast component diffusion-weighted MR imaging

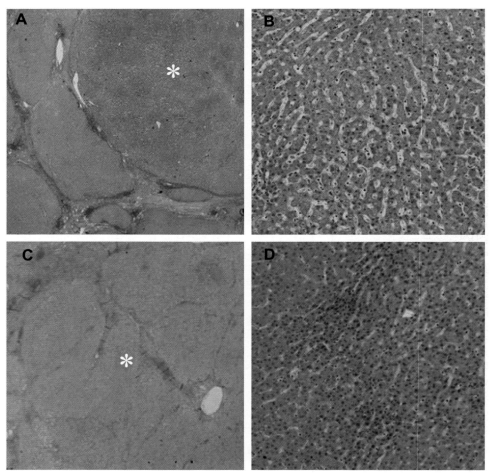

Fig. 16. Photomicrographs (Azan-Mallory stain, original magnification ×20 and ×100) in a patient with HCV shows low-grade dysplastic nodule (*asterisk*) (*A, B*) and high-grade dysplastic nodule (*asterisk*) (*C, D*). (*Courtesy of* Osamu Nakashima, MD, Department of Pathology, Kurume University School of Medicine, Japan.)

obtained with low b values may provide information related to microperfusion changes in diffuse liver disease whereas the slow component diffusion-weighted MR imaging obtained with high b values has been suggested to reflect a decrease in water proton diffusion.[43] The principles of diffusion-weighted MR imaging is discussed further in this presentation on functional MR imaging techniques.

In vivo MR spectroscopy (MRS) is most commonly used to assess signals from hydrogen (^{1}H) and phosphorus (^{31}P). Although ^{1}H-based MRS allows for the quantification of certain metabolites and lipids, ^{31}P-based MRS provides insights on processes, including cell turnover and energy state, based on the substantial ^{31}P concentrations within hepatocytes.[44] Previous studies have suggested MRS may be useful in detecting hepatic fibrosis.[45,46] An increased levels of hepatic phosphomonoesters (PME) have been reported in patients with established cirrhosis,[45,46] and an increasing PME to phosphodiester (PDE) ratio has been reported to correlate with worsening necroinflammatory and fibrosis scores on liver histology.[47] It has also been suggested that a PME and PDE ratio 0.2 or less is correlated with mild hepatitis and 0.3 or greater is correlated with cirrhosis in a study involving patients with chronic hepatitis C.[48] Despite some preliminary promising data, ^{31}P-based MRS is not widely used due to specific technical requirements. The role of MRS in the detection of liver inflammation and fibrosis requires further investigation.

CIRRHOSIS-ASSOCIATED HEPATOCELLULAR NODULES
Regenerative Nodules

Regenerative nodules form in response to necrosis, altered circulation, or other stimuli,[49] and may progress along a well-described carcinogenetic pathway to become dysplastic nodules or hepatocellular carcinomas.[50] These nodules are present in all cirrhotic livers and are surrounded by fibrous septa (see Fig. 10).[16] The nodules may be monoacinar or multiacinar, depending on

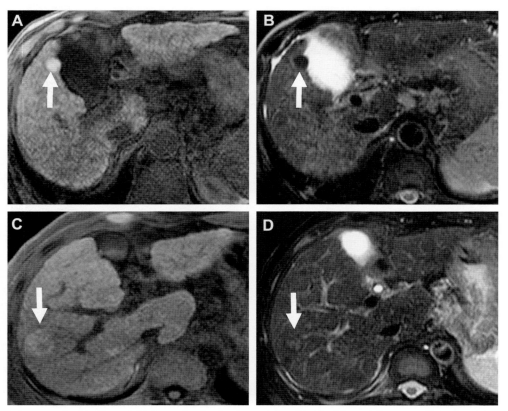

Fig. 17. Low-grade (*A*, *B*) and high-grade dysplastic nodules (*C*, *D*). All nodules were hyperintense on T1-weighted fat-saturated 3D GRE images (TR/TE = 3.6/1.7 ms, flip angle = 15°) (*A*, *C*) (*arrows*). In T2-weighted fat-saturated TSE images, in contrast, a low-grade dysplastic nodule is observed as hypointense (*B*) (*arrow*), whereas a high-grade nodule is observed as slightly hyperintense (*D*) (*arrow*).

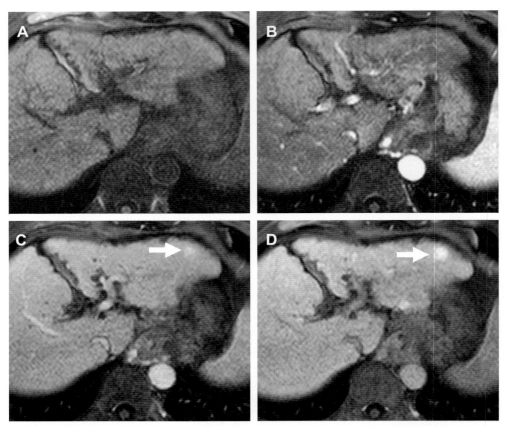

Fig. 18. Dynamic enhancement patterns of a high-grade dysplastic nodule in axial T1-weighted fat-saturated 3D GRE images (TR/TE = 3.6/1.7 ms, flip angle = 15°), presenting before (*A*) and in the arterial phase (30 s) (*B*), portal phase (90 s), and (*C*) equilibrium phase (4 min), and (*D*) after intravenous injection of Gd-EOB-DTPA. Portal and equilibrium phases (*arrow*) show increased enhancement of high-grade dysplastic nodule.

whether they contain one or more terminal portal tracts, and can also be classified by size as of the micronodular (≤3 mm) (**Fig. 14**), macronodular (>3 mm) (see **Fig. 14**), or mixed type (features of both micro- and macronodular types).[51]

MR imaging demonstrates regenerative nodules with greater sensitivity than any other imaging modality. These nodules usually appear isointense to hypointense (**Fig. 15**) on T2-weighted images relative to the surrounding inflammatory fibrous septa, and isointense to hyperintense (see **Fig. 15**) relative to background liver parenchyma on T1-weighted images.[52] The accumulation of iron within regenerative nodules (siderotic nodules) may cause hypointensity on both T1- and T2-weighted images (see **Fig. 15**) owing to susceptibility effects.[53] With regard to blood supply on dynamic imaging, regenerative nodules are usually enhanced to the same or greater degree than the background liver in the portal venous phase,[54] owing to the large contribution from the portal vein, with minimal contribution from the hepatic artery (**Table 4**).[55]

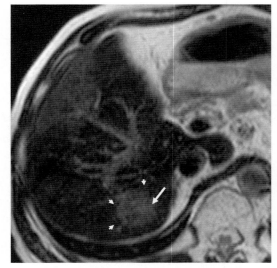

Fig. 19. T2-weighted TSE image shows an iso- to slightly high-signal–intensity nodule (*arrowheads*) with a focus of higher signal intensity (*arrow*) within the nodule. This higher signal intensity focus within the nodule shows the presence of HCC.

Dysplastic Nodules

Dysplastic nodules are considered an intermediate, premalignant step along the hepatocarcinogenesis process, and can also be classified by the degree of dysplasia as low- or high-grade.[56]

Low-grade dysplastic nodules are sometimes vaguely nodular but are often distinct from the surrounding cirrhotic liver because of the presence of peripheral fibrous scar.[56] This nodule is not a true capsule, but rather condensation of scarring as is seen around all cirrhotic nodules. Low-grade dysplastic nodules show mild increase in cell density with a uniform pattern, and without cytologic atypia.[56] Architectural changes beyond clearly regenerative features are not present; these lesions do not contain pseudoglands or markedly thickened trabeculae (**Fig. 16**).[56] High-grade dysplastic nodules may also be distinctly or vaguely nodular in the background of cirrhosis, although they also lack a true capsule, similar to low-grade dysplastic nodules; however, they are more likely to show a vaguely nodular pattern than low-grade dysplastic nodules.[56] A high-grade dysplastic nodule is defined as having architectural and/or cytologic atypia, but the atypia is insufficient for a diagnosis of HCC.[56] These lesions most often show increased cell density, sometimes more than 2 times higher than the surrounding nontumoral liver, often with an irregular trabecular pattern (see **Fig. 16**).[56] On MR imaging, dysplastic nodules have variable

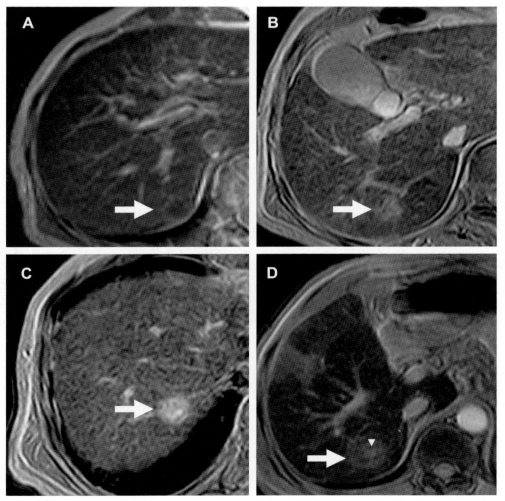

Fig. 20. T2-weighted GRE images (TE, 9.5 ms) after administration of SPIO in well-differentiated hepatocellular carcinoma (HCC) shows various signal intensities depending on Kupffer cell function within the nodule (*A−D*) (*arrow*). A dysplastic nodule with a central focus of HCC is observed as "a nodule within a nodule" (*D*) (*arrowhead*).

appearances, and their signal intensity character-istics overlap with those of regenerative nodules and well-differentiated HCC. On T2-weighted images, most dysplastic nodules are usually hypo-intense, and only rarely hyperintense (**Fig. 17**) It has been suggested that high-grade dysplastic nodules tend to have slightly higher signal intensity on T2-weighted images (see **Fig. 17**)[57]; however, the distinction from HCC and a high-grade dysplastic nodule may be difficult even on pathology. On T1-weighted images dysplastic nodules characteristically demonstrate high signal intensity, which may be related to deposition of copper, Fe^{3+}, or glycogen, or a high protein or lipid content (see **Fig. 17**).[58,59] However, the appear-ance on T1-weighted images cannot be used to distinguish low- and high-grade dysplastic nodules because both display variable (low, iso-, or high) signal intensity.[57]

With regard to blood supply, dysplastic nodules are typically hypovascular lesions with predomi-nantly portal venous blood supply, although increased arterial flow is seen in a small minority of cases (**Fig. 18**) (see **Table 4**).[60] The signal inten-sity characteristics of some high-grade dysplastic nodules that receive increasing supply from the hepatic artery may overlap with those of HCC nodules during the process of hepatocarcinogen-esis.[61] The hepatocarcinogenesis theory has been supported by the description of a dysplastic nodule with a central focus of HCC on T2-weighted images as "a nodule within a nodule."[62] The classic MR appearance is a focus of high signal intensity within a low-signal–intensity nodule on T2-weighted images (**Fig. 19**). This focus of HCC may also be enhanced in the arterial phase.[63] Despite the possibility of HCC devel-oping within dysplastic nodules, the development of this tumor may not be a linear process because HCC is recognized to occur in patients with chronic HBV but without cirrhosis.

Liver-Specific MR Contrast Agents (SPIO, Gd-EOB-DTPA) for Liver Nodules

Because the density of Kupffer cells within regen-erative nodules is similar to that in the surrounding nonneoplastic hepatic parenchyma, these nodules take up SPIO through Kupffer cell phagocytosis. On T2-weighted GRE and T2-weighted spin-echo sequences after administration of SPIO, regenerative nodules show the same signal inten-sity as that of surrounding hepatic parenchyma. In contrast, because Kupffer cell density within

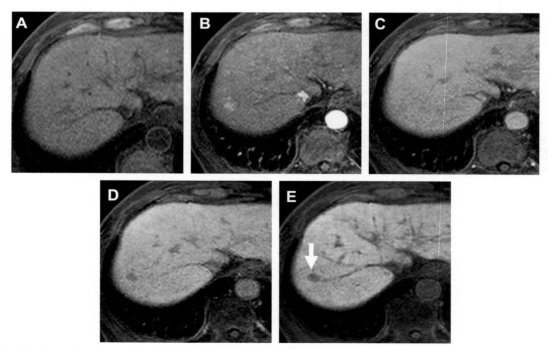

Fig. 21. Dynamic enhancement patterns of well-differentiated HCC in axial 3D fat-saturated T1-weighted GRE images (TR/TE = 3.6/1.7 ms, flip angle = 15°), presenting before (*A*) and in the arterial phase (*B*), portal phase (*C*), equilibrium phase (*D*), and hepatocyte-selective phase (*E*) after intravenous injection of Gd-EOB-DTPA. Well-differentiated HCC is commonly observed as hypointense in the hepatocyte-selective phase (*arrow*).

dysplastic nodules and well-differentiated HCC is variable, the signal intensity of these nodules may also vary after administration of SPIO.[57,64] It has been suggested that the extent of SPIO uptake may reflect the degree of Kupffer cell function (Fig. 20).[65] Signal intensity characteristics of dysplastic nodules after administration of SPIO also overlap with those of regenerative nodules and well-differentiated HCC, and uptake of SPIO into these nodules may cause a decrease in detection.

Regenerative nodules generally have normal hepatocellular function and therefore demonstrate uptake of hepatocellular contrast agents such as Gd-EOB-DTPA. As dedifferentiation proceeds, the number of expressed organic anion transporters decreases, with a resulting progressive decrease in the uptake of hepatocellular agents.[66] It is considered that the appearance of HCC at hepatocyte-selective phases with hepatocellular agents is dependent on the degree of tumor differentiation. However, hepatocytes in well-differentiated HCC may retain enough hepatocellular function to take up hepatocellular agents, and hence may be overlooked at this phase of imaging, or appear similar to a regenerative or dysplastic nodule (see Table 4).

In the authors' experience, most well-differentiated HCCs diagnosed by needle biopsy are clearly observed as hypointense to liver at hepatocyte-selective phases on Gd-EOB-DTPA–enhanced MR imaging (Fig. 21). Nevertheless, some well-differentiated HCCs are observed as isointense or hyperintense. Conclusive differentiation of dysplastic nodules from well-differentiated HCCs appears difficult (Fig. 22). Moreover, the diagnostic differentiation of dysplastic nodules from other cirrhosis-associated hepatocellular nodules may be difficult even on histopathologic analysis, and the use of molecular genetics-based techniques may be necessary in future.[61]

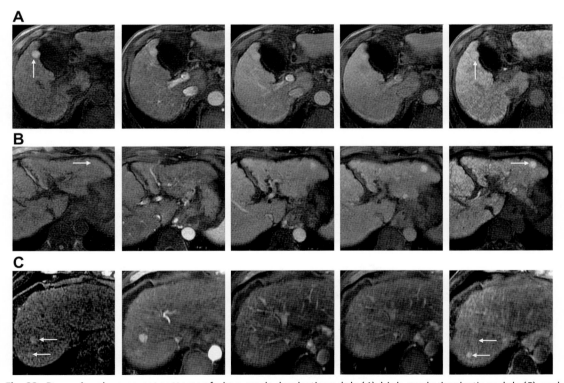

Fig. 22. Dynamic enhancement patterns of a low-grade dysplastic nodule (A), high-grade dysplastic nodule (B), and well-differentiated HCCs (C) in axial T1-weighted fat-saturated 3D GRE images (TR/TE = 3.6/1.7 ms, flip angle = 15°), presenting before and in the arterial phase, portal phase, equilibrium phase, and hepatocyte-selective phase after intravenous injection of Gd-EOB-DTPA. In the hepatocyte-selective phase, each nodule is observed as isointense or hyperintense owing to the uptake of hepatocellular agents (arrows). In series (C), both nodules were well-differentiated HCCs. In the hepatocyte-selective phase, both HCCs are observed as isointense and hyperintense, respectively. All these HCCs were diagnosed by needle biopsy.

REFERENCES

1. Mortele KJ, Ros PR. MR imaging in chronic hepatitis and cirrhosis. Semin Ultrasound CT MR 2002;23(1): 79–100.
2. Popper H. Pathologic aspects of cirrhosis. A review. Am J Pathol 1978;87:228–58.
3. Garcia-Tsao G, Lim JK. Members of Veterans Affairs Hepatitis C Resource Center Program. Management and treatment of patients with cirrhosis and portal hypertension: recommendations from the Department of Veterans Affairs Hepatitis C Resource Center Program and the National Hepatitis C Program. Am J Gastroenterol 2009;104(7):1802–29.
4. Sorrell MF, Belongia EA, Costa J, et al. National Institutes of Health Consensus Development Conference Statement: management of hepatitis B. Ann Intern Med 2009;150:104–10.
5. Global surveillance and control of hepatitis C. Report of a who consultation organized in collaboration with the viral hepatitis prevention board, Antwerp, Belgium. J Viral Hepat 1999;6:35–47.
6. Davis GL, Albright JE, Cook SF, et al. Projecting future complications of chronic hepatitis C in the United States. Liver Transpl 2003;9:331–8.
7. Afdhal NH. The natural history of hepatitis C. Semin Liver Dis 2004;24(Suppl 2):3–8.
8. Maher JJ. Alcoholic liver disease. In: Feldman M, Friedman LS, Sleisenger MH, editors. Gastrointestinal and liver disease, vol. II. Philadelphia: Saunders; 2002. p. 1375–91.
9. Breitkopf K, Nagy LE, Beier JI, et al. Current experimental perspectives on the clinical progression of alcoholic liver disease. Alcohol Clin Exp Res 2009; 33:1647–55.
10. Greenfield V, Cheung O, Sanyal AJ. Recent advances in nonalcoholic fatty liver disease. Curr Opin Gastroenterol 2008;24(3):320–7.
11. Itoh H, Sakai T, Takahashi N, et al. Periportal high intensity on T2-weighted MR images in acute viral hepatitis. J Comput Assist Tomogr 1992;16:564–7.
12. Matsui O, Kadoya M, Takashima T, et al. Intrahepatic periportal abnormal intensity on MR images: an indication of various hepatobiliary diseases. Radiology 1989;171:335–8.
13. Fisher MR, Gore RM. Computed tomography in the evaluation of cirrhosis and portal hypertension. J Clin Gastroenterol 1985;7:173–81.
14. Ito K, Mitchell DG, Gabata T. Enlargement of hilar periportal space: a sign of early cirrhosis at MR imaging. J Magn Reson Imaging 2000;11:136–40.
15. Ito K, Mitchell DG. Imaging diagnosis of cirrhosis and chronic hepatitis. Intervirology 2004;47:134–43.
16. Ito K, Mitchell DG, Siegelman ES. Cirrhosis: MR imaging features. Magn Reson Imaging Clin N Am 2002;10:75–92.
17. Lafortune M, Matricardi L, Denys A, et al. Segment 4 (the quadrate lobe): a barometer of cirrhotic liver disease at US. Radiology 1998;206:157–60.
18. Ito K, Mitchell DG, Gabata T, et al. Expanded gallbladder fossa: simple MR imaging sign of cirrhosis. Radiology 1999;211:723–6.
19. Ito K, Mitchell DG, Kim MJ, et al. Right posterior hepatic notch sign: a simple diagnostic MR finding of cirrhosis. J Magn Reson Imaging 2003;18:561–6.
20. Okazaki H, Ito K, Fujita T, et al. Discrimination of alcoholic from virus-cirrhosis on MR imaging. AJR Am J Roentgenol 2000;175:1677–81.
21. Ito K, Mitchell DG, Outwater EK, et al. Primary sclerosing cholangitis: MR imaging features. AJR Am J Roentgenol 1999;172(6):1527–33.
22. Brancatelli G, Federle MP, Ambrosini R. Cirrhosis: CT and MR imaging evaluation. Eur J Radiol 2007; 61(1):57–69.
23. Wenzel JS, Donohoe A, Ford KL 3rd, et al. Primary biliary cirrhosis: MR imaging findings and description of MR imaging periportal halo sign. AJR Am J Roentgenol 2001;176:885–9.
24. Kobayashi S, Matsui O, Gabata T, et al. MRI findings of primary biliary cirrhosis: correlation with Scheuer histologic staging. Abdom Imaging 2005;30(1): 71–6.
25. Martí-Bonmatí L. MR contrast agents in hepatic cirrhosis and chronic hepatitis. Semin Ultrasound CT MR 2002;23(1):101–13.
26. Vilgrain V. Ultrasound of diffuse liver disease and portal hypertension. Eur Radiol 2001;11:1563–77.
27. Van Beers BE, Leconte I, Materne R, et al. Hepatic perfusion parameters in chronic liver disease: dynamic CT measurements correlated with disease severity. AJR Am J Roentgenol 2001;176:667–73.
28. Semelka RC, Chung JJ, Hussain SM, et al. Chronic hepatitis: correlation of early patchy and late linear enhancement patterns on gadolinium-enhanced MR images with histopathology: initial experience. J Magn Reson Imaging 2001;13:385–91.
29. Faria SC, Ganesan K, Mwangi I, et al. MR imaging of liver fibrosis: current state of the art. Radiographics 2009;29(6):1615–35.
30. Yeh MM, Brunt EM. Pathology of nonalcoholic fatty liver disease. Am J Clin Pathol 2007;128(5):837–47.
31. Bedossa P, Dargere D, Paradis V. Sampling variability of liver fibrosis in chronic hepatitis C. Hepatology 2003;38:1449–57.
32. Blci NC, Semelka RC. Contrast agents for MR imaging of the liver. Radiol Clin North Am 2005; 43(5):887–98.
33. Lucidarme O, Baleston F, Cadi M, et al. Non-invasive detection of liver fibrosis: Is superparamagnetic iron oxide particle-enhanced MR imaging a contributive technique? Eur Radiol 2003;13(3):467–74.
34. Aguirre DA, Behling CA, Alpert E, et al. Liver fibrosis: noninvasive diagnosis with double contrast

material-enhanced MR imaging. Radiology 2006; 239:425–37.

35. Marti-Bonmatí L, Lonjedo E, Poyatos C, et al. MnDPDP enhancement characteristics and differentiation between cirrhotic and noncirrhotic livers. Invest Radiol 1998;33(10):717–22.

36. Murakami T, Baron RL, Federle MP, et al. Cirrhosis of the liver: MR imaging with mangafodipir trisodium (Mn-DPDP). Radiology 1996;198(2):567–72.

37. Muthupillai R, Lomas DJ, Rossman PJ, et al. Magnetic resonance elastography by direct visualization of propagating acoustic strain waves. Science 1995;269:1854–7.

38. Muthupillai R, Ehman RL. Magnetic resonance elastography. Nat Med 1996;2:601–3.

39. Yin M, Talwalkar JA, Glaser KJ, et al. Assessment of hepatic fibrosis with magnetic resonance elastography. Clin Gastroenterol Hepatol 2007;5(10): 1207–13.

40. Taouli B, Tolia AJ, Losada M, et al. Diffusion-weighted MRI for quantification of liver fibrosis: preliminary experience. AJR Am J Roentgenol 2007;189:799–806.

41. Boulanger Y, Amara M, Lepanto L, et al. Diffusion-weighted MR imaging of the liver of hepatitis C patients. NMR Biomed 2003;16:132–6.

42. Luciani A, Vignaud A, Cavet M, et al. Liver cirrhosis: intravoxel incoherent motion MR imaging—pilot study. Radiology 2008;249:891–9.

43. Koinuma M, Ohashi I, Hanafusa K, et al. Apparent diffusion coefficient measurements with diffusion-weighted magnetic resonance imaging for evaluation of hepatic fibrosis. J Magn Reson Imaging 2005;22:80–8.

44. Jalan R, Taylor-Robinson SD, Hodgson HJF. In vivo hepatic magnetic resonance spectroscopy: clinical or research tool? J Hepatol 1999;25:414–24.

45. Khan SA, Cox IJ, Hamilton G, et al. In vivo and in vitro nuclear magnetic resonance spectroscopy as a tool for investigating hepatobiliary disease: a review of H and P MRS applications. Liver Int 2005;25:273–81.

46. Munakata T, Griffiths RD, Martin PA, et al. An in vivo ^{31}P MRS study of patients with liver cirrhosis: progress towards a non-invasive assessment of disease severity. NMR Biomed 1993;6:168–72.

47. Van Wassenaer-van Hall HN, van der Grond J, van Hattum J, et al. [31]P magnetic resonance spectroscopy of the liver: correlation with standardized serum, clinical, and histological changes in diffuse liver disease. Hepatology 1995;21:443–9.

48. Menon DK, Sargentoni J, Taylor-Robinson SD, et al. Effect of functional grade and etiology on in vivo hepatic phosphorus-31 magnetic resonance spectroscopy in cirrhosis: biochemical basis of spectral appearances. Hepatology 1995; 21:417–27.

49. Cho SG, Kim MY, Kim HJ, et al. Chronic hepatitis: in vivo proton MR spectroscopic evaluation of the liver and correlation with histopathologic findings. Radiology 2001;221:740–6.

50. Coleman WB. Mechanisms of human hepatocarcinogenesis. Curr Mol Med 2003;3(6):573–88.

51. Lee RG. Fibrosis and cirrhosis. In: Lee RG, editor. Diagnostic liver pathology. St Louis (MO): Mosby-Year Book, Inc; 1994. p. 281–308.

52. Krinsky GA, Lee VS. MR imaging of cirrhotic nodules. Abdom Imaging 2000;25:471–82.

53. Zhang J, Krinsky GA. Iron-containing nodules of cirrhosis. NMR Biomed 2004;17(7):459–64.

54. Seale MK, Catalano OA, Saini S, et al. Hepatobiliary-specific MR contrast agents: role in imaging the liver and biliary tree. Radiographics 2009;29(6): 1725–48.

55. Lim JH, Kim EY, Lee WJ, et al. Regenerative nodules in liver cirrhosis: findings at CT during arterial portography and CT hepatic arteriography with histopathologic correlation. Radiology 1999;210(2): 451–8.

56. International Consensus Group for Hepatocellular Neoplasia. Pathologic diagnosis of early hepatocellular carcinoma: a report of the international consensus group for hepatocellular neoplasia. Hepatology 2009;49(2):658–64.

57. Hanna RF, Aguirre DA, Kased N, et al. Cirrhosis-associated hepatocellular nodules: correlation of histopathologic and MR imaging features. Radiographics 2008;28(3):747–69.

58. Amano S, Ebara M, Yajima T, et al. Assessment of cancer cell differentiation in small hepatocellular carcinoma by computed tomography and magnetic resonance imaging. J Gastroenterol Hepatol 2003; 18:273–9.

59. Ebara M, Fukuda H, Kojima Y, et al. Small hepatocellular carcinoma: relationship of signal intensity to histopathologic findings and metal content of the tumor and surrounding hepatic parenchyma. Radiology 1999;210:81–8.

60. Matsui O, Kadoya M, Kameyama T, et al. Benign and malignant nodules in cirrhotic livers: distinction based on blood supply. Radiology 1991;178:493–7.

61. Willatt JM, Hussain HK, Adusumilli S, et al. MR Imaging of hepatocellular carcinoma in the cirrhotic liver: challenges and controversies. Radiology 2008; 247(2):311–30.

62. Mitchell DG, Rubin R, Siegelman ES, et al. Hepatocellular carcinoma within siderotic regenerative nodules: appearance as a nodule within a nodule on MR images. Radiology 1991;178(1):101–3.

63. Goshima S, Kanematsu M, Matsuo M, et al. Nodule-in-nodule appearance of hepatocellular carcinomas: comparison of gadolinium-enhanced and ferumoxides-enhanced magnetic resonance imaging. J Magn Reson Imaging 2004;20(2):250–5.

64. Lim JH, Choi D, Cho SK, et al. Conspicuity of hepato-cellular nodular lesions in cirrhotic livers at ferumoxides-enhanced MR imaging: importance of Kupffer cell number. Radiology 2001;220(3):669–76.

65. Tonan T, Fujimoto K, Azuma S, et al. Evaluation of small (< or = 2 cm) dysplastic nodules and well-differentiated hepatocellular carcinomas with ferucarbotran-enhanced MRI in a 1.0-T MRI unit: utility of T2*-weighted gradient echo sequences with an intermediate-echo time. Eur J Radiol 2007; 64(1):133–9.

66. Gandi SN, Brown MA, Wong JG, et al. MR contrast agents for liver imaging: what, when, how. Radio-graphics 2006;26:1621–36.

MR Imaging of Benign Focal Liver Lesions

Ahmed Ba-Ssalamah, MD[a],*, Susanne Baroud, MD[a],
Nina Bastati, MD[a], Aliya Qayyum, MD, MRCP, FRCR[b]

KEYWORDS
- Benign focal liver lesions • MRI • 1.5T and 3T
- MRI techniques • MRI contrast material

IMAGING OF FOCAL LIVER LESIONS

With the increased use of cross-sectional imaging modalities, focal liver lesions are more often detected incidentally or seen on surveillance scans, especially in patients with underlying oncologic diseases. Recent advances in CT and MR imaging technology allow the acquisition of thinner sections, resulting in the detection of hepatic lesions measuring in the millimeter range.[1] Although a high prevalence of benign liver lesions measure 1 cm or less, substantial limitations remain regarding the confident characterization of these small hepatic lesions, particularly in patients with a clinical history of cancer.[2] Furthermore, benign focal liver lesions can have an atypical appearance that can mimic metastases.[3–5] Therefore, further characterization is desirable, because the presence of hepatic metastases or other malignant lesions may substantially alter patient prognosis and therapy. Given that most small focal liver lesions are benign in patients without obvious liver metastases, immediate further evaluation and definitive characterization of a benign lesion offer marked benefits beyond peace of mind for both patient and physician. Thus, from a clinical and socioeconomic point of view (eg, avoiding biopsy, multistep diagnosis, long-term follow-up), noninvasively establishing a confident diagnosis of focal liver lesions is very important.

Recent technical advances in the hard- and software of MR imaging technology, including the increased use of 3 Tesla MR imaging in the daily clinical routine, has led to better temporal and spatial resolution, particularly for contrast-enhanced, T1-weighted three-dimensional images, allowing near-isotropic imaging.[6–8] Because the noninvasive characterization of focal liver lesions is largely based on their morphologic appearance or enhancement patterns on contrast-enhanced dynamic imaging, the use of various nonspecific and liver-specific contrast agents has significantly expanded the role of MR imaging in the diagnosis of focal liver lesions. These lesions can now be characterized based on their morphology, vascularity, and specific functional features on a cellular basis, through a tailored examination that leads to a confident and noninvasive diagnosis.[9] The introduction of new MR imaging pulse sequences, such as diffusion-weighted imaging (DWI), into routine clinical practice may further improve the noninvasive diagnostic workup of focal liver lesions.[10]

This article describes the most commonly encountered benign focal liver lesions, including simple cysts, biliary hamartoma, hemangioma, focal nodular hyperplasia (FNH), and adenoma. Their typical and atypical appearance and their enhancement pattern are illustrated, and how a confident noninvasive diagnosis can be achieved using the above-mentioned MR imaging techniques in combination with various available contrast agents is explained.

TECHNICAL CONSIDERATIONS AND CONTRAST AGENTS

Currently, liver MR imaging examinations are performed routinely using either 1.5 or 3 Tesla

[a] Department of Radiology, Medical University of Vienna, Waehringer Guertel 18-20, A-1090 Vienna, Austria
[b] Department of Radiology and Biomedical Imaging, University of California San Francisco, 505 Parnassus Avenue, San Francisco, CA 94143, USA
* Corresponding author.
E-mail address: ahmed.ba-ssalamah@meduniwien.ac.at

Magn Reson Imaging Clin N Am 18 (2010) 403–419
doi:10.1016/j.mric.2010.08.001
1064-9689/10/$ — see front matter © 2010 Elsevier Inc. All rights reserved.

machines.[6,7] Further recent developments in MR imaging technology include stronger gradient systems, multichannel coils, navigator triggering, and parallel imaging.[11] Because of these remarkable technical innovations that lead to faster pulse sequences, the entire liver can be examined rapidly within a single breath-hold. Thus, multiphase, T1-weighted volume interpolated or three-dimensional gradient-echo (GRE), with almost isotropic voxel imaging and a slice thickness of 1 to 2 mm using VIBE (volumetric interpolated breath-hold examination) or THRIVE (T1W high-resolution isotropic volume examination), sequences for dynamic imaging of the liver and injection of gadolinium chelate contrast agent can be performed easily.[8,12] This technique improves the detection and characterization of focal liver lesions based on their vascularity or typical enhancement pattern.

However, a high spatial resolution is indispensable for abdominal imaging, which necessitates longer acquisition times. New techniques to compensate for breathing motion artifacts, such as breath-triggering and navigator-triggering technology, offer a possible solution to this dilemma. Thus, high-resolution T2- and diffusion-weighted respiratory-triggered sequences are now feasible with increased high spatial and temporal resolution, leading to a marked improvement in the detection and characterization of focal liver lesions. The introduction of different liver-specific contrast agents has further established the role of MR imaging in liver imaging. Although dynamic gadolinium chelate—enhanced MR imaging is crucial in the detection and characterization of focal liver lesions, some limitations exist to the use of these contrast agents that have pharmacokinetics similar to those of the iodine contrast media used in CT.[13]

Particular difficulties occur with liver tumors that show an atypical morphology and vascularity, or that show an overlapping enhancement pattern.[9,14,15] Compared with extracellular contrast media, liver-specific MR contrast media are selectively taken up by the normal liver parenchyma through specific and well-known uptake mechanisms. Currently, two main groups of liver-specific contrast media are used in clinical practice.[9,16] The first group includes superparamagnetic iron-oxide particles (SPIO) (ie, ferumoxide [Endorem], and ferucarbotran [Resovist]). These substances are transported out of the blood circulation and taken up by the reticuloendothelial system (or Kupffer cells of the liver) through phagocytosis.[17] These particles cause magnetic field inhomogeneities with shortening of T2 relaxation time, leading to a decrease in the signal of the normal liver parenchyma on T2-weighted sequences, best seen on T2* or GRE sequences for lesion detection. However, for lesion characterization T2-weighted turbo spin-echo (TSE) sequences or HASTE (half-Fourier acquisition single-shot turbo spin-echo) sequences are more sensitive for evaluating signal intensity loss. Depending on the content of the Kupffer cells, benign hepatocellular lesions show uptake of these contrast agents.[17,18] Hemangiomas present an exception for SPIO contrast media uptake because of their relatively large, slow-flowing blood pool that allows the effect of the SPIO particles to occur and therefore, although lacking Kupffer cells, show a decrease in signal on T2-weighted images.[9,17]

Lesions that do not contain Kupffer cells (eg, malignant lesions, metastases) do not take up SPIO contrast agents, rendering them bright against the background of the dark liver parenchyma on T2-weighted post-SPIO sequences. The resulting increase in contrast between the liver and a lesion of nonhepatic origin increases the detection rate compared with unenhanced images and allows an easy distinction from benign hepatic lesions.[18] Unfortunately, one of these agents (ferucarbotran) will no longer be available after the beginning of 2011.

The second group of liver-specific contrast agents includes the hepatobiliary contrast media, which are selectively taken up by hepatocytes and excreted through the biliary tracts.[9,19] This activity results in an increase in signal of the normal liver parenchyma on T1-weighted sequences. Malignant lesions show washout, appearing hypointense, and thus become more conspicuous. Mangafodipir (Mn-DPDP), gadobenate dimeglumine (Gd-BOPTA), and gadoxetate (Gd-EOB-DTPA) belong to this group of contrast media. The manganese-based contrast agent Mn-DPDP (formerly known as *mangafodipir trisodium* or *teslascan*) is a contrast medium that enhances the liver parenchyma and bile ducts through this pathway of excretion on T1-weighted sequences. This contrast agent was unfortunately discontinued recently. The gadolinium-based bimodal contrast agents show combined perfusion- and hepatocyte-specific properties.[9] The subgroup of gadolinium-based contrast material comprises gadobenate dimeglumine (MultiHance, Bracco Diagnostics, Princeton, NJ, USA) and gadoxetate (Primovist, Bayer Schering Pharma, Berlin, Germany). These substances are administered intravenously as a bolus for dynamic imaging in the arterial, portal venous, and delayed phases, allowing the evaluation of morphology, vascularity, and functional properties within a single examination.

CYSTS

Hepatic cysts are the most common benign focal liver lesions, with an incidence of 2% to 7%.[20] They can be further differentiated into simple cysts, cysts in autosomal dominant polycystic kidney disease, ciliated hepatic foregut cysts, and parasitic (hydatid) cysts.

Simple Cysts

Simple cysts are well-defined, round, or oval lesions. They are lined with very thin or imperceptible layers of fibrous tissue and show no communication to the biliary tree.[21,22] The origin of simple hepatic cysts is unclear, but developmental and acquired causes that lead to the retention of bile are postulated. On MR imaging, these cysts show homogenous low signal intensity on T1-weighted images. In the rare condition that these cysts become hemorrhagic or contain protein, they show an increase in signal intensity on T1-weighted images. Because of the very long T2-time of fluid, cysts retain signal on sequences with long echo times (eg, >120 ms), showing very high signal intensity on T2-weighted images.

In autosomal dominant polycystic kidney disease, hepatic cysts are found in 40% of the cases,[22–24] with the liver the primary site for extra-renal cyst manifestation. These cysts tend to be multiple and varied in size (usually <2 cm) (**Fig. 1**). Intercystic hemorrhage is rare but is encountered more often than in simple hepatic cysts without this underlying disease.[22]

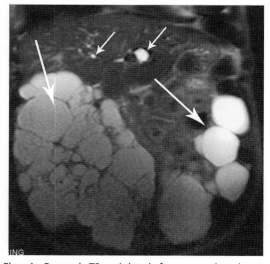

Fig. 1. Coronal T2-weighted fat saturation image shows multiple small liver cysts (*small arrows*) in a patient with autosomal dominant polycystic kidney disease (*large arrows*). The cysts appear strongly hyperintense.

Ciliated Hepatic Foregut Cyst

Ciliated hepatic foregut cysts are very rare benign congenital solitary lesions believed to arise from the embryonic foregut.[21,25] They are usually unilocular, smaller than 3 cm, and are most often situated in the left liver lobe at the anterosuperior liver margin or intersegmentally, where they tend to bulge the outer contour of the liver. The content can show various viscosities, from serous to mucinous, which affects the MR signal intensity, especially in T1-weighted images. The signal intensity can be low or high or anywhere in between. On T2-weighted imaging, the cyst content is homogenously hyperintense (**Fig. 2A**).[26]

Using DWI, simple and ciliated hepatic foregut cysts and liver cysts in polycystic kidney disease show a signal intensity decrease with increasing b-values, and are strongly hyperintense and homogeneous on analog-to-digital (ADC) sequences (**Fig. 2B–D**).[27–29] After application of contrast material, either gadolinium chelate or liver-specific contrast agents, the fluid content of hepatic cysts never shows uptake of contrast material, this being a useful feature in differentiating hepatic cysts from poorly vascularized malignant cystic lesions (**Fig. 2E**).[22,23]

Echinococcal Cysts

Echinococcus granulosus is a parasite that causes hydatid cysts, predominantly in the liver and lung and, less commonly, the heart and spleen.[30] Hydatid cysts are usually round in shape, have a fibrous capsule, and are unilocular or multiseptated.[31] Because of the frequent presence of smaller daughter cysts within the periphery of the mother cyst, the hydatid cyst often appears multicystic. The fluid component of the hydatid cyst is typically low on T1-weighted and high on T2-weighted images. In the presence of interluminal debris, the signal intensity can become moderately inhomogeneous on both T1- and T2-weighted images. Degenerated cysts decrease in size and appear heterogeneous, solid, or pseudo-tumor-like, whereas dead cysts are characterized by a thickened calcified wall.[31] The fibrous capsule and internal septa appear hypointense on T2-weighted images and show enhancement in the post-gadolinium phase (**Fig. 3**); however, these structures are better visualized on ultrasound than MR imaging or CT, whereas capsular calcifications are better depicted with CT than with MR imaging.

The parasite *E multilocularis* produces multilocular alveolar cysts in any body organ or tissue, but the liver is the site most commonly affected,

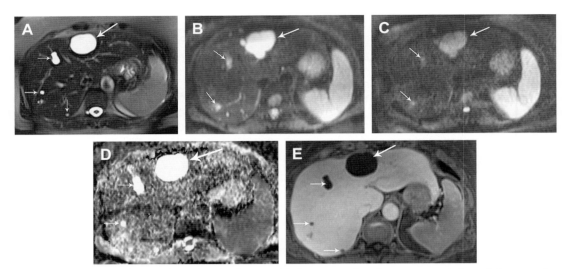

Fig. 2. (*A*) Axial T2-weighted turbo spin-echo image with fat suppression shows a strongly hyperintense, unilocular, ciliated hepatic foregut cyst approximately 3 cm in diameter (*large arrow*) in the left liver lobe with a slight bulge of the outer contour of the liver and multiple small simple cysts (*small arrows*). Axial diffusion-weighted images with b value of 50 (*B*), 600 (*C*), and ADC (*D*). All cysts show a high signal intensity in the diffusion-weighted image, with a b-value of 50, and a marked decrease in b-value of 600 (*white arrows*), and appear again strongly hyperintense on the ADC map, this is very characteristic for liver cysts (*white arrows*). (*E*) Gadolinium-enhanced axial T1 gradient-recalled echo three-dimensional sequence. All cysts show no enhancement after injection of contrast material and are well-delineated.

which leads to hepatic alveolar echinococcosis (HAE).[31,32] HAE cysts are, in contrast to hydatid cysts, not true cysts. HAE cysts are solitary, multilocular, or confluent; 1 to 10 mm in diameter; resemble alveoli; and can grow to between 15 and 20 cm. HAE cysts show irregular margins, lack a fibrous capsule, and have cystic and solid components (coagulation necrosis, granuloma, and calcification). HAE cysts tend to involve extensive regions of the liver, with a propensity for the porta hepatis, causing stenoses of bile ducts, portal, and hepatic veins, and can lead to portal hypertension. These lesions are hypointense on T1- weighted images and can be hypo-, iso-, or hyperintense on T2-weighted imaging (**Fig. 4**).[31] In post-gadolinium images, these lesions appear inhomogeneous. As the lesion heals, it begins to calcify, first in a scattered form, and eventually becomes a large calcified mass. Again, calcification is better depicted with CT.[33] DWI of hydatid cysts shows the same characteristics as the simple cysts and hepatic foregut cysts.[29,34] The appearance of HAE cysts in DWI is inhomogeneous when calcifications are present.

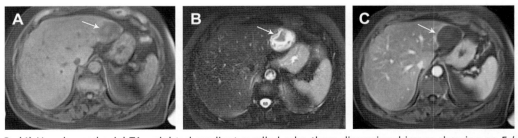

Fig. 3. (*A*) Unenhanced axial T1-weighted gradient-recalled echo three-dimensional image showing an *Echinococcus granulosus* cyst, which appears round in shape and moderately hypointense. The fibrous capsule and internal septae appear inhomogeneous on T1-weighted images. (*B*) Axial T2-weighted turbo spin-echo image with fat suppression shows an *E granulosus* cyst, which appears round in shape and moderately hyperintense (*arrow*). The fibrous capsule and internal septae appear hypointense. (*C*) Gadolinium-enhanced axial T1-weighted gradient-recalled echo three-dimensional image shows an enhancement of the fibrous capsule in the interstitial phase after contrast injection (*arrow*).

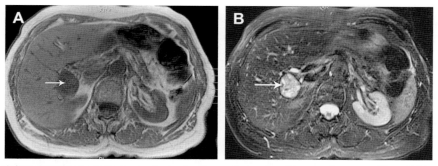

Fig. 4. (*A*) Axial T1-weighted gradient-recalled echo three-dimensional image shows a solitary *Echinococcus multilocularis*, about 3 cm in diameter, located in the porta hepatis, which appears round in shape and inhomogeneous on T1-weighted images, in this case because of calcifications (*arrow*). (*B*) On axial T2-weighted turbo spin-echo image with fat suppression, the lesion appears inhomogeneously hyperintense because of internal and rim calcifications (*arrow*).

BILIARY HAMARTOMA/BILE DUCT HAMARTOMA

Bile duct hamartomas, also known as *biliary microharmatomas* or *von Meyenburg complexes*, are rare, benign, cystic lesions that are thought to arise from ductal plate malformations of the small interlobular bile ducts.[35] At histopathology, these lesions appear as a collection of small, sometimes dilated, irregular and branching bile ducts, embedded in a fibrous stoma. They are usually less than 1 cm in diameter, can be numerous, and are usually incidental radiologic findings.[35,36] Bile duct hamartomas are well-defined lesions that show low signal intensity on T1-weighted imaging and appear strongly hyperintense on T2-weighted imaging (**Fig. 5**A).[37] On post-gadolinium images, these cystic lesions

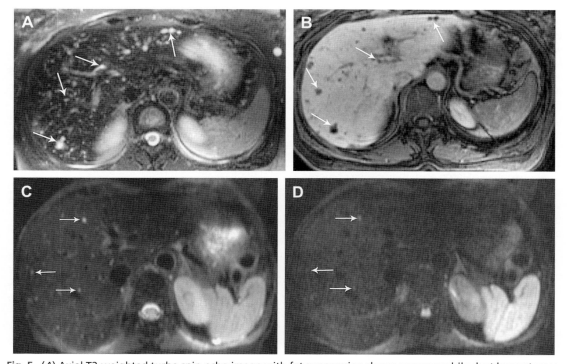

Fig. 5. (*A*) Axial T2-weighted turbo spin-echo image with fat suppression shows numerous bile duct hamartomas, which appear strongly hyperintense (*arrows*). (*B*) On axial T1-weighted gradient-recalled echo three-dimensional image, the bile duct hamartomas are well defined and show low signal intensity (*arrows*). (*C*) Axial DWI image (b-value 50) shows numerous bile duct hamartomas, which appear strongly hyperintense (*arrows*). (*D*) Axial DWI image (b-value 600) shows numerous bile duct hamartomas, which show marked signal intensity loss (*arrows*).

show no internal enhancement; however, thin rim enhancement on early and late post-gadolinium images is typical (**Fig. 5B**). The enhancing rim consists of compressed adjacent hepatic parenchyma and should not be mistaken for a fibrous capsule. This rim enhancement may lead to the misinterpretation of a metastatic lesion; however, biliary hamartomas, as opposed to metastases, do not show perilesional contrast enhancement or progressive centripetal fill-in on equilibrium-phase after administration of gadolinium contrast. Biliary hamartomas also do not show uptake of liver-specific contrast agents, because these lesions do not communicate with the bile ducts. On DWI, biliary hamartomas show the typical features of cystic lesions because of the significant signal intensity loss with increasing b-values (**Fig. 5C, D**), and appear strongly hyperintense on the ADC sequences.

HEMANGIOMA

Hemangioma is the most common benign liver neoplasm, with a prevalence of up to 20%.[5,38] It is usually an incidental finding in patients at any age, but is up to five times more common in women, and can be found as a solitary lesion or as multiple lesions.[20] Hemangiomas are thought to be hamartomatous lesions[39] and are usually well contained within the liver. On rare occasions, however, hemangiomas can cause a bulge of the liver surface, showing exophytic or even extrahepatic growth, with only a thin stalk connecting them to the liver, as in a pedunculated hemangioma (**Fig. 6**).[40] However, this has no effect on the appearance on unenhanced MR images or the contrast enhancement pattern. On rare occasions, hemangiomas can become symptomatic when, because of large size, they cause compression of adjacent structures, and in 1% to 4% of cases may rupture and bleed into the peritoneum.[41] A pedunculated hemangioma may undergo torsion and infarction.[42]

At histopathology, hemangiomas appear as multiple vascular channels lined by a single layer of endothelial cells, and can be classified into two predominant types according to the size of their vascular spaces. The most common is the cavernous hemangioma, consisting of numerous large vascular channels separated by thin fibrous septae. The second most common is the capillary hemangioma (16%),[39,43] which differs from the cavernous type by the presence of narrower vascular spaces with regard to the numerous capillary channels. Hemangiomas can also be classified according to their size.[44] A capillary

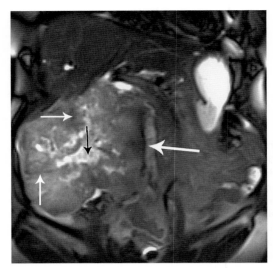

Fig. 6. Coronal T2-weighted turbo spin-echo image with fat suppression shows a giant hemangioma with exophytic growth that bulges the liver surface (*large white arrow*) and has a central area of high signal intensity (*black arrow*), and a network of multiple fibrous septae of low signal intensity (*small white arrows*).

hemangioma has a size ranging from 1 to 2 cm, whereas the cavernous hemangioma can measure up to 5 cm, and a giant hemangioma is classified as a lesion greater than 5 cm in diameter.[9,45] At unenhanced MR imaging, hemangiomas are seen as well-delineated lesions that are round in shape when small and tend to show lobular borders when larger. Because of their very long T2 time, hemangiomas retain signal on heavily T2-weighted images (echo time>120 ms),[5,39] consequently appearing homogeneously hyperintense, and conversely, showing low signal intensity on T1-weighted MR images (**Fig. 7**). On T2-weighted images, giant hemangiomas frequently show a central area of either bright, dark, or mixed signal intensity and a network of multiple fibrous septae of low signal intensity (see **Fig. 6**). At histopathology, the bright central area corresponds to hypocellular myxoid tissue. Furthermore, hemorrhage, small areas of thrombosis, calcification, and areas of extensive fibrosis can rarely be seen in giant hemangiomas.[46] Depending on the uptake of contrast material, hemangiomas show three typical enhancement patterns on post-gadolinium dynamic images.[9]

Type 1

Type 1 pattern is characterized by uniform, fast, and intense enhancement in the arterial phase, showing isointense or slightly hyperintense signal compared with the normal liver parenchyma on

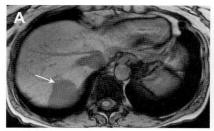
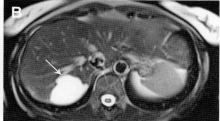

Fig. 7. (A) Axial T1-weighted gradient-recalled echo three-dimensional image shows a moderate-sized hemangioma with lobular borders, which appears as a well-delineated hypointense lesion (*arrow*). (B) Axial T2-weighted turbo spin-echo image with fat suppression shows a moderate-sized hemangioma with lobular borders, which appears as a well-delineated, strongly hyperintense lesion (*arrow*).

the later post-gadolinium images (**Fig. 8**A). In rare cases, fast-enhancing (type 1) small hemangiomas can present a diagnostic challenge if a perilesional high signal is present on T2-weighted images and perilesional enhancement is seen on post-gadolinium images, for example mimicking carcinoid or renal cell cancer metastases. This imaging feature in hemangiomas likely reflects high flow in efferent perilesional veins. However, type 1 hemangiomas typically remain hyperintense to surrounding liver parenchyma on later post—contrast-enhanced images (**Fig. 8**B). Unlike hemangiomas, metastases appear hypointense to the surrounding liver parenchyma

Type 2

Type 2 pattern is characterized by peripheral, discontinuous nodular enhancement on arterial phase post-gadolinium images, with centripetal progressive confluent enhancement on portal venous phase images (70 s) and homogeneous fill-in on delayed post-gadolinium (3—5 minutes) imaging (**Fig. 9**).

Type 3

Type 3 pattern has the same enhancement pattern as type 2 in the arterial phase post-gadolinium

images; however, show failure to completely fill and no enhancement of the central scar, even on very delayed images up to 15 minutes after injection of contrast material (**Fig. 10**).

The enhancement pattern is related to hemangioma size. Small hemangiomas most commonly show a type 1 enhancement pattern, but may show a type 2 pattern. Medium-sized hemangiomas tend to show the classical type 2 enhancement, and, less frequently, a type 1 enhancement pattern. Giant hemangiomas almost always show a type 3 enhancement pattern.[9,47]

With bimodal contrast agents, gadobenate and gadoxetate, hemangiomas show the same dynamic imaging characteristics on the arterial and portal venous phase as the non—tissue-specific extracellular gadolinium chelates. However, on the very delayed phase images (20- to 60-minute hepatocyte phase images), hemangiomas appear homogeneously hypointense compared with the normal liver parenchyma because they lack hepatocytes (**Fig. 11**).[9] Hemangiomas do not show uptake of Manganese-based contrast agents (Mn-DPDP).[9] Although hemangiomas lack Kupffer cells and no reticuloendothelial uptake of SPIO agents occurs, hemangiomas may show a moderate to significant signal intensity loss on the T2-weighted images 10 minutes after

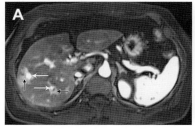
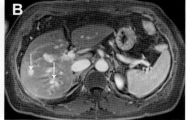

Fig. 8. (A) Axial gadolinium-enhanced T1-weighted gradient-recalled echo three-dimensional image in the arterial phase shows a type 1 hemangioma with a uniform, fast, and intense enhancement (*white arrows*) with perilesional enhancement reflecting high flow in efferent, perilesional veins (*small black arrows*). (B) Axial gadolinium-enhanced T1-weighted gradient-recalled echo three-dimensional image in the delayed phase shows a type 1 hemangioma, which is still moderately hyperintense to surrounding liver parenchyma (*arrow*).

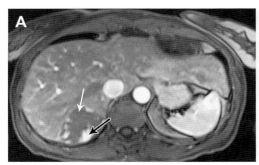
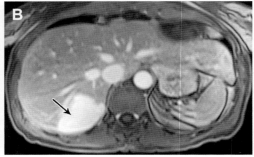

Fig. 9. (A) Axial gadolinium-enhanced T1-weighted gradient-recalled echo three-dimensional image in the arterial phase shows a type 2 hemangioma (*white arrow*) with peripheral, discontinuous nodular enhancement (*black arrow*). (B) Axial gadolinium-enhanced T1-weighted gradient-recalled echo three-dimensional image on delayed (3 minutes) post-gadolinium image shows centripetal confluent enhancement progression, and homogeneous fill-in (*arrow*). (Same patient as in Fig. 7.)

ferucarbotran or 40 minutes after ferumoxide because of the blood-pool phase of these agents (Fig. 12).[9,48]

In most cases a confident diagnosis of hemangioma can be made based on the combination of T2-weighted images and the described enhancement patterns using extracellular gadolinium chelates. However, a confident diagnosis based on morphology, signal intensity on T2-weighted imaging, and post-gadolinium imaging alone can be a challenge in atypical appearing hemangiomas,[5,39] especially when evaluating patients with an underlying hypervascular primary malignancy (eg, neuroendocrine tumors) or in patients with a cystic primary malignancy if gadolinium contrast is not administered (eg, ovarian cancer, colorectal cancer).[49] Thus, although hemangiomas posses several distinctive features, the

dependence on any single sequence characteristic may lead to misdiagnosis.

A further potential pitfall is the failure to recognize the rather rare hyalinized or sclerosed hemangioma, which is believed to represent the end stage of hemangioma involution. The replacement of vascular spaces through hyalinized fibrotic tissue leads to marked modifications of the typical imaging features of hemangioma, with a loss of the characteristic high signal intensity on T2-weighted images and of the typical nodular enhancement on contrast-enhanced T1-weighted images (Fig. 13A, B).[50] These changes may be observed in cirrhosis, with the potential misdiagnosis of hepatocellular carcinoma (HCC), and therefore the identification of the hemangioma on prior images is extremely helpful. In patients without cirrhosis, metastases represent the main

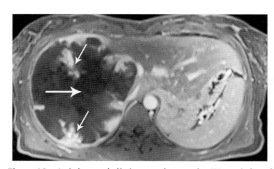

Fig. 10. Axial gadolinium-enhanced T1-weighted gradient-recalled echo three-dimensional image on a very delayed post-gadolinium phase of a giant hemangioma that shows the same enhancement pattern as type 2 in the periphery (*small arrows*), but no enhancement of the central scar, even on very delayed images up to 15 minutes after injection of contrast material (*large arrow*).

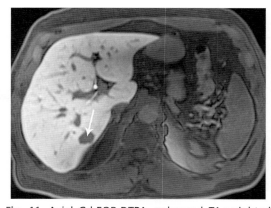

Fig. 11. Axial Gd-EOB-DTPA–enhanced T1-weighted gradient-recalled echo three-dimensional image on hepatospecific phase 20 minutes after contrast media injection shows a small hypointense lesion in the right liver lobe (*arrow*), relative to the normal liver parenchyma due to the absence of hepatocytes.

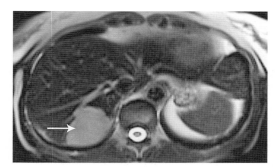

Fig. 12. Axial SPIO-enhanced, T2-weighted turbo spin-echo image with fat suppression after intravenous administration of 1.4 mL of ferucarbutran shows a signal intensity loss compared with the precontrast, T2-weighted image in Fig. 7B (same patient), because of the blood pooling effect (arrow). (Same patient as in Fig. 7.)

differential consideration, especially in the context of a known primary malignancy.

In these more challenging cases, the use of an SPIO contrast agent can often elucidate the diagnosis, because metastases will not show uptake of the SPIO contrast agent due to the lack of Kupffer cells, and thus, will not show change in signal intensity on T2-weighted images.[9] The pooling effect of SPIO contrast material within the hemangiomas, even of the sclerosed or hyalinized type, however, will lead to a significant, measurable signal intensity loss, allowing a confident diagnosis (see Fig. 13).[9] In contrary, the blood pooling effect in metastases is negligible and therefore causes no signal intensity loss.

On DWI, hemangiomas show signal intensity loss with increased b-values and typically show

high signal intensity on the ADC map. However, a confident differentiation between cystic metastases and hemangioma cannot be achieved solely with this single pulse sequence and should be interpreted in conjunction with contrast-enhanced images (Fig. 14).[10,28,51]

FNH

FNH is the second most common benign solid liver tumor, with a prevalence of 3% to 5%[52] and a 2:1 predilection in women of reproductive age.[22,53] The histologic structure of FNH is very similar to the normal liver parenchyma, with pseudo-lobules of normal hepatocytes that are abnormally aligned around a central scar (10%–49% of cases) consisting of an arteriovenous malformation.[54] If present, vessels in the central scar receive their blood supply from the hepatic artery. FNH contains exuberant bile ducts without a connection to the biliary tree, and fibrous septae that radiate from the central scar.[55] The central scar is a characteristic feature of FNH, but can be absent in up to 50% of cases.[56] FNHs are usually less than 5 cm in diameter; however, lesions of more than 10 cm in diameter have been described.

The origin of FNH is not fully understood. Current concepts suggest that FNH is a hyperplastic response of hepatocytes to an underlying congenital vascular anomaly, such as an arteriovenous malformation. This theory is supported by the propensity of FNH to be associated with hepatic cavernous hemangiomas.[57] Two types of FNH have been described: the more common solid type, characterized by a central scar, and the

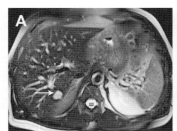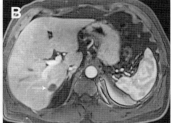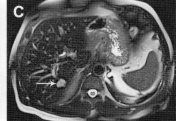

Fig. 13. (A) Axial T2-weighted turbo spin-echo with fat suppression image shows the same partially sclerosed hemangioma, which appears moderately and inhomogeneously hyperintense in the right liver lobe in segment 7 subcapsularly (arrow), in a patient with a clinical history of colon cancer of the mucinous type. (B) Axial gadolinium-enhanced T1-weighted gradient-recalled echo three-dimensional image of the arterial post-gadolinium phase shows a partially sclerosed hemangioma of approximately 1.5 cm in diameter. The hemangioma appears as a hypointense lesion in the right liver lobe in segment 7 subcapsularly, without the typical enhancement pattern for hemangioma (arrow), even in the portal and delayed phase (not shown) in a patient with a clinical history of colon cancer. (C) Axial SPIO-enhanced, T2-weighted turbo spin-echo image with fat suppression image after administration of 1.4 mL ferucarbutran shows a signal intensity loss of the lesion compared with the precontrast, T2-weighted image because of the blood pooling in the partially sclerosed hemangioma (arrow). Thus, a metastasis can be excluded.

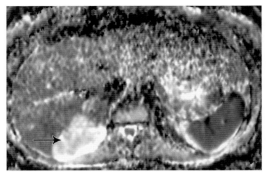

Fig. 14. Axial ADC image shows a hemangioma of approximately 4 cm in diameter in the right liver lobe in segment 7 subcapsularly (*arrow*) (same patient as in Fig. 7), which appears hyperintense and inhomogeneous. The ADC value was about 1 to 2.40×10^{-3} mm^2/s cm/s.

telangiectatic type that shows central, dilated, blood-filled spaces.[58] Recently, some authors classified the latter type as a subtype of adenoma, the so-called inflammatory adenoma.[59]

The multiple FNH syndrome is a separate entity, consisting of a complex of pathologies and multiple lesions, such as liver hemangiomas, meningioma, astrocytoma, dysplastic systemic arteries, and portal vein atresia.[60]

FNH is seen on MR imaging as a well-circumscribed lesion, appearing iso- to minimally hypointense to the normal liver parenchyma on unenhanced T1-weighted MR images and iso- to slightly hyperintense on unenhanced T2-weighted images. The central scar appears hypointense on T1-weighted and hyperintense on T2-weighted images (Fig. 15A, B).[4,9,61]

On nonspecific, gadolinium chelate–enhanced, dynamic T1-weighted MR imaging, FNH shows intense homogeneous enhancement in the arterial phase (Fig. 15C) that rapidly washes out in the portal venous and equilibrium phase (Fig. 15D), appearing isointense to the surrounding liver parenchyma. If present, the central scar shows a slow, progressive contrast uptake, and therefore appears hypointense in the arterial and venous phases and iso- to hyperintense in the later phases.[4,9] The slower uptake and contrast material accumulation in the central scar can help distinguish FNH from the central necrosis often encountered in malignant tumors. Furthermore, the central scar of FNH appears hyperintense on T2-weighted images, whereas the central scar of fibrolamellar hepatocellular carcinoma appears hypointense on T2-weighted images.[56]

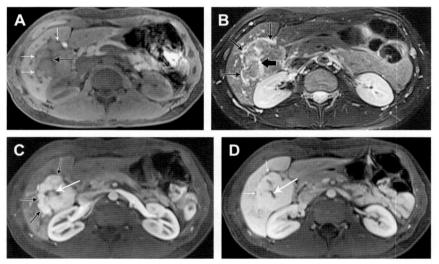

Fig. 15. (*A*) Axial, unenhanced, T1-weighted gradient-recalled echo three-dimensional image shows an FNH that is approximately 5 cm in diameter, which appears as an isointense lesion in the right liver lobe in segment 6 subcapsularly. Note the hypointense central scar (*black arrow*) and the pseudocapsule (*small white arrows*). (*B*) Axial T2-weighted image shows the same FNH as in Fig. A, which appears isointense. Note the hyperintense central scar (*wide black arrow*), and the hyperintense pseudocapsule (*thin black arrows*). (*C*) Axial gadolinium-enhanced T1-weighted gradient-recalled echo three-dimensional image in the arterial phase showing strong and vigorous enhancement of the FNH in the right liver lobe in segment 6 subcapsularly. Note the hypointense central scar (*white arrow*), and the hypointense pseudocapsule (*black arrows*). (*D*) Axial gadolinium-enhanced T1-weighted gradient-recalled echo three-dimensional image 3 minutes after contrast material injection in the equilibrium phase shows the FNH, which shows homogeneous enhancement like the surrounding liver parenchyma. Note the hypointense central scar (*white arrow*) and the hypointense pseudocapsule (*small white arrows*).

Immediate post-gadolinium images are especially important in the detection of small FNH (<1.5 cm) that are isointense on unenhanced on T1- and T2-weighted MR images. A uniform early enhancement, however, is also commonly observed with adenoma and HCC and must be interpreted cautiously. Furthermore, FNH, adenoma and HCC characteristically show contrast washout and appear hypointense on portal venous and delayed-phase images. Because FNH can show atypical features, such as heterogeneous or weak early enhancement, or can lack the central scar (**Fig. 16**A), the hepatospecific contrast agents have been very helpful in establishing the diagnosis.[4] With gadobenate- and gadoxetate-enhanced dynamic imaging, FNH shows a very similar arterial enhancement pattern to that of nonspecific gadolinium chelates. However, on delayed or hepatospecific phase T1-weighted images, a substantial hepatocellular enhancement can be observed within the lesion while the central scar commonly remains hypointense (**Fig. 16**B).[9] FNH shows marked uptake of the manganese-based contrast agent, Mn-DPDP, in the same amount or even more than the surrounding liver tissue.[9]

Because FNH contains a variable amount of Kupffer cells, uptake of SPIO contrast agents is observed that results in a loss of signal intensity in T2-weighted images. However, this usually occurs to a lesser degree than the decrease of signal intensity in the normal surrounding liver parenchyma[9] (**Fig. 17**). Administration of either hepatobiliary or SPIO contrast agents may be helpful for differentiating between FNH and fibrolamellar HCC because the latter shows no uptake of these contrast agents.[9]

As a solid tumor, FNH shows slightly high signal intensity with increasing b-values on DWI, and is again hypo-intense on ADC, with a reported ADC value between 1 and 1.40 × 10^{-3} mm^2/s cm/s. However, the ADC values may overlap with those of other solid lesions, including adenoma and malignant lesions (**Fig. 18**),[10,28] and therefore cannot be relied on for lesion characterization.

HEPATOCELLULAR ADENOMA

Hepatocellular adenoma (HCA) is a benign, focal neoplasm of the liver, predominantly seen in otherwise healthy women in their third to fifth decade, who use an estrogen- or androgen-containing medication,[62] or in patients who have an abnormal carbohydrate metabolism (ie, glycogen storage disease, familial diabetes mellitus, galactosemia).[63] Cessation of steroid hormone intake usually results in a spontaneous involution of the lesions. HCA, however, can also occur in patients in the absence of predisposing factors.

Histologically, HCA is composed of clusters of benign hepatocytes separated by dilated sinusoids, has varying numbers of Kupffer cells, and is associated with an accumulation of lipids. A characteristic feature of HCA is the lack of bile ducts and portal veins within this lesion.[64] Hepatic adenomas are vascularized solely by the hepatic arteries. HCAs are grossly 1 to 10 cm in diameter, and solitary in 70% to 80% of cases. *Adenomatosis* is the term used to describe the presence of multiple (4–10) lesions, which is predominantly associated with glycogen storage diseases.[65] Although at histopathology the adenomas in adenomatosis are similar to solitary adenomas, they are not steroid-dependent.[66]

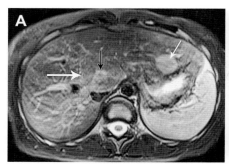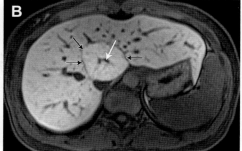

Fig. 16. (*A*) Axial T2-weighted turbo spin-echo image with fat suppression shows two focal liver masses, the first one in the left liver lobe, about 2.5 cm in diameter, that appears moderately hyperintense, without a central scar (not typical for FNH) (*small white arrow*). The second mass, in segment 4b, about 4 cm in diameter, appears iso-intense (*big white arrow*) with a hyperintense central scar (*black arrow*). (*B*) Axial Gd-EOB-DTPA–enhanced T1-weighted gradient-recalled echo three-dimensional image, 20 minutes after injection of contrast material in the hepatospecific phase, showing homogeneous enhancement of the two FNH lesions in segments 3 and 4b. The lesion in segment 4b shows a hypointense central scar (*white arrow*) and pseudocapsule (*black arrows*).

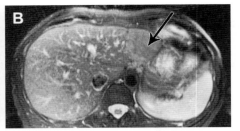
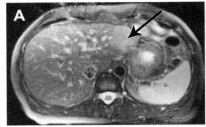

Fig. 17. (*A*) Axial T2-weighted turbo spin-echo image with fat suppression shows a slightly hyperintense FNH in segment five of the right liver lobe, about 4 cm in diameter (*arrow*). (*B*) Axial SPIO-enhanced, T2-weighted turbo spin-echo image with fat suppression after administration of 1.4 mL of ferucarbutran shows a moderate signal intensity loss of the FNH compared with the precontrast, T2-weighted image, because of the uptake through the Kupffer cells (*arrow*). Also note the signal intensity loss of the surrounding liver parenchyma.

Most patients with fewer than five small- to medium-sized adenomas are clinically asymptomatic and the lesions are incidental findings. Large or multiple lesions can cause right upper-quadrant discomfort or pain. Large adenomas show central degenerative changes that can lead to hemorrhage and sudden abdominal pain.[67] A serious complication of large adenomas is sudden rupture and bleeding into the peritoneal cavity, a condition that calls for immediate emergency intervention.[51,68]

Malignant transformation of hepatocellular adenoma may occur but is rare (up to 7% as reported in the literature).[67,69] Recently, some authors suggested a pathomolecular classification (phenotyping) and categorization of HCA into subgroups using immunohistochemical markers that may affect the management strategies for hepatocellular adenomas in the future.[70,71] One study suggests that 35% to 40% of HCA show inactivated mutations of the *HNF1A* gene. *HNF1A*-inactivated HCAs display characteristic pathologic features, such as marked steatosis. In that study, 10% to 15% of HCA presented with a β-catenin mutation, which, for example, can be characterized by an overexpression of glutamine synthetase. This subtype is associated with a higher risk for malignant transformation and is difficult to differentiate from well-differentiated HCC. Fifty percent of HCAs were classified into a different subtype of inflammatory HCA, defined by the presence of inflammatory infiltrates, sinusoidal dilatation, and thick-walled arteries. In the past, this subtype was defined as telangiectatic FNH.[69] Fewer than 10% of HCAs were categorized into a subgroup of unclassified HCA, which did not show any of the phenotypic markers.[68,71]

On MRI, adenomas may exhibit substantial fat, which can best be visualized by the drop in signal intensity on out-of-phase, T1-weighted gradient echo sequences, compared with in-phase images (**Fig. 19**A, B).[70] Because of the heterogeneity of adenomas,[69] the signal intensity on T1-weighted images varies among mildly hypointense, isointense, and moderately hyperintense (see **Fig. 19**A). On T2-weighted images, hepatic adenoma generally appear mildly hyperintense, but can also be isointense to normal liver parenchyma (**Fig. 19**C).[72] Although, homogeneous arterial phase enhancement may also occur, adenomas characteristically show heterogeneous arterial phase enhancement that fades to near isointensity after 1 minute (**Fig. 19**D). The heterogeneity of the signal intensity is especially seen in very large adenomas because of pronounced intralesional degenerative changes (**Fig. 19**E).

After administration of hepatocyte-specific contrast agents, such as gadobenate (Gd-BOPTA) and gadoxetate (Gd-EOB-DTPA), adenomas typically appear hypointense on T1-weighted,

Fig. 18. Axial ADC map shows a 5-cm FNH (same patient as in **Fig. 15**), which appears as a lobulated, hypointense lesion in the right liver lobe (subcapsular in segment 6). Note the hyperintense central scar (*large black arrow*) and the hyperintense pseudocapsule (*small black arrows*).

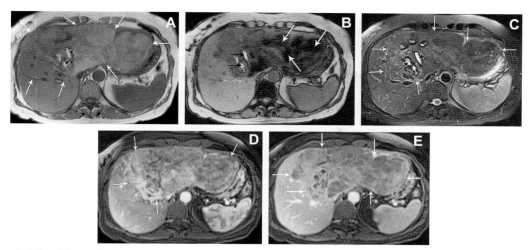

Fig. 19. (*A*) Axial unenhanced T1-weighted gradient-recalled echo two-dimensional in-phase image shows a large adenoma that is 10 cm in diameter, which appears inhomogeneous and slightly hyperintense in the left liver lobe in segments 2 and 3 subcapsularly (*white arrows*) because of the fatty content. Note the hemorrhagic areas (*black arrows*), which appear markedly hyperintense. (*B*) Axial unenhanced T1-weighted gradient-recalled echo two-dimensional opposed-phase image showing the large adenoma, which appears inhomogeneous and, to a large extent, markedly hypointense (*white arrows*) because of the signal loss of the fatty content. Note the hemorrhagic areas (*black arrows*), which appear markedly hyperintense. (*C*) Axial T2-weighted turbo spin-echo image with fat suppression showing the large adenoma, which appears inhomogeneous and slightly hyperintense (*white arrows*), with hemorrhagic areas (*black arrows*) that appear markedly hyperintense with a dark hemosiderin rim. (*D*) Gadolinium-enhanced axial T1-weighted gradient-recalled echo three-dimensional image in the arterial phase shows the large adenoma, which appears as an inhomogeneous and slightly hyperintense mass in the left liver lobe in segments 2 and 3 subcapsularly (*white arrows*). (*E*) Gadolinium-enhanced axial T1-weighted gradient-recalled echo three-dimensional image in the portal venous phase, showing the large adenoma, which appears as an inhomogeneous hypointense mass because of wash-out (*white arrows*).

delayed-phase images. Although adenomas contain hepatocytes, the lack of hepatic phase enhancement with liver-specific contrast agents is thought to be from the absence of specific cellular receptors responsible for the active uptake of these contrast agents through the adenoma's cellular surface (**Fig. 20**A, B).[73] Conversely, hepatocyte-specific Mn-DPDP is taken up by adenomas, usually rendering them isointense or slightly hyperintense to normal liver (**Fig. 20**C).[74]

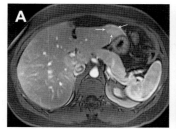
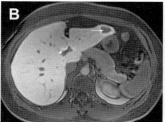
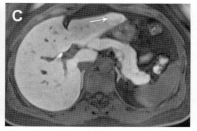

Fig. 20. (*A*) Axial T1-weighted gradient-recalled echo three-dimensional image in the arterial phase after administration of Gd-EOB-DTPA shows a moderately hyperintense 3 cm adenoma in the left liver lobe in segment 2 subcapsularly (*white arrows*). (*B*) Axial T1-weighted gradient-recalled echo three-dimensional image in the hepatocyte-specific phase (20 minutes after administration of Gd-EOB-DTPA) shows the adenoma as a hypointense lesion (*white arrow*) because of wash-out of this contrast agent. (*C*) Axial T1-weighted gradient-recalled echo three-dimensional image in the hepatospecific phase 30 minutes after administration of mangafodipir shows the adenoma in segment 3, which appears inhomogeneously hyperintense because of the active uptake of this contrast agent (*white arrow*). Note also the biliary excretion of contrast (*arrow*).

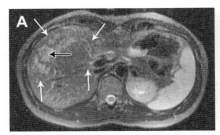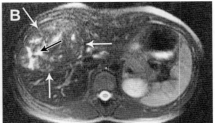

Fig. 21. (*A*) Axial T2-weighted turbo spin-echo with fat suppression, showing a large adenoma that is approximately 8 cm in diameter, which appears inhomogeneous and slightly hyperintense to isointense in the right liver lobe in segment 8 (*white arrows*), with necrotic areas (*black arrow*) that appear slightly hyperintense. (*B*) SPIO-enhanced axial T2-weighted turbo spin-echo with fat saturation, after administration of 1.4 mL of ferucarbutran intravenously, showing marked signal intensity loss of the liver parenchyma and also of the large adenoma that is 8 cm in diameter, which appears inhomogeneous in the right liver lobe in segment 8 (*white arrow*), with necrotic areas (*black arrow*) that appear hyperintense.

The difference in uptake of these two types of hepatobiliary contrast agents may be attributed to different cellular uptake mechanisms, with the cellular uptake mechanism of Gd-BOPTA and Gd-EOB-DTPA perhaps performed by a similar receptor, but with Mn-DPDP uptake involving a different receptor. This difference in hepatocyte-specific contrast uptake may be used to distinguish between FNH and adenoma, and between adenoma and metastases or lymphoma.[9,10]

Regarding uptake of SPIO contrast agents (ferucarbotran, or ferumoxide), adenomas may show an isointense signal loss consistent with healthy liver parenchyma, or remain hyperintense on T2-weighted images (**Fig. 21**). The extent of signal intensity loss with SPIO contrast agents is caused by the extremely variable number of Kupffer cells within these lesions, and typically the uptake of iron oxides is moderate at best.[75] As a solid tumor, an adenoma shows slight signal intensity increase with increasing b-values on DWI and appears hypointense on ADC maps. The ADC value ranges between 1 and 1.40×10^{-3} mm²/s cm/s. However, the ADC values may overlap with FNH, HCC, and other malignant solid lesions (**Fig. 22**).[34]

SUMMARY

Using the recent developmental techniques in MRI, such as high-field-strength (3 Tesla), in combination with parallel imaging and dynamic, contrast-enhanced, isotropic T1-weighted three-dimensional gradient-recalled echo sequences, and DWI and T2-weighted sequences, a higher detection rate for focal liver lesions can be achieved. Through combining these modern techniques with a tailored administration of liver-specific contrast agents, benign focal liver lesions can be accurately characterized, and unnecessary biopsy avoided.

Fig. 22. Axial ADC map showing a 3-cm adenoma in the left liver lobe in segment 2 subcapsularly (*white arrows*) (same patient as in **Fig. 20**), which shows a heterogeneous slightly hyper- to isointense signal. The ADC value is about 1 to 1.40×10^{-3} mm²/s cm/s. However, this may overlap with FNH, HCC, and other malignant solid lesions.

REFERENCES

1. Winterer JT, Kotter E, Ghanem N, et al. Detection and characterization of benign focal liver lesions with multislice CT. Eur Radiol 2006;16(11):2427–43.
2. Schwartz LH, Gandras EJ, Colangelo SM, et al. Prevalence and importance of small hepatic lesions found at CT in patients with cancer. Radiology 1999; 210(1):71–4.
3. Mueller GC, Hussain HK, Carlos RC, et al. Effectiveness of MR imaging in characterizing small hepatic lesions: routine versus expert interpretation. AJR Am J Roentgenol 2003;180(3):673–80.

4. Ba-Ssalamah A, Schima W, Schmook MT, et al. Atypical focal nodular hyperplasia of the liver: imaging features of nonspecific and liver-specific MR contrast agents. AJR Am J Roentgenol 2002; 179(6):1447–56.

5. Caseiro-Alves F, Brito J, Araujo AE, et al. Liver haemangioma: common and uncommon findings and how to improve the differential diagnosis. Eur Radiol 2007;17(6):1544–54.

6. Baudendistel KT, Heverhagen JT, Knopp MV. Clinical MR at 3 Tesla: current status. Radiologe 2004; 44(1):11–8 [in German].

7. Choi JS, Kim MJ, Choi JY, et al. Diffusion-weighted MR imaging of liver on 3.0-Tesla system: effect of intravenous administration of gadoxetic acid disodium. Eur Radiol 2010;20(5):1052–60.

8. Dobritz M, Radkow T, Nittka M, et al. VIBE with parallel acquisition technique - a novel approach to dynamic contrast-enhanced MR imaging of the liver. Rofo 2002;174(6):738–41 [in German].

9. Ba-Ssalamah A, Uffmann M, Saini S, et al. Clinical value of MRI liver-specific contrast agents: a tailored examination for a confident non-invasive diagnosis of focal liver lesions. Eur Radiol 2009; 19(2):342–57.

10. Qayyum A. Diffusion-weighted imaging in the abdomen and pelvis: concepts and applications. Radiographics 2009;29(6):1797–810.

11. Griswold MA, Jakob PM, Heidemann RM, et al. Generalized autocalibrating partially parallel acquisitions (GRAPPA). Magn Reson Med 2002;47(6):1202–10.

12. Lee VS, Lavelle MT, Rofsky NM, et al. Hepatic MR imaging with a dynamic contrast-enhanced isotropic volumetric interpolated breath-hold examination: feasibility, reproducibility, and technical quality. Radiology 2000;215(2):365–72.

13. Semelka RC, Helmberger TK. Contrast agents for MR imaging of the liver. Radiology 2001;218(1):27–38.

14. Ba-Ssalamah A, Happel B, Kettenbach J, et al. MRT of the liver. Clinical significance of nonspecific and liver-specific MRT contrast agents. Radiologe 2004; 44(12):1170–84 [in German].

15. Bluemke DA, Weber TM, Rubin D, et al. Hepatic MR imaging with ferumoxides: multicenter study of safety and effectiveness of direct injection protocol. Radiology 2003;228(2):457–64.

16. Gandhi SN, Brown MA, Wong JG, et al. MR contrast agents for liver imaging: what, when, how. Radiographics 2006;26(6):1621–36.

17. Ba-Ssalamah A, Heinz-Peer G, Schima W, et al. Detection of focal hepatic lesions: comparison of unenhanced and SHU 555 A-enhanced MR imaging versus biphasic helical CTAP. J Magn Reson Imaging 2000;11(6):665–72.

18. Ba-Ssalamah A, Fakhrai N, Matzek WK, et al. Magnetic resonance imaging of liver malignancies. Top Magn Reson Imaging 2007;18(6):445–55.

19. Seale MK, Catalano OA, Saini S, et al. Hepatobiliary-specific MR contrast agents: role in imaging the liver and biliary tree. Radiographics 2009;29(6):1725–48.

20. Horton KM, Bluemke DA, Hruban RH, et al. CT and MR imaging of benign hepatic and biliary tumors. Radiographics 1999;19(2):431–51.

21. Mortele KJ, Ros PR. Cystic focal liver lesions in the adult: differential CT and MR imaging features. Radiographics 2001;21(4):895–910.

22. Elsayes KM, Narra VR, Yin Y, et al. Focal hepatic lesions: diagnostic value of enhancement pattern approach with contrast-enhanced 3D gradient-echo MR imaging. Radiographics 2005;25(5):1299–320.

23. Mosetti MA, Leonardou P, Motohara T, et al. Autosomal dominant polycystic kidney disease: MR imaging evaluation using current techniques. J Magn Reson Imaging 2003;18(2):210–5.

24. Bae KT, Tao C, Zhu F, et al. MRI-based kidney volume measurements in ADPKD: reliability and effect of gadolinium enhancement. Clin J Am Soc Nephrol 2009;4(4):719–25.

25. Kadoya M, Matsui O, Nakanuma Y, et al. Ciliated hepatic foregut cyst: radiologic features. Radiology 1990;175(2):475–7.

26. Fang SH, Dong DJ, Zhang SZ. Imaging features of ciliated hepatic foregut cyst. World J Gastroenterol 2005;11(27):4287–9.

27. Quan XY, Sun XJ, Yu ZJ, et al. Evaluation of diffusion weighted imaging of magnetic resonance imaging in small focal hepatic lesions: a quantitative study in 56 cases. Hepatobiliary Pancreat Dis Int 2005;4(3): 406–9.

28. Koike N, Cho A, Nasu K, et al. Role of diffusion-weighted magnetic resonance imaging in the differential diagnosis of focal hepatic lesions. World J Gastroenterol 2009;15(46):5805–12.

29. Inan N, Arslan A, Akansel G, et al. Diffusion-weighted imaging in the differential diagnosis of simple and hydatid cysts of the liver. AJR Am J Roentgenol 2007;189(5):1031–6.

30. Garcia-Diez AI, Ros Mendoza LH, Villacampa VM, et al. MRI evaluation of soft tissue hydatid disease. Eur Radiol 2000;10(3):462–6.

31. Czermak BV, Akhan O, Hiemetzberger R, et al. Echinococcosis of the liver. Abdom Imaging 2008;33(2): 133–43.

32. Parsak CK, Demiryurek HH, Inal M, et al. Alveolar hydatid disease: imaging findings and surgical approach. Acta Chir Belg 2007;107(5):572–7.

33. Sezgin O, Altintas E, Saritas U, et al. Hepatic alveolar echinococcosis: clinical and radiologic features and endoscopic management. J Clin Gastroenterol 2005;39(2):160–7.

34. Kilickesmez O, Bayramoglu S, Inci E, et al. Value of apparent diffusion coefficient measurement for discrimination of focal benign and malignant hepatic masses. J Med Imaging Radiat Oncol 2009;53(1):50–5.

35. Cook JR, Pfeifer JD, Dehner LP. Mesenchymal hamartoma of the liver in the adult: association with distinct clinical features and histological changes. Hum Pathol 2002;33(9):893–8.

36. Zen Y, Terahata S, Miyayama S, et al. Multicystic biliary hamartoma: a hitherto undescribed lesion. Hum Pathol 2006;37(3):339–44.

37. Ryu Y, Matsui O, Zen Y, et al. Multicystic biliary hamartoma: imaging findings in four cases. Abdom Imaging August 15, 2009. [Epub ahead of print].

38. Volk M, Strotzer M, Lenhart M, et al. Frequency of benign hepatic lesions incidentally detected with contrast-enhanced thin-section portal venous phase spiral CT. Acta Radiol 2001;42(2):172–5.

39. Vilgrain V, Boulos L, Vullierme MP, et al. Imaging of atypical hemangiomas of the liver with pathologic correlation. Radiographics 2000;20(2):379–97.

40. Bader TR, Braga L, Semelka RC. Exophytic benign tumors of the liver: appearance on MRI. Magn Reson Imaging 2001;19(5):623–8.

41. Cappellani A, Zanghi A, Di Vita M, et al. Spontaneous rupture of a giant hemangioma of the liver. Ann Ital Chir 2000;71(3):379–83.

42. Belli G, D'Agostino A, Fantini C, et al. Surgical treatment of giant liver hemangiomas by enucleation using an ultrasonically activated device (USAD). Hepatogastroenterology 2009;56(89):236–9.

43. Hanafusa K, Ohashi I, Himeno Y, et al. Hepatic hemangioma: findings with two-phase CT. Radiology 1995;196(2):465–9.

44. Nelson RC, Chezmar JL. Diagnostic approach to hepatic hemangiomas. Radiology 1990;176(1):11–3.

45. Danet IM, Semelka RC, Braga L, et al. Giant hemangioma of the liver: MR imaging characteristics in 24 patients. Magn Reson Imaging 2003;21(2):95–101.

46. Semelka RC, Brown ED, Ascher SM, et al. Hepatic hemangiomas: a multi-institutional study of appearance on T2-weighted and serial gadolinium-enhanced gradient-echo MR images. Radiology 1994;192(2):401–6.

47. Montet X, Lazeyras F, Howarth N, et al. Specificity of SPIO particles for characterization of liver hemangiomas using MRI. Abdom Imaging 2004;29(1):60–70.

48. McNicholas MM, Saini S, Echeverri J, et al. T2 relaxation times of hypervascular and non-hypervascular liver lesions: do hypervascular lesions mimic haemangiomas on heavily T2-weighted MR images? Clin Radiol 1996;51(6):401–5.

49. Aibe H, Hondo H, Kuroiwa T, et al. Sclerosed hemangioma of the liver. Abdom Imaging 2001;26(5):496–9.

50. Sandrasegaran K, Akisik FM, Lin C, et al. The value of diffusion-weighted imaging in characterizing focal liver masses. Acad Radiol 2009;16(10):1208–14.

51. Nguyen BN, Flejou JF, Terris B, et al. Focal nodular hyperplasia of the liver: a comprehensive pathologic study of 305 lesions and recognition of new histologic forms. Am J Surg Pathol 1999;23(12):1441–54.

52. Giannitrapani L, Soresi M, La Spada E, et al. Sex hormones and risk of liver tumor. Ann N Y Acad Sci 2006;1089:228–36.

53. Powers C, Ros PR, Stoupis C, et al. Primary liver neoplasms: MR imaging with pathologic correlation. Radiographics 1994;14(3):459–82.

54. Wanless IR, Mawdsley C, Adams R. On the pathogenesis of focal nodular hyperplasia of the liver. Hepatology 1985;5(6):1194–200.

55. Kim T, Hori M, Onishi H. Liver masses with central or eccentric scar. Semin Ultrasound CT MR 2009;30(5):418–25.

56. Toshikuni N, Kawaguchi K, Miki H, et al. Focal nodular hyperplasia coexistent with hemangioma and multiple cysts of the liver. J Gastroenterol 2001;36(3):206–11.

57. Attal P, Vilgrain V, Brancatelli G, et al. Telangiectatic focal nodular hyperplasia: US, CT, and MR imaging findings with histopathologic correlation in 13 cases. Radiology 2003;228(2):465–72.

58. Wanless IR, Albrecht S, Bilbao J, et al. Multiple focal nodular hyperplasia of the liver associated with vascular malformations of various organs and neoplasia of the brain: a new syndrome. Mod Pathol 1989;2(5):456–62.

59. Kapp N, Curtis KM. Hormonal contraceptive use among women with liver tumors: a systematic review. Contraception 2009;80(4):387–90.

60. Lee PJ. Glycogen storage disease type I: pathophysiology of liver adenomas. Eur J Pediatr 2002;161(Suppl 1):S46–9.

61. Rummeny E, Weissleder R, Sironi S, et al. Central scars in primary liver tumors: MR features, specificity, and pathologic correlation. Radiology 1989;171(2):323–6.

62. Shortell CK, Schwartz SI. Hepatic adenoma and focal nodular hyperplasia. Surg Gynecol Obstet 1991;173(5):426–31.

63. Greaves WO, Bhattacharya B. Hepatic adenomatosis. Arch Pathol Lab Med 2008;132(12):1951–5.

64. Grazioli L, Federle MP, Ichikawa T, et al. Liver adenomatosis: clinical, histopathologic, and imaging findings in 15 patients. Radiology 2000;216(2):395–402.

65. Wiener Y, Dushnitzky T, Slutzki S, et al. Synchronous bleeding of liver adenomatosis and possible relation to acoustic trauma. HPB (Oxford) 2001;3(4):267–9.

66. Santambrogio R, Marconi AM, Ceretti AP, et al. Liver transplantation for spontaneous intrapartum rupture of a hepatic adenoma. Obstet Gynecol 2009;113(2 Pt 2):508–10.

67. Farges O, Dokmak S. Malignant transformation of liver adenoma: an analysis of the literature. Dig Surg 2010;27(1):32–8.

68. Bioulac-Sage P, Balabaud C, Zucman-Rossi J. Subtype classification of hepatocellular adenoma. Dig Surg 2010;27(1):39–45.

69. Zucman-Rossi J, Jeannot E, Nhieu JT, et al. Geno-type-phenotype correlation in hepatocellular adenoma: new classification and relationship with HCC. Hepatology 2006;43(3):515—24.

70. Prasad SR, Wang H, Rosas H, et al. Fat-containing lesions of the liver: radiologic-pathologic correlation. Radiographics 2005;25(2):321—31.

71. Bioulac-Sage P, Laumonier H, Couchy G, et al. Hepatocellular adenoma management and pheno-typic classification: the Bordeaux experience. Hepatology 2009;50(2):481—9.

72. Barbier C, Denny P, Becker S, et al. MRI aspect of hepatic adenomatosis. J Radiol 1997;78(12): 1281—4 [in French].

73. Grazioli L, Morana G, Kirchin MA, et al. Accurate differentiation of focal nodular hyperplasia from hepatic adenoma at gadobenate dimeglumine-enhanced MR imaging: prospective study. Radiology 2005;236(1):166—77.

74. Chung JJ, Kim MJ, Kim KW. Mangafodipir trisodium-enhanced MRI for the detection and characterization of focal hepatic lesions: is de-layed imaging useful? J Magn Reson Imaging 2006;23(5):706—11.

75. Vogl TJ, Hammerstingl R, Schwarz W, et al. Superpar-amagnetic iron oxide—enhanced versus gadolinium-enhanced MR imaging for differential diagnosis of focal liver lesions. Radiology 1996;198(3):881—7.

MR Imaging of Hepatocellular Carcinoma

Gaurav Khatri, MD, Laura Merrick, BA, Frank H. Miller, MD*

KEYWORDS

- Hepatocellular carcinoma
- Magnetic Resonance Imaging • HCC • MRI

Hepatocellular carcinoma (HCC) accounts for 85% to 90% of all primary liver malignancies. It is one of the most common cancers and the third leading cause of cancer mortality worldwide. Among American men, it is the fastest growing cause of cancer death. The incidence is at least twice as high in males as in females.[1,2] A recent study showed that the incidence of HCC in the United States has tripled since 1975 from 1.5 per 100,000 to 4.9 per 100,000. Although mortality rates from HCC have also continued to rise with rising incidence of the tumor, 1-year survival rates have nearly doubled since 1992 from 25% to 47%. This may be in part related to more active screening programs and aggressive therapies.[3]

The development of HCC is related to chronic liver inflammation that leads to fibrosis and cirrhosis. Although HCC can be seen in noncirrhotic patients with chronic viral hepatitis (HBV), toxin exposure, or other chronic liver diseases such as hemochromatosis,[4,5] 70% to 90% of detected cases are seen in the setting of cirrhosis.[1] Among patients with cirrhosis, the annual incidence of HCC is between 2% and 6%.[6] Cirrhosis is a major underlying risk factor regardless of its etiology, although cirrhosis from viral hepatitis or hereditary hemochromatosis confers the highest risk among cirrhotic patients.[5,7] Within the United States, hepatitis C virus (HCV) infection is the major underlying etiology of cirrhosis and subsequent development of HCC. It accounts for 50% of cases of HCC in the United States and Europe and up to 70% of cases in Japan.[5] Alcoholic cirrhosis confers similar risk as that of other causes of cirrhosis, such as cryptogenic cirrhosis and primary biliary cirrhosis; however, alcohol abuse in the setting of chronic viral hepatitis or other chronic liver disease compounds the risk of HCC.[1,5,7] Obesity is another compounding risk factor for the development of HCC in the setting of cirrhosis.[1,5,7]

Hepatitis B virus (HBV) is the single most important risk factor for HCC worldwide.[6] Although most HCCs related to HBV infection develop on a background of cirrhosis, HBV infection is an independent risk factor even without cirrhosis.[1,5] Coinfection with HIV in the setting of HBV or HCV infection is associated with more rapid progression of the liver disease and development of HCC.[8] The risk of development of HCC in the setting of certain other conditions such as autoimmune hepatitis (AIH) is debated.[5,7–11] Nonalcoholic steatohepatitis and alpha1-antitrypsin deficiency are categorized as high-risk conditions for the development of HCC,[8] although associated HBV or HCV infection may play a larger role in patients with alpha1-antitrypsin deficiency than the metabolic disorder itself.[7] There is also an association between HCC and Budd-Chiari syndrome; however, the prevalence of HCC in this population is variable, suggesting that other factors, such as viral infection, play a role in the development of HCC in these patients as well.[12]

Financial disclosures/conflicts of interest: The authors have nothing to disclose.
Department of Radiology, Northwestern University Feinberg School of Medicine, 676 North St Clair Street, Suite 800, Chicago, IL 60611, USA
* Corresponding author.
E-mail address: fmiller@northwestern.edu

Magn Reson Imaging Clin N Am 18 (2010) 421–450
doi:10.1016/j.mric.2010.08.002

mri.theclinics.com

HCC SCREENING

The median survival period after diagnosis of HCC has been reported as less than 1 year.[13] Unfortunately, prognosis after the onset of cancer-related symptoms is poor with 5-year survival being 0 to 10%.[8] HCC lesions diagnosed at screening are generally smaller, more often subclinical and resectable, and have a significantly higher survival rate than those diagnosed without a screening program.[14,15] One study demonstrated a 37% reduction in mortality attributable to biannual screening.[15] Surveillance is generally recommended for populations where the risk of HCC is 1.5% per year or greater in non–hepatitis B carriers or 0.2% per year in hepatitis B carriers. The American Association for the Study of Liver Diseases (AASLD) recommended time interval for surveillance for HCC is 6 to 12 months. Patients on the transplant waiting list should also be screened at regular intervals because it may determine their transplant wait list status. The development of HCC in a patient on the transplant list provides increased priority as long as tumor burden is within the transplant criteria.[8]

IMAGING OF HCC

Imaging of the cirrhotic liver can be performed with ultrasound, CT, or MRI. Although relatively high accessibility and low cost have made ultrasound the most widely used modality for screening and surveillance of HCC, ultrasound has its limitations. Besides being operator dependant, ultrasound is limited by markedly heterogeneous hepatic echo-texture in the setting of cirrhosis and has limited utility in depicting small HCCs that can have variable appearances.[8] The presence of fatty deposition and fibrosis in the liver and ascites in the abdomen make evaluation for liver masses on ultrasound very difficult. Without the approval of sonographic contrast material in the United States, detection and characterization of focal liver lesions, especially small lesions, is difficult because evaluation of arterial hypervascularity to suggest HCC cannot be performed. As will be discussed, evaluation of flow dynamics to a lesion in the setting of cirrhosis is critical in the characterization process.

Although CT has the advantage of being able to use intravenous contrast, and arterial and portal venous imaging can be performed, MRI is superior in that it has the ability to obtain multiple phases of enhancement rapidly following contrast without the associated radiation exposure. MRI also has greater sensitivity to contrast material and improved contrast resolution. It is imperative to

be able to correctly time the contrast bolus and image acquisitions. Imaging times can be highly variable among patients because of cirrhosis, portal hypertension, volume status, and other causes. Consequently, standard timing may not be optimal and methods such as fluoroscopy preparation or bolus tracking should be used to determine the correct acquisition time for the different phases in each patient after contrast infusion. Another challenge, regardless of the modality, is the background heterogeneity of the cirrhotic liver, which makes it difficult to identify small lesions. As is discussed, the radiologist should assess for imaging features on T2-weighted and unenhanced and contrast-enhanced T1-weighted sequences that might suggest the presence of HCC. Our institutional protocol for liver MRI is shown in **Table 1**.

LESIONS IN CIRRHOSIS

When evaluating liver lesions, it is critical to consider the patient population. In the general noncirrhotic patient population, hemangiomas and cysts are the most common hepatic lesions. In young and middle-aged women, focal nodular hyperplasia (FNH) and hepatic adenomas are additional benign lesions in the differential diagnosis. In patients with known malignancies, hepatic metastases should be considered. In contrast, "nothing likes to live in the cirrhotic liver" (Richard Baron, MD, University of Chicago, personal communication, 2009) and the differential considerations become more limited and include regenerative and dysplastic nodules, and hepatocellular carcinomas.[16]

Regenerative Nodules

Regenerative nodules are cirrhotic nodules that are surrounded by fibrosis[17,18] and form as a result of necrosis or changes in hepatic circulation. They are usually multiple and scattered throughout the parenchyma,[16,17] but may be difficult to detect, as they may blend with other regenerative nodules or with the surrounding fibrosis.[18] The nodules in cirrhosis can be micronodules (<3 mm) or macronodules ($\geq$ 3 mm) based on size, and either mono-acinar or multiacinar based on the number of portal tracts they contain.[16,17] Alcohol-related cirrhosis is typically micronodular, although over time may progress to a macronodular or mixed pattern.[19,20] Macronodular cirrhosis is usually seen with chronic viral hepatitis, but may also be seen with autoimmune and metabolic disorders.[19,21] Most regenerative nodules are small (<2 cm); however, larger regenerative nodules can be seen in the setting of Budd-Chiari

Table 1
Northwestern University MR liver protocol
Transverse and coronal T2-weighted half-Fourier acquisition single-shot turbo spin echo (HASTE): repetition time/echo time (TR/TE), 1000/60; flip angle, 150°; matrix, 256×256; slice thickness, 5 mm; gap 1 mm; rectangular field of view (FOV), 36–40 cm; number of signals acquired, 1
Transverse T1-weighted gradient echo in and opposed phase: TR/TE, 150-200/2.3 (opposed phase) - 4.6 (in phase); flip angle, 70°; matrix, 256×256; section thickness, 5 mm; gap, 1.8 mm; rectangular field of view, 36–40 cm; number of signals acquired, 1
Breath hold T2-weighted turbo spin-echo (TSE) with fat suppression: TR/TE, 4000/100; flip angle, 150°; matrix, 256×194; section thickness, 6 mm; gap 1.8 mm; rectangular field of view, 36–40 cm; number of signals acquired, 1
Diffusion weighted imaging b50, b500, and b1000 sec/mm^2: single-shot spin-echo echo-planar imaging (EPI) with spectral prostration attenuated inversion-recovery (SPAIR) fat-suppressed pulse. Integrated parallel imaging techniques (pat) using generalized autocalibrating partially parallel acquisitions (GRAPPA) are used with a twofold acceleration time. TR/TE, 5000/80; matrix of 192×192; bandwidth, 1446 Hz/px; section thickness, 6 mm; gap, 1.8 mm; FOV, 300–400 mm; partial Fourier factor 6/8; averages, 2; parallel imaging factor of 2
Unenhanced fat-suppressed T1-weighted gradient echo images: TR/TE, 189-217/1.9; flip angle, 70°; slice thickness, 6 mm; gap, 1.8 mm; matrix, 256×189; rectangular field of view, 36–40 cm; 23 slices acquired in breath hold of 20 seconds
Fluoro-preparation timing run
Dynamic gadolinium-enhanced gradient echo fat-suppressed T1-weighted images using shared prepulses (SHARP) in arterial, venous (45–60 s and coronal 90 s), and 2–5 minutes—same parameters as unenhanced T1-weighted GRE images
Optional sequences: MR choliangiopancreatography; T2 gradient echo for hemochromatosis; MR elastography for cirrhosis

syndrome[12,22] as well as cirrhosis from autoimmune hepatitis.[23]

Regenerative nodules have a similar vascular profile to the surrounding cirrhotic liver and draw their blood supply from the portal venous system.[24–26] Consequently, they are typically isointense to liver following contrast administration, although they may be hypointense (**Fig. 1**). Additionally, hepatobiliary function is generally preserved in regenerative nodules and they take up hepatobiliary contrast agents.[16] For these reasons, small lesions are difficult to detect on CT or MR imaging. Regenerative nodules demonstrate variable signal on T1-weighted images.[16,20,21,25,27,28] On T2-weighted MR imaging, typical regenerative nodules are isointense to hypointense (see **Fig. 1**).[16,20,27,28] They are almost never hyperintense on T2-weighted imaging unless they undergo infarction or occur in the setting of Budd-Chiari syndrome.[12,20] Low signal intensity of regenerative nodules on T1- and T2-weighted sequences can be attributed to the presence of iron.[20,28,29] The susceptibility effect of iron within the nodules is increased with increasing echo time (TE) on gradient echo (GRE) sequences such that they demonstrate more hypointense signal intensity on in-phase GRE

sequences (TE = 4.2 msec) than the opposed-phase GRE sequences (TE = 2.1 msec).[29] Consequently, GRE pulse sequences with longer TE have a higher sensitivity for detection of siderotic nodules (see **Fig. 1**).[29] Although some investigators hypothesize a causal relationship between siderotic nodules and HCC,[30] other studies have shown no significant increase in the incidence of HCC in livers with siderotic nodules.[29]

Dysplastic Nodules

A dysplastic nodule is a nodular hepatocellular region that contains dysplastic features without histologic evidence for malignancy.[17,31] Dysplastic nodules may contain architectural derangement, high nuclear density, atypia, and abnormal vascular profile.[16,32] They are considered premalignant and may be low or high grade.[16,21,31] Low-grade dysplastic nodules are difficult to distinguish histologically from regenerative nodules[16,17] and have low malignant potential.[33] High-grade dysplastic nodules demonstrate more advanced architectural distortion, atypia, and associated vascular abnormalities.[16,21,31,32] They are more likely to progress to hepatocellular carcinoma than are low-grade dysplastic nodules.[33] A dysplastic nodule that

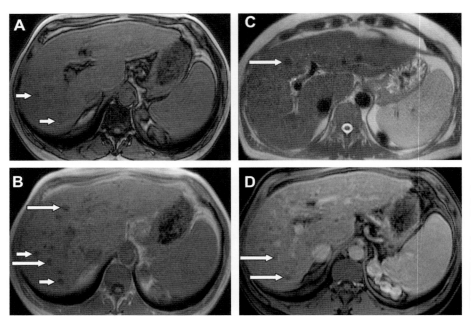

Fig. 1. Regenerative siderotic nodules. (*A*) Axial T1-weighted (T1W) GRE opposed-phase (TE = 2.1 msec) image shows multiple hypointense lesions (*arrows*). (*B*) Axial T1W GRE in-phase image with longer TE (4.2 msec) shows additional lesions (*arrows*) because of the longer TE and resultant greater T2 weighting. The nodules are iron-containing (siderotic) regenerative nodules. (*C*) Axial T2W image demonstrates the lesions to be hypointense owing to the presence of iron (*arrow*). (*D*) Axial gadolinium-enhanced T1FS image shows that the lesions hypo-enhance (*arrows*) because of their portal venous blood supply and lack of arterial blood supply.

contains a microscopic focus of HCC is called "dysplastic nodule with subfocus of HCC."[31] Dysplastic nodules are seen in 15% to 25% of patients with cirrhosis,[20,21,34] although are not seen on imaging as frequently,[35] possibly because they appear similar to regenerative nodules or the surrounding liver.

Dysplastic nodules may have a variable MRI appearance; however, are classically high signal intensity on T1-weighted imaging[21,31] and low signal intensity on T2-weighted images (**Fig. 2**),[16,21,31,34] although they may be isointense to the liver on T1- and T2-weighted images similar to regenerative nodules.[28] Dysplastic nodules predominately have a venous blood supply from the portal vein,[20,26,28,31] and, as such, low-grade dysplastic nodules may be indistinguishable from regenerative nodules based on enhancement characteristics. High-grade dysplastic nodules are associated with increased hepatic arterial blood supply and therefore may demonstrate hypervascularity mimicking HCC.[26,28,34,36] Dysplastic nodules may also contain iron, in which case they follow imaging features of siderotic nodules as discussed previously (in the "Regenerative Nodules" section). MRI cannot reliably

differentiate siderotic nodules that are regenerative from those that are dysplastic.[31,37] The distinction may not be critical compared with the diagnosis of HCC. Furthermore, because HCC can sometimes demonstrate high T1-weighted and low T2-weighted signal intensity, it may be difficult to differentiate dysplastic nodules from HCC on unenhanced MRI.[20,21,31] Unlike HCC, dysplastic nodules only rarely demonstrate hyperintense T2 signal intensity,[20,21,34] and focal masses with increased T2 signal intensity in high-risk patients are generally considered suspicious for HCC with the exception of cysts or hemangiomas. A further distinguishing feature of dysplastic nodules from HCC is that dysplastic nodules typically lack a capsule.[21,38] However, the overlap in imaging features may make the distinction between dysplastic nodules and HCC challenging. The difficulty in distinguishing between high-grade dysplastic and well-differentiated HCC on imaging studies is paralleled in their histologic appearance.[8] Dysplastic nodules generally remain stable or in rare cases regress in size on follow-up imaging; however, those that demonstrate increase in size are more likely to progress to HCC.[39,40]

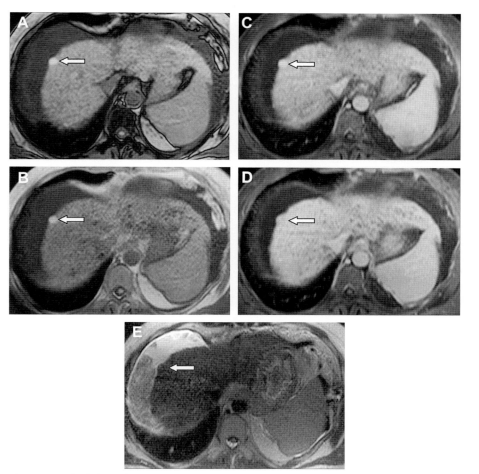

Fig. 2. Dysplastic nodule. (*A*) Axial T1W GRE opposed-phase image shows a focal hyper-intense hepatic nodule (*arrow*). (*B*) Axial T1W GRE in-phase image shows increased signal intensity within the nodule (*arrow*). In addition, multiple additional hypointense lesions are seen on the in-phase images, which were not seen on the opposed-phase image. These multiple liver lesions are most likely from siderotic nodules. (*C*) Axial gadolinium-enhanced arterial-phase T1FS GRE image shows enhancement within the lesion (*arrow*); however, assessment for enhancement is difficult given the unenhanced T1 hyperintense signal intensity. (*D*) Axial delayed gadolinium-enhanced T1FS GRE image shows the lesion (*arrow*) is isointense and does not washout relative to the liver. (*E*) Axial T2W image shows the lesion is not high in signal intensity (*arrow*). The features on MR are most consistent with a dysplastic nodule.

Hepatocellular Carcinoma

Microscopic invasion of stroma and portal tracts is the primary diagnostic feature used to differentiate well-differentiated HCC from dysplastic nodules.[16,17] One pathway of carcinogenesis suggests that HCC develops as a result of a multi-step process. Chronic inflammation related to cirrhosis induces nodular regeneration, which predisposes hepatocytes to genetic mutations and resultant abnormal proliferation and dysplasia. Low-grade dysplastic nodules undergo further mutations and growth, and progress to high-grade dysplastic nodules that eventually develop foci of malignancy.[16] This may be followed by vascular invasion and metastasis.[41] As there is progression along this pathway, there is a corresponding decrease in hepatocyte function and Kupffer cell density.[16,41] Although well-differentiated HCCs may retain some biliary function, poorly or de-differentiated HCCs generally do not. There is also progressive sinusoidal capillarization and recruitment of unpaired arterioles,[16,24,32,41] which results in the characteristic arterial hypervascularity of hepatocellular carcinomas seen on imaging studies. Arterial hypervascularity and other imaging features of HCC are discussed separately.

A coexistent alternative pathway for HCC development has also been suggested. Yu and colleagues[42] studied 152 newly diagnosed HCCs and observed that only a minority of these lesions had precancerous findings on retrospective analysis. Furthermore, it is known that HCC may arise in the absence of liver cirrhosis as is classically observed with chronic HBV-related liver disease. Such observations indicate a de novo pathway, in which a single progenitor cell or a group of cells undergoes malignant transformation into a small HCC that then progresses to large HCC.[16,27,42]

IMAGING FEATURES OF HEPATOCELLULAR CARCINOMA
Characteristic MR Features of HCC

Arterial enhancement
As dysplastic nodules progress to develop malignant foci, the tumor recruits unpaired arteries and sinusoidal capillaries[16,24,32,41] with resultant avid arterial enhancement[28] that is best detected on the arterial phase. Approximately 80% to 90% of HCCs are hypervascular during the arterial phase (**Fig. 3**).[16] HCCs measuring 1.5 cm or smaller may actually be seen only on the arterial-phase images.[43] Contrast-enhanced thin-section T1-weighted imaging alone has been shown to be equivalent in accuracy to the combination of T2-weighted and contrast-enhanced thin-section T1-weighted imaging for the detection of HCC.[44] It is this arterial enhancement that is the most important feature in the diagnosis of hepatocellular carcinoma. When seen in lesions larger than 2 cm in conjunction with delayed washout, arterial enhancement is diagnostic of HCC in the setting of cirrhosis and biopsy confirmation is not considered necessary.[8]

The characteristic arterial enhancement of HCC emphasizes the importance of optimizing techniques to image in the arterial phase. If imaged

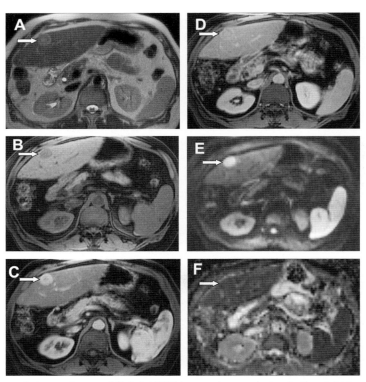

Fig. 3. Typical hepatocellular carcinoma. (*A*) Axial T2W image shows a lesion in the right hepatic lobe with mild increased signal intensity (*arrow*). (*B*) Axial unenhanced T1W GRE image shows low signal intensity within the lesion (*arrow*). (*C*) Axial gadolinium-enhanced arterial-phase T1FS GRE image shows hypervascularity typical of HCC (*arrow*). (*D*) Axial delayed gadolinium-enhanced T1FS GRE image shows washout of lesion with capsular enhancement (*arrow*). (*E*) Axial DWI (b500) shows lesion is increased signal intensity owing to restricted diffusion (*arrow*). (*F*) Axial ADC map shows lesion (*arrow*) is decreased in signal intensity proving that the high signal intensity on DWI is not from T2 shine-through, but from truly restricted diffusion.

too early in the arterial phase when the aorta is initially opacified, the images may be optimal to obtain an MR angiogram but there may not be sufficient opacification of the liver. As a result, HCCs will not appear hypervascular and may not be detected easily. Consequently, arterial-phase images should be obtained during the late arterial phase or portal venous inflow phase. Imaging in the arterial phase can be obtained with a variety of methods including using a test bolus to determine the appropriate acquisition time.[34,44] We use a fluoroscopic-prep timing sequence that allows us to individualize the arterial phase scan time to the patient. Other investigators have suggested obtaining multiple arterial-phase

sequences through the liver to circumvent differences in blood flow kinetics and tumor characteristics[45]; however, these sequences may compromise spatial resolution to obtain optimal temporal resolution. Subtraction techniques can also be applied to improve detection for enhancement within the lesion.[28,44]

About 10% to 20% of HCCs may be hypovascular to the surrounding parenchyma on the immediate gadolinium-enhanced images.[16] This is generally seen in smaller tumors and may be related to lack of arterialization of the tumor.[28,46] Large HCCs may also be hypovascular on the arterial phase and may appear more heterogeneous in enhancement (**Fig. 4**).

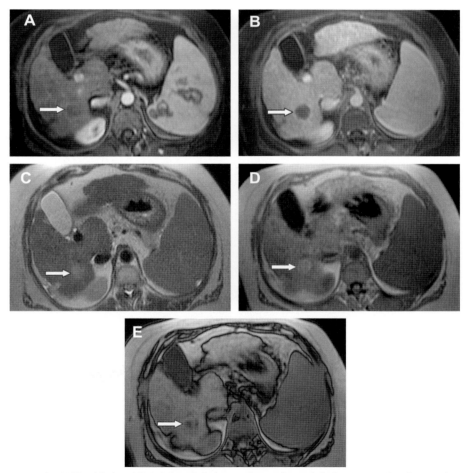

Fig. 4. Hypovascular HCC with fat. (*A*) Axial gadolinium-enhanced arterial-phase T1FS GRE image shows a hypovascular lesion (*arrow*). (*B*) Axial delayed gadolinium-enhanced T1FS GRE image shows the lesion (*arrow*) remains hypovascular to the liver. (*C*) On the axial T2W image, the lesion is increased in signal intensity (*arrow*), which is more typical of HCC than dysplastic nodule. (*D*) Axial T1W GRE in-phase image shows that the lesion (*arrow*) is increased in signal intensity. (*E*) Axial T1W GRE opposed-phase image shows that the lesion (*arrow*) drops in signal intensity because of the presence of fat. The high T2 signal intensity and presence of fat in a lesion in a cirrhotic liver suggests HCC.

Washout

Hypointensity relative to the surrounding paren-chyma on the portal venous and delayed contrast-enhanced phases is called "washout" and is highly suggestive of HCC (see **Fig. 3**) with a specificity of 95% to 96%.[47] Although delayed hypointensity of an arterially enhancing lesion increases diagnostic accuracy for diagnosis of HCC,[28,47,48] the lack of washout does not exclude malignancy. Occasionally, HCC may stay hyperin-tense or isointense to the background liver on the venous and delayed phases.[16,28,38,49] In a series by Lutz and colleagues,[49] 47% of HCCs were hy-pointense on the portal-venous phase images whereas 28% were hyperintense and 25% isoin-tense; 58% of HCCs were hypointense on the de-layed equilibrium phase images whereas 3% were hyperintense and 39% were isointense on the de-layed equilibrium phase images.

Capsule

A tumor capsule is most often seen in large HCCs and may be present in 24% to 90% of cases in the Asian population and 12% to 42% of cases in the non-Asian population.[43,50–52] When present, a capsule or pseudocapsule strongly suggests a diagnosis of HCC. Larger tumors tend to demonstrate thicker capsules. The capsule may be hypointense on T1- and T2-weighted images; however, can rarely be hyperintense on T2-weighted images.[43,52] Histologically, the capsule consists of an inner fibrous layer and an outer layer composed of compressed vessels and bile ducts[16,52] and may demonstrate persistent or delayed enhancement (see **Fig. 3**; **Fig. 5**).[16,38,43] Lower grade tumors are more likely to be encapsulated.[51] Transarterial chemoembolization (TACE) is reportedly more effective in HCCs with a capsule than in unencapsulated HCCs.[53] Ishiga-mi and colleagues[53] demonstrated that some HCCs that show an enhancing rim on dynamic MRI actually do not have a true fibrous capsule histologically. In these cases, the "pseudocap-sule" seen on MRI represents prominent hepatic sinusoids and/or peritumoral fibrosis. They showed that there is no significant difference in tumor size, tumor grade, and incidence of vascular invasion between tumors with a pseudocapsule and tumors with a true histologic fibrous capsule. Pseudocapsules also appear hypointense on T1- and T2-weighted imaging[54] and thus are not distinguishable from a true capsule on MRI.

Extracapsular extension has been shown to be a negative prognostic factor seen pathologically

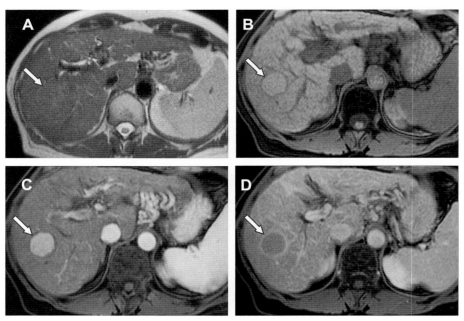

Fig. 5. HCC isointense on T2W images. (*A*) Axial T2W image shows a 2.5-cm lesion (*arrow*) that is isointense to the liver and difficult to visualize. (*B*) Axial unenhanced T1FS GRE image shows the lesion has increased signal inten-sity relative to the liver (*arrow*). The findings may suggest a dysplastic nodule but evaluation is incomplete without assessment of the enhancement pattern. (*C*) Axial gadolinium-enhanced arterial-phase T1FS GRE image shows that the lesion is hypervascular (*arrow*). (*D*) Axial delayed gadolinium-enhanced T1FS GRE image shows washout of the lesion and capsular enhancement typical of HCC (*arrow*).

in 43% to 77% of HCCs. MRI is sensitive in detecting extracapsular extension, which usually manifests as projection of tumor into the surrounding parenchyma as well as appearance of small satellite nodules adjacent to the main lesion.[16,55] More aggressive HCCs may demonstrate not only extracapsular extension, but also extrahepatic spread with invasion of adjacent structures such as the diaphragm or abdominal wall.[16]

Increased T2-weighted/decreased T1-weighted signal intensity

Hepatocellular carcinomas typically demonstrate mild to moderate increased signal intensity on T2-weighted sequences (see **Fig. 3**).[21,43] The high T2-weighted signal intensity may allow differentiation from dysplastic nodules that rarely exhibit this finding[20,21,31,34,38]; however, this feature is not seen in all HCCs. Some well-differentiated hepatocellular carcinomas may demonstrate isointense or hypointense T2-weighted signal intensity.[31,34,43,56] Consequently, the absence of high T2 signal intensity in a lesion should not exclude HCC especially when other suggestive features are present (see **Fig. 5**). Furthermore, in the setting of cirrhosis, heterogeneity and nodularity of the background liver may make it difficult to detect HCC on T2-weighted images.[28,35,56] Consequently, T2-weighted images have been shown to be helpful in the diagnosis of focal lesions in the noncirrhotic liver,[57–59] but have been shown to have less utility in the setting of cirrhosis.[44,56]

On T1-weighted images, HCCs are more commonly hypointense.[43] Although T1 hyperintensity within a cirrhotic nodule is more typical of dysplastic nodules, it can also been seen in HCCs.[31,43] Kelekis and colleagues[43] reported 42 (12%) of 354 HCCs were hyperintense on T1-weighted images. T1 hyperintensity in HCC has been attributed to the presence of fat, copper, proteins, melanin, hemorrhage, and glycogen within the lesion.[16,21,35,60,61] It has been suggested that HCCs with higher T1-weighted signal intensity may be associated with higher grades of differentiation.[60] However, because signal intensity on MR imaging is a relative rather than an absolute entity, the presence of zinc or iron will reduce signal intensity of the background liver, which will result in the relative hyperintense appearance of HCCs.[60]

Restricted diffusion

Diffusion-weighted imaging (DWI) has been used more frequently in abdominal MR imaging in recent years. Studies have shown that DWI can help differentiate cysts and hemangiomas from solid lesions, but differentiating among different solid lesions such as HCC, focal nodular hyperplasia, and adenoma may be difficult based on apparent diffusion coefficient (ADC) values alone.[62,63] A mass in the cirrhotic liver with restricted diffusion favors a solid lesion, and would be confirmatory for HCC especially when other MRI features of HCC are present (see **Fig. 3**). Conversely, not all HCCs demonstrate restricted diffusion. Eleven of 125 HCCs in a series by Nasu and colleagues[64] demonstrated hypo- to isointense signal on DWI. The absence of restricted diffusion in a hepatic mass that otherwise demonstrates MR imaging features of hepatoma should not sway the diagnosis away from HCC. It should also be noted that the background cirrhotic liver also has restricted diffusion and is reported to demonstrate a reduced ADC relative to nonfibrotic livers.[65] Consequently, identification of restricted diffusion in HCC in the setting of cirrhosis may be more difficult to identify visually than in the setting of a noncirrhotic background liver in our opinion. DWI has been used to monitor response to therapies such as TACE and radioembolization[66–68]; however, utility of DWI to differentiate grades of tumor is not clearly established.[64,69]

Vascular invasion

Vascular invasion is frequently seen in the setting of HCC and has been reported to occur in as many as 6.5% to 48.0% of cases.[43,50,51,70,71] It has been found to be more common in patients with tumors that are larger or of higher grade. Tumor thrombus has also been observed to be more common in the setting of cirrhosis, and a greater incidence has been suggested with alcoholic cirrhosis compared with viral hepatitis.[51] Vascular extension involves the portal venous system more frequently than the hepatic veins.[43,50,51] However, involvement of the hepatic veins predisposes to tumor thrombus extension into the inferior vena cava and right atrium (**Fig. 6**).[43] The distinction between tumor and bland thrombus is critical because of the associated management implications. Malignant tumor thrombus is typically seen in contiguity with or in close proximity to the primary tumor and characteristically expands the involved vessel.[16,28,72] Malignant thrombus usually exhibits similar imaging features as the primary tumor. In contrast to bland thrombus, it may demonstrate T2 hyperintense signal intensity and arterial enhancement with washout, as well as restricted diffusion.[16,27,28,38,71,72] A recent study demonstrated the utility of DWI imaging in differentiating tumor thrombus from bland thrombus based on the

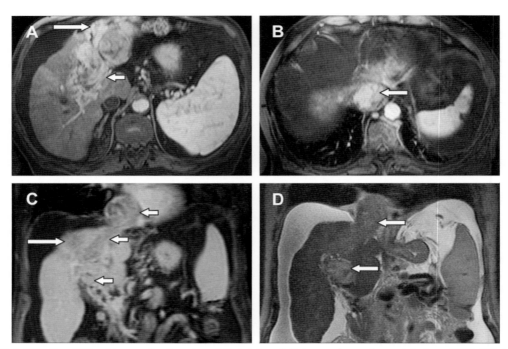

Fig. 6. Infiltrative HCC with vascular invasion. (*A*) Axial gadolinium-enhanced arterial-phase T1FS GRE image shows enhancing thrombus within the portal vein that appears expanded (*short arrow*). The presence of tumor thrombus suggests an underlying mass. Patchy enhancement is seen in the adjacent left hepatic lobe consistent with infiltrative HCC (*long arrow*). (*B*) Axial gadolinium-enhanced arterial-phase T1FS GRE image just cranial to the liver demonstrates enhancing thrombus extending into the right atrium (*arrow*). (*C*) Coronal delayed gadolinium-enhanced T1FS GRE image demonstrates washout of the infiltrative HCC (*long arrow*), as well as tumor thrombus within the portal vein, hepatic vein, and right atrium (*short arrows*). (*D*) Coronal T2W image shows mildly T2 hyperintense signal intensity within the tumor thrombus (*arrows*).

finding that bland thrombus demonstrates a considerably higher ADC value than the underlying HCC as opposed to tumor thrombus, which demonstrates a low ADC similar to the tumor itself.[71] In cases of diffuse or infiltrating HCC, the presence of tumor thrombus may be the only clue to suggest that there is an underlying malignancy, especially if the background parenchyma is very cirrhotic and heterogeneous (see **Fig. 6**). As mentioned previously, it is important to diagnose tumor thrombus, as it is associated with a worse patient prognosis. Patients with tumor thrombus are typically not candidates for surgical resection or transplant. Vascular invasion is one of the contraindications for TACE, as these patients are at higher risk of liver failure and death.[5,6,8] Targeted intra-arterial treatment with Yttrium-90 (Y-90) is associated with fewer complications in patients with portal vein occlusion.[73,74]

Mosaic appearance

HCCs can exhibit a mosaic appearance as manifested by variable unenhanced and contrast-enhanced T1- and T2-weighted signal intensity areas within a single lesion (**Fig. 7**). This appearance has been seen in 28% to 63% of cases and is more common in larger tumors.[51,52,70] Pathologically, the mosaic appearance reflects multiple confluent areas of tumor nodularity interspersed with fibrous septations, necrosis, hemorrhage, copper deposition, and fatty infiltration, as well as varying degrees of histologic differentiation.[16,27,51,52,75] T2-weighted images are more sensitive to the mosaic appearance than T1-weighted images[52]; however, the mosaic appearance may also be evident on contrast-enhanced T1-weighted images, as some higher grade poorly differentiated HCCs may have decreased arterial blood supply,[76] whereas other large atypical well-differentiated HCCs may be characterized by areas of portal perfusion.[77]

Uncommon Features of Hepatocellular Carcinoma

Diffuse infiltrative hepatocellular carcinoma

Diffuse infiltrating HCCs are uncommon with a reported incidence of 13% in one study.[78] The

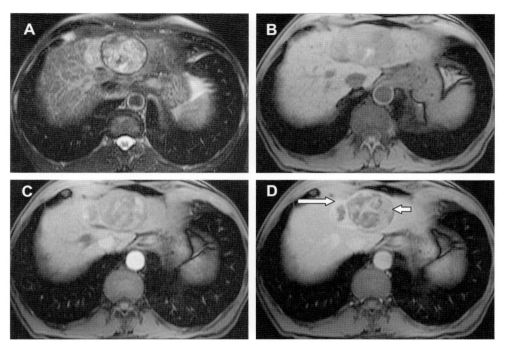

Fig. 7. HCC with mosaic enhancement. (*A*) Axial T2W image shows HCC with heterogeneous signal intensity. (*B*) Axial unenhanced T1FS GRE image also shows heterogeneous signal intensity within the lesion. (*C*) Axial gadolinium-enhanced arterial-phase T1FS GRE image demonstrates a heterogeneous mosaic enhancement pattern within the lesion. (*D*) Axial gadolinium-enhanced delayed phase T1FS GRE image also demonstrates heterogeneous mosaic enhancement pattern. There is washout (*short arrow*) of areas that were avidly enhancing on the arterial phase. Delayed capsular enhancement is also present (*long arrow*).

infiltrating lesions are poorly marginated and demonstrate variable T1- and T2-weighted appearance (usually mild to moderate T1 hypointensity and mild to moderate T2 hyperintensity). Although typically thought of as heterogeneous appearing, diffuse infiltrative HCCs can demonstrate homogeneous signal.[78,79] On gadolinium-enhanced images, diffuse infiltrative HCC may appear hypovascular[79] or demonstrate "patchy or miliary enhancement" on the arterial phase, reflecting enhancement of tumor micronodules within the lesion.[78] On the portal-venous or more delayed postcontrast phases, the lesions may demonstrate heterogeneous reticular or homogeneous hypointensity.[78,79] Tumor thrombus within the portal vein is extremely common in cases of diffuse HCC (see **Fig. 6**).[78,79] Consequently, visualization of tumor thrombus within the portal vein should prompt close examination of the parenchyma for the presence of diffuse infiltrating HCC, as these tumors can be difficult to diagnose because of their heterogeneous appearance, which is similar to the background cirrhotic liver parenchyma. A serologic clue of diffuse or infiltrating HCCs is the commonly associated marked elevation in serum alpha-fetoprotein levels.[78]

Fatty metamorphosis

HCCs may sometimes contain fat.[51,52,80,81] In these cases, the tumors may appear iso-to hyperintense on T1-weighted imaging. HCCs contain intracellular lipid more often than macroscopic fat, which results in loss of signal intensity on the opposed phase GRE T1-weighted images (see **Fig. 4**). Macroscopic fat, on the other hand, would exhibit loss of signal on fat-saturated images and low attenuation on CT images.[80,82] Other processes such as hemorrhage, melanin, and copper or glycoprotein accumulation can also lead to hyperintense T1 signal intensity.[16,21,35,60,61] The presence of fat within a lesion favors a primary HCC. Other hepatic lesions that contain fat include adenomas, rarer tumors such as angiomyolipomas, lipomas, and certain metastases such as those from liposarcomas, teratomas, ovarian dermoids, Wilms tumors, and certain renal cell carcinomas.[80–82] Although fatty components have been described in regenerative nodules[16] and focal nodular hyperplasia, such an observation is rare and possibly related to underlying liver steatosis.[82] In the cirrhotic liver, a fat-containing lesion should raise suspicion for HCC over these other lesions, which are not typically seen in cirrhotic livers.[16] Although a fat-containing HCC may appear otherwise relatively nonspecific on MRI, and may not show the typical arterial-phase hypervascularity or capsular enhancement,[81] all lesions in the cirrhotic liver with signal intensity drop-off on the opposed phase images should be considered suspicious for HCC.

Nodule within nodule appearance

When foci of HCC develop within a preexisting dysplastic nodule, the typical appearance of a high T2 signal intensity nodule within a low T2 signal intensity nodule is termed a "nodule within nodule" appearance.[16,31,83] The appearance on T1-weighted imaging may be of a T1 hypointense HCC within a T1 hyperintense dysplastic nodule.[31] If the focus of HCC develops within a sideriotic nodule, T1-weighted imaging may demonstrate a markedly low signal intensity outer nodule with a relatively isointense or hyperintense to liver central focus of HCC.[83] The internal nodule of HCC will demonstrate typical arterial enhancement, whereas the outer dysplastic nodule will typically remain hypovascular.[16] HCC that occurs within a preneoplastic focus and exhibits such imaging features has been shown to have potential for rapid growth.[84] A different nodule-in-nodule appearance can also be seen on gadolinium-enhanced imaging when necrotic hepatocellular carcinomas contain foci of viable enhancing tumor.[16]

Appearance with Hepatobiliary Contrast Agents

Hepatobiliary contrast agents are taken up by hepatocytes and excreted in the biliary tract.[41] They are useful to evaluate lesion vascularity as well as hepatocellular function within the lesion.[16] Gadobenate dimeglumine (Gd-BOPTA) and gadoxetate disodium (Gd-EOB-DTPA) are the 2 hepatobiliary contrast agents that are approved by the Food and Drug Administration (FDA) in the United States. Approximately 5% of the administered dose of Gd-BOPTA and 50% of the administered dose of Gd-EOB-DTPA are excreted in the bile. On the early postcontrast phase, both are nonspecific extracellular contrast agents, but on the delayed contrast-enhanced phases (40 to 120 minutes for Gd-BOPTA and 10 to 20 minutes for Gd-EOB-DTPA), they are hepatocyte-specific agents.[41,85] Images acquired with a hepatobiliary contrast agent will demonstrate uptake of the agent by normal hepatocytes on delayed postcontrast phases. Although more experience is needed, preliminary studies suggest that well-differentiated HCCs often behave similar to hepatocytes and are isointense or sometimes hyperintense on delayed imaging with a hepatobiliary agent. Poorly differentiated HCCs on the other hand typically do not accumulate the hepatobiliary contrast agent and appear relatively hypointense on the delayed contrast-enhanced images.[41,85] In a recent study on lesion detection with Gd-EOB-DTPA by Sun and colleagues,[86] 42 of 44 HCCs demonstrated low signal intensity on the delayed hepatobiliary phase. This was in contrast to arterial-enhancing pseudolesions, 94% of which were isointense to the liver on the delayed hepatobiliary phase. Although the accumulation of contrast in a lesion does not exclude HCC, if the HCC does accumulate a hepatobiliary contrast agent, it is postulated to be well differentiated.[41,85] The use of hepatobiliary agents poses additional challenges including acquisition of good arterial-enhanced images especially because the current approved dose of Gd-EOB-DTPA in the United States is smaller than other gadolinium-based agents, a relative high cost of the contrast agents, and prolonged scan time. The incremental benefit of hepatocyte-specific agents in the assessment of HCC remains under investigation. In their study correlated with explant liver pathology, Choi and colleagues[87] reported that Gd-BOPTA had a sensitivity of 80% to 85% and a positive predictive value of only 65% to 66% for detection of HCC. Furthermore, Gd-BOPTA had limited value in the detection and characterization of lesions smaller than 1 cm in diameter. Other studies comparing sensitivity of Gd-EOB-DTPA and Gd-BOPTA enhanced MRI to multiphasic multidetector CT (MDCT) suggest that it may improve lesion detection, particularly for small lesions.[88–90]

HCC in the Noncirrhotic Liver

The overall prevalence of HCC in the noncirrhotic liver has been reported to be between 6.7% and 54.0%.[91] Such HCCs are often larger and diagnosed at a later stage, likely related to lack of screening of noncirrhotic individuals. They are more commonly solitary, well circumscribed, and may contain areas of necrosis.[27,38,92,93] Additionally, some of these HCCs may develop from large preexisting hepatic adenomas.[93] Although a major differential consideration is fibrolamellar HCC, conventional HCC in noncirrhotic livers may be distinguished because they rarely contain calcification, fibrosis, or a true central scar, and are more likely to be associated with elevated serum tumor markers than fibrolamellar HCC.[93] In the absence of underlying cirrhosis, biopsy is often required for the diagnosis of HCC, as the imaging features are more nonspecific and the differential diagnosis is broader.

Hemochromatosis and HCC

Hereditary hemochromatosis (HH) is associated with liver disease leading to cirrhosis and HCC. The condition carries a 20- to 200-fold higher risk for development of HCC.[5,7] The 5-year cumulative incidence of HCC in patients with hereditary hemochromatosis is 21%.[7] On abdominal MR imaging, patients with primary hemochromatosis demonstrate iron deposition outside the reticuloendothelial system such as within hepatocytes of the liver and in the pancreas. As a result, the liver and pancreas may be hypointense on T2-weighted images. The dark liver serves as a negative background on which lesions that do not accumulate iron, such as HCC, may be more easily detected as relatively hyperintense foci.[94] However, the relative increased signal intensity of the HCC in hemochromatosis may reduce conspicuity of lesion enhancement after gadolinium (Fig. 8). In this situation, true enhancement can be assessed using region of interest measurements on unenhanced and contrast-enhanced images. Subtraction of the unenhanced images from the postcontrast images may also be helpful in demonstrating enhancement, although enhancement characteristics may not be typical.[94]

Hepatocellular Carcinoma Mimics

Although FNH and adenomas are usually hypervascular on the arterial phase like HCC, they are extremely uncommon in the cirrhotic liver. The entities listed in the following sections are those that may pose a diagnostic challenge in the setting of cirrhosis.

Hemangiomas

Although common in the general population, hemangiomas occur less frequently in the setting of cirrhosis. Preexisting hemangiomas likely undergo obliteration from fibrosis and necrosis.[18] When hemangiomas do occur in the cirrhotic liver, they are commonly solitary.[95] Either related to fibrosis[18,96] or alterations in blood flow,[95] hemangiomas in cirrhotic livers have also been shown to progressively decrease in size and display more atypical imaging characteristics, including loss of the peripheral nodular enhancement.[96] Atypical or sclerosing hemangiomas (Fig. 9) may demonstrate only mild or moderate T2 hyperintensity[21,97] in contrast to typical hemangiomas that exhibit high signal intensity on T2-weighted imaging. Hemangiomas in the cirrhotic patient may also be associated with adjacent capsular

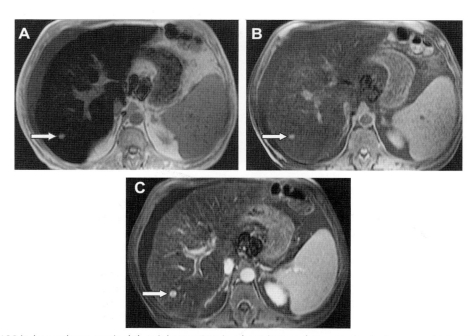

Fig. 8. HCC in hemochromatosis. (A) Axial T1W GRE in-phase image shows markedly low signal intensity within the liver from iron deposition. A small hyperintense lesion is present in the right hepatic lobe (arrow). The lesion was also hyperintense against a background of dark liver on the T2W images (not shown). (B) Axial unenhanced T1FS GRE image again shows the hyperintense lesion (arrow) against a background of dark liver. (C) Axial gadolinium-enhanced T1FS GRE image shows high signal intensity within the lesion (arrow) but enhancement characteristics are difficult to evaluate because of hyperintense signal intensity on the unenhanced images. In the setting of hemochromatosis and cirrhosis, this lesion is suspicious for HCC.

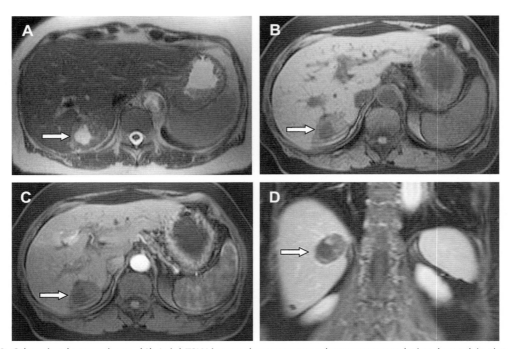

Fig. 9. Sclerosing hemangioma. (*A*) Axial T2W image demonstrates a heterogeneous lesion (*arrow*) in the right hepatic lobe with mild signal hyperintensity peripherally and more high signal intensity centrally. (*B*) Axial unenhanced T1FS GRE image shows the heterogeneous lesion (*arrow*) has low signal intensity centrally. (*C*) Axial gadolinium-enhanced arterial-phase T1FS GRE image demonstrates minimal to no enhancement in the lesion (*arrow*). (*D*) Coronal delayed gadolinium-enhanced T1FS GRE image demonstrates minimal "bright dots" (*arrow*) of enhancement within the lesion. There is no appreciable enhancement centrally. The imaging features of heterogeneous T1- and T2-weighted signal intensity and minimal enhancement are nonspecific and can be seen with atypical hemangiomas or hypovascular mosaic HCC. Core biopsy demonstrated hyalinized tissue consistent with sclerosing hemangioma.

retraction,[96,98,99] although this appearance is more commonly seen with peripheral cholangiocarcinoma, epithelioid hemangioendothelioma, metastasis, or confluent fibrosis.[98,99] Small flash-filling hemangiomas may simulate HCC, as they demonstrate early homogeneous arterial-phase enhancement.[35,95,100,101] Persistent enhancement on delayed images rather than washout is suggestive of hemangioma; however, these may be associated with minimal central enhancement.[101,102] HCC should be considered more likely than hemangioma in cirrhosis if the nodular area of enhancement demonstrates washout, and may be confirmed by evidence of interval growth on a 2- to 3-month follow-up scan. Peliotic change within HCC is rare but may lead to misdiagnosis as hemangioma. Peliotic HCC contains multiple blood-filled sinusoids, which may result in T2-hyperintensity and persistent peripheral enhancement that progresses centrally.[52,103] The potential for overlapping MR imaging features of hemangiomas and HCC may necessitate a tissue diagnosis or follow-up imaging. Prior imaging

(predevelopment of cirrhosis) showing more typical hemangioma features and stability or sclerosis of the lesion over time facilitates diagnosis. Alternatively, if an indeterminate lesion demonstrates interval increase in size in a cirrhotic liver, HCC should be suspected (**Fig. 10**).

Regenerative nodules

As discussed earlier, regenerative nodules are generally small and hypovascular following contrast administration. However, in the setting of Budd-Chiari syndrome with cirrhosis, regenerative nodules can have features suggestive of HCC, including a size larger than 2 cm, increased T2 signal intensity, and arterial-phase enhancement.[12,22,104] Such hypervascular regenerative nodules have also been shown to have a central scar.[104] On portal venous phase of enhancement, the appearance may be variable (hypointense or hyperintense signal). A hypointense regenerative nodule rim has also been reported in patients with Budd-Chiari.[12] The incidence of HCC in patients with Budd-Chiari is variable, ranging

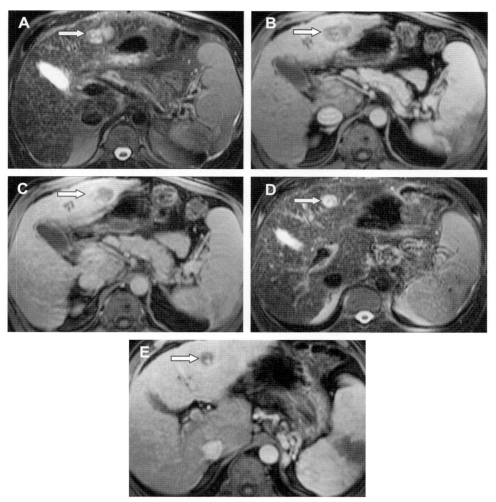

Fig. 10. HCC mimicking hemangioma. (*A*) Axial T2FS image shows a mild to moderate T2 hyperintense lesion (*arrow*) in a cirrhotic liver. (*B*) Axial gadolinium-enhanced arterial-phase T1FS GRE image shows mild enhancement (*arrow*). (*C*) Axial gadolinium-enhanced delayed T1FS GRE image shows filling in of the lesion (*arrow*), a finding that can be seen with hemangioma. (*D*) Axial T2FS image 3 months prior shows a hyperintense lesion mimicking hemangioma (*arrow*) that was smaller than on the current study. (*E*) Axial gadolinium-enhanced arterial T1FS GRE image 3 months prior also shows that the lesion was smaller, but demonstrated only minimal peripheral enhancement (*arrow*). Based on the interval growth, a biopsy was recommended for suspected HCC. Results of the tissue sampling were consistent with HCC.

from 6.4% in a Japanese study to 48.0% in a population from South Africa.[12] Vilgrain and colleagues[12] suggest that although HCC and regenerative nodules may be difficult to distinguish based on imaging characteristics in the setting of Budd-Chiari, the presence of more than 10 nodules measuring up to 4 cm in diameter should favor the diagnosis of regenerative nodules.

Arterially enhancing regenerative nodules have also been demonstrated by Qayyum and colleagues[23] on multiphase CT in patients with autoimmune hepatitis without superimposed viral infection. Some of these lesions demonstrated enhancement also on portal-venous phase imaging, whereas others demonstrated washout on the portal-venous images similar to HCC. Bilaj and colleagues[105] also demonstrated hypervascular nodules on MRI in 22% of their study population of patients with autoimmune hepatitis, although they suggest these represented dysplastic nodules. They also described a separate population of regenerative nodules that although large (>2 cm), demonstrated more typical imaging features of regenerative nodules in that they were isointense to the liver on T1- and T2-weighted images and showed similar enhancement pattern to the surrounding liver. Although regenerative nodules in autoimmune hepatitis may mimic hepatocellular carcinoma, none of the lesions shown by Qayyum and colleagues[23] showed a persistent hyperdense rim that is more typical of HCC and such delayed capsular enhancement can possibly be used as a distinguishing feature to suggest HCC. Furthermore, autoimmune hepatitis without superimposed viral infection has been shown to have a relatively low incidence of hepatocellular carcinoma.[10]

Confluent hepatic fibrosis

Confluent hepatic fibrosis is typically seen in the setting of advanced cirrhosis,[28] most commonly in cases secondary to primary sclerosing cholangitis (PSC).[18] Hepatic fibrosis usually demonstrates high T2-weighted and low T1-weighted signal intensity.[18,35,106] Although it typically exhibits delayed enhancement,[18,99,106] hepatic fibrosis can occasionally enhance in the arterial phase.[107] Hepatic fibrosis may present as a confluent mass,[18,35] or may be poorly marginated, mimicking infiltrating HCC.[34] A differentiating feature is that hepatic fibrosis is generally wedge-shaped, has linear margins, and is typically seen in the anterior segment of the right lobe and medial segment of the left lobe (segments 8 and 4). It characteristically demonstrates volume loss with focal capsular retraction of the adjacent liver surface,[18,35,99,106] unlike hepatocellular carcinoma, which generally has mass effect and often expands the contour. In troublesome cases where confluent masslike fibrosis simulates a neoplasm, biopsy may be necessary for differentiation.[18] Because hepatic fibrosis and cholangiocarcinoma share features such as delayed or persistent enhancement, associated capsular retraction, and common occurrence in patients with PSC, these two entities may also be confused. However, the characteristic location and geographic morphology[18,35,99,106] in conjunction with the absence of biliary duct dilation may help to distinguish confluent fibrosis from cholangiocarcinoma in cirrhosis.[99]

Intrahepatic cholangiocarcinoma

Intrahepatic cholangiocarcinoma (IHC) may sometimes be difficult to distinguish from HCC, particularly diffuse infiltrating HCC. Although there is overlap of imaging features, IHC is more likely to appear as a discrete mass than diffuse infiltrating HCC. IHCs typically demonstrate heterogeneous T2-weighted signal intensity and may contain areas of strong hyperintense or even areas of hypointense signal intensity. In contrast, HCC reportedly demonstrates more homogeneous and less hyperintense T2-weighted signal.[79] Contrast enhancement characteristics may provide the strongest differentiation between the two entities. IHCs usually exhibit thick irregular peripheral enhancement with progressive central enhancement on more delayed images (**Fig. 11**), which is a pattern that is rarely seen in HCC.[70,79] The persistent enhancement seen with IHC is generally a function of the fibrotic nature of the tumor. Unlike hemangiomas, the peripheral enhancement of IHCs is not nodular or cloudlike and is not similar to the blood pool enhancement. There may be associated peripheral biliary ductal dilatation secondary to mass effect from the IHCs. Although biliary ductal dilatation is not commonly associated with HCCs, if present, it may be mild and may actually be intratumoral. The pattern of vascular involvement also differs between the two tumors. IHCs are more likely to encase and compress the portal vein rather than directly invade it or result in tumor thrombus, a finding seen very commonly with diffuse infiltrating HCC.[79] History of PSC or other cholangitides should also raise suspicion for IHC over HCC. Finally, IHC is more commonly associated with volume loss and capsular retraction than HCC.[99] Rare tumors can have a mixed histology, demonstrating features of both HCC and cholangiocarcinoma.[70] Although delayed enhancement and associated capsular retraction are common features of both IHC and confluent hepatic fibrosis, IHC should be suspected in the case of a mass with bulging margins rather than the straight wedge-shaped morphology of hepatic fibrosis with linear margins,[18,35,99,106] as mentioned earlier. Furthermore, biliary ductal dilatation, although seen in the peripheral liver secondary to mass effect from IHC, is rarely seen in hepatic fibrosis.

Transient hepatic intensity differences

Transient hepatic intensity differences (THIDs) are a common finding seen in the cirrhotic liver on arterial-phase MR images. They are the MR equivalent to CT transient hepatic attenuation differences (THADs).[108] They are typically seen as well-defined areas of enhancement only on the arterial phase and not on other phases. Although not usually seen on the T2-weighted images, they can occasionally have a corresponding area of hyperintensity on the T2-weighted images when intense.[108] THIDs are usually triangular or fan-shaped, peripherally located, and have straight margins. They may follow the segmental anatomy of the liver. THIDs

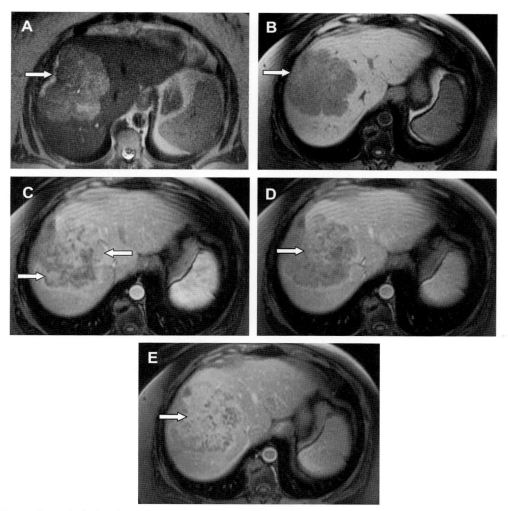

Fig. 11. Intrahepatic cholangiocarcinoma. (*A*) Axial T2W image demonstrates a large mass with adjacent capsular retraction (*arrow*) favoring cholangiocarcinoma over HCC. There are areas of variable T2 hyperintensity within the mass. (*B*) Axial unenhanced T1FS GRE image demonstrates the mass (*arrow*) to be hypointense to the surrounding liver. (*C*) Axial gadolinium-enhanced arterial-phase T1FS GRE image demonstrates thick irregular peripheral enhancement within the lesion (*arrows*). (*D*) Axial gadolinium-enhanced portal-venous phase T1FS GRE image demonstrates increased central enhancement within the lesion (*arrow*). (*E*) Axial gadolinium-enhanced delayed venous phase T1FS GRE image demonstrates persistent central enhancement (*arrow*) rather than washout within the lesion. Findings are consistent with cholangiocarcinoma.

may be caused by underlying focal lesions because of a siphoning or sump effect of the lesion, from portal hypoperfusion either attributable to compression or thrombosis from the lesion, or because of arterioportal shunting related to the lesion causing diversion of flow.[108] THIDs can also be induced by portal hypoperfusion attributable to nontumoral causes, anomalous blood supply, or arterioportal shunting not related to focal lesions, and inflammation of biliary vessels or adjacent organs.[109]

Occasionally these arterial phenomena can appear round and mimic a hypervascular lesion; however, unlike most hepatocellular carcinomas, THIDs characteristically do not have corresponding T1 and T2 signal abnormality, do not demonstrate delayed postcontrast washout, do take up hepatobiliary contrast on the delayed hepatocyte phase, and may have normal vessels coursing through them.[109,110] The waxing and waning of the size of a hypervascular lesion in cirrhosis at 2- to 3-month follow-up imaging also favors a THID or pseudolesion. Because HCC is the most common primary hepatic tumor associated with a THID,[110] even when an arterially enhancing focus is deemed to be a THID, in the setting of cirrhosis, the radiologist should look closely for an associated HCC.

ENHANCING LESIONS SEEN ONLY ON THE HEPATIC ARTERIAL PHASE ON MR IMAGING

Enhancing lesions seen only on the hepatic arterial phase on MR imaging are a daily challenge. These are generally small lesions that are not seen on T1- and T2-weighted images or other phases. Although small HCCs smaller than or equal to 1.5 cm in size are frequently isointense on T1- and T2-weighted sequences and may only be seen as diffuse homogeneously enhancing lesions on the arterial enhanced phase,[43] it is important to not consider such arterially enhancing lesions as specific for hepatocellular carcinoma. In a study by Holland and colleagues[111] of 16 patients with explanted liver, correlation of the 45 hepatic arterial-phase–enhancing ("HAPE")-only lesions seen, 93% were benign; there were only 3 (7%) "neoplastic" lesions: 1 HCC, 1 HCC within a dysplastic nodule, and 1 high-grade dysplastic nodule. Most of the lesions had no correlative pathology. Of note, all 3 "neoplastic" lesions were seen in patients with concomitant hepatocellular carcinoma. All 3 neoplastic HAPE-only lesions in this study were oval in shape.[111] Using size and interval growth on follow-up imaging as a predictor of malignancy, another study also found a higher percentage of arterial-enhancing lesions were suspicious in patients with HCC (32.5%) versus in patients without HCC (5%).[112] In a published study by Shimizu and colleagues[113] of 158 small (<2 cm) early-enhancing hepatic lesions, 31 (20%) were suspicious for HCC based on pathology or interval growth on follow-up imaging. Of these 31, 29 were round or oval; however, 75 other round or oval lesions were not suspicious for HCC.[113] This study and additional investigators[111] suggest that although a round or oval lesion may have more likelihood of being neoplastic than a wedge-shaped, geographic, or triangular lesion, round or oval lesions as a group are still more likely to not be neoplastic. Additionally, of the 31 suspicious lesions seen by Shimizu and colleagues,[113] 17 (55%) were not visible on T2-weighted images and 15 (48%) were not visible on delayed postcontrast images. Another study, by Jeong and colleagues,[114] showed 13% of such arterially enhancing lesions without T2 hyperintensity to represent hepatocellular carcinoma. In contrast to these prior reports where the incidence of a non–T2-hyperintense arterial-enhancing lesion being suspicious for HCC ranged from 7% to 20%,[111–114] a recent study of patients with mild cirrhosis and hepatitis B[115] showed 44 (67%) of 66 lesions seen only on the arterial phase to be suspicious for HCC based on pathology, imaging findings, or elevated serum alpha-fetoprotein (AFP). The investigators point out that this contradiction to prior reports may be related to selection bias in the study population because most of the patients had multiphasic MDCT before the MRI and those with definitively benign lesions on MDCT, such as classic arterioportal shunts, were not included in the study. Additionally, the study population had only mild cirrhosis in which arterioportal shunts may be less common than in more severe cirrhosis. Finally, the investigators also attribute the contradiction to different underlying etiologies for the cirrhosis in their patient population (hepatitis B) versus that of the prior studies (hepatitis C).[115]

Yu and colleagues[42] found that 55 of 152 newly diagnosed HCCs showed a focal abnormality on retrospective analysis of the prior study. The most common abnormality was homogeneous arterial-phase enhancement, which was seen in 33 patients. However, this pre-HCC homogeneous arterial enhancement could not be differentiated from small noncancerous arterioportal shunting. Furthermore, lesions with this finding on retrospective review had the shortest doubling time. Our approach to hepatic lesions seen on the arterial phase is to check the other phases and sequences to confirm that they are only seen on the hepatic arterial phase and do not have other features of hepatocellular carcinoma such as washout, capsular enhancement, restricted diffusion, loss of signal intensity on opposed phase images suggesting microscopic fat, or increased signal intensity on T2-weighted images. When the abnormality is peripheral, wedge-shaped, and seen only on the hepatic arterial phase, it is more likely to represent a perfusional phenomenon. Identification of a supplying and draining vessel is suggestive of a vascular shunt. However, if the abnormality is round, oval, or masslike in shape, but small (<2 cm), and seen only on the arterial phase without other features of hepatocellular carcinoma, close interval follow-up MR examination (3 to 6 months) may be considered to assess for growth or features more suggestive of HCC on follow-up examination. Other investigators have recommended similar approaches.[28] Besides shunts and perfusional abnormalities, hemangiomas and high-grade dysplasias are differential consideration for small arterial-phase–enhancing foci.[109,110,114]

HCC TREATMENT

Treatment of HCC is based on multiple factors, including burden of liver disease, tumor stage, and performance status to name a few. The Barcelona Clinic Liver Cancer (BCLC) staging system takes into account these factors and is considered the most accurate predictive system for making therapeutic decisions in patients with HCC.[6,8]

The treatment of choice in noncirrhotic patients is resection[5,6,8]; however, noncirrhotic patients account for only about 5% of patients with HCC in Western countries and about 40% of patients with HCC in Asia, except Japan.[6,8] Applicability of strict selection criteria for resection among cirrhotic patients yields a resectability rate of 5% to 10%.[6] Liver resection has limitations in patients with cirrhosis as the liver lacks functional reserve. In contrast to normal liver, the cirrhotic liver does not regenerate as well following resection. In addition, the residual cirrhotic liver remains at risk for hepatocellular carcinoma. Tumor recurrence rates exceed 70% at 5 years after resection.[5,6,8] The AASLD practice guidelines recommend surgical resection in patients with a single lesion if they are noncirrhotic patients or if they are cirrhotic patients with well-preserved liver function.[8]

For unresectable cases of HCC, liver transplantation has emerged as a viable option. In addition to potentially curing the malignancy, it ameliorates the underlying chronic liver disease.[6] Patients with up to 3 lesions, each 3 cm or smaller, or a single lesion 5 cm or smaller had a 75% 5-year survival rate for transplantation based on the Milan criteria.[116] University of California San Francisco showed similar survival rates in patients with 1 lesion measuring 6.5 cm or smaller or up to 3 lesions, each 4.5 cm or smaller (with a total tumor diameter of 8 cm or smaller).[117] Although these expanded criteria have been validated in subsequent studies,[118] other analyses of expanded criteria have had mixed results[119,120] and the AASLD guidelines do not make a recommendation regarding the expansion of criteria beyond the Milan criteria.[8]

Treatment options for patients who are not candidates for either resection or transplantation include localized therapies such as cryoablation, percutaneous ethanol ablation (PEA), radiofrequency ablation (RFA), microwave ablation, or

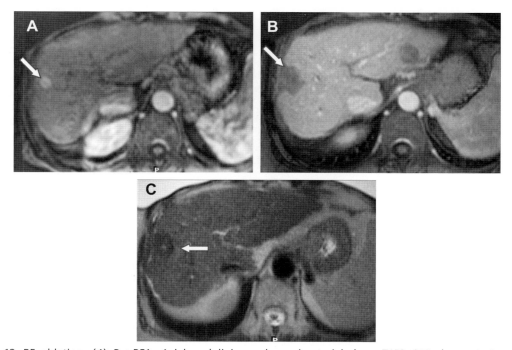

Fig. 12. RF ablation. (*A*) Pre-RFA: Axial gadolinium-enhanced arterial-phase T1FS GRE demonstrates solid enhancing lesion (*arrow*) that washed out on the delayed phase (not shown). (*B*) Post-RFA: Axial gadolinium-enhanced T1FS GRE arterial-phase image demonstrates a nonenhancing ablation cavity (*arrow*) that is larger than the original pre-RFA lesion. (*C*) Post-RFA: Axial T2W image demonstrates a T2 hypointense ablation cavity that is larger than the original pre-RFA lesion. There may be mild surrounding increased T2 signal intensity representing reactive change in the adjacent parenchyma (*arrow*).

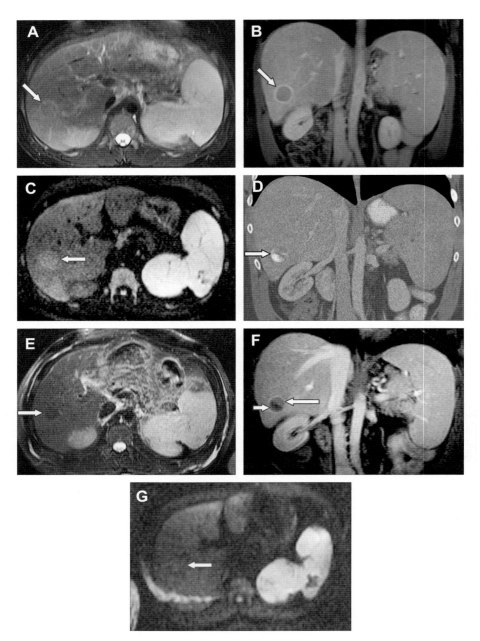

Fig. 13. TACE. (*A*) Pre-TACE: Axial T2FS image demonstrates a centrally isointense HCC in the right hepatic lobe (*arrow*). (*B*) Pre-TACE: Coronal gadolinium-enhanced delayed T1FS GRE image demonstrates the lesion to have capsular enhancement (*arrow*). The central portion of the tumor is enhancing, but has washed out relative to the surrounding normal hepatic parenchyma as expected of HCC. (*C*) Pre-TACE: Axial DWI (b1000) demonstrates restricted diffusion within the lesion (*arrow*) that was confirmed on the ADC map (not shown). (*D*) Post-TACE: Coronal reformatted contrast-enhanced CT image demonstrates increased density within the lesion (*arrow*) that could correspond to either lipiodol accumulation or enhancement. (*E*) Post-TACE: Axial T2FS image demonstrates hypointense signal intensity within the lesion (*arrow*) relative to the pre-TACE appearance. The lesion also appears smaller. (*F*) Post-TACE: Coronal enhanced delayed phase T1FS GRE image demonstrates necrosis within the more caudal portion of the lesion (*short arrow*), but there is some residual enhancement along the cranial and medial aspect of the lesion (*long arrow*). (*G*) Post-TACE: Axial DWI (b1000) shows no evidence of restriction within the caudal portion of the lesion corresponding to necrosis on the delayed enhanced T1FS image.

intravascular therapies such as TACE or radioem-bolization with Y-90 microspheres. Although some of these options serve as definite therapy, others are used to downstage patients before definitive therapies. The AASLD recommends local ablation with alcohol or RFA in unresectable cases or as a bridge to transplantation, noting that RFA may be more efficacious in larger lesions (>2 cm), and although equally efficacious in smaller lesions (<2 cm), may require fewer treatment sessions. TACE is recommended by the AASLD as first-line noncurative therapy for patients who are not surgical or ablative candidates and have large or multifocal HCC without vascular invasion or extra-hepatic spread. Contraindications to TACE include advanced liver disease and portal vein thrombosis, especially lobar or segmental, as this puts the patient at risk for necrosis and liver failure.[5,6,8] Ra-dioembolization with Y-90 reportedly has fewer complications compared with TACE and has been safely performed in patients with portal vein occlusion.[73,74] External beam radiotherapy has been used in patients who are not candidates for

other localized therapies. Although systemic chemotherapy does not currently play a major role in treatment of HCC, trials with targeted molecular therapy with sorafenib have shown some positive results.[6]

IMAGING OF TREATED HCC

Localized therapies include but are not limited to RFA, cryoablation, PEA, TACE, and Y-90 micro-spheres. Knowledge of posttreatment appearance of HCC is imperative to assess response, which can often be challenging.

Although uneven coagulation necrosis and thermal injury may yield heterogeneous T1- and T2-weighted signal intensity within lesions treated with RFA,[121] other investigators report homoge-neous low T2-weighted and high T1-weighted signal intensity associated with the necrosis and hemorrhagic or proteinaceous material.[122,123] The hyperintense T1-weighted signal intensity can persist for months or years.[28] It may also be normal to see a high signal intensity peripheral

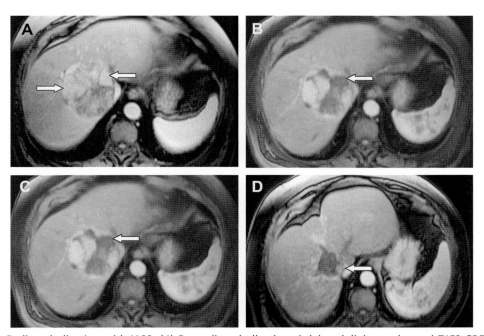

Fig. 14. Radioembolization with Y-90. (*A*) Pre-radioembolization: Axial gadolinium-enhanced T1FS GRE image demonstrates a large HCC with areas of arterial enhancement (*arrows*). The lesion measured approximately 10 cm, precluding liver transplantation. (*B*) At 1.5 months after radioembolization, axial gadolinium-enhanced T1FS GRE image demonstrates decrease in size of lesion as well as increased necrosis within the lesion (*arrow*). There are some persistent areas of enhancement medially and laterally. (*C*) At 7 months after radioembolization, axial gadolinium-enhanced T1FS GRE image demonstrates further decrease in size of lesion and resolution of enhancement seen within the lateral aspect of the lesion on the initial follow-up, but with persistent focal enhancement along the medial aspect (*arrow*). (*D*) At 4 months after retreatment with bland embolization, axial gadolinium-enhanced T1FS GRE image demonstrates further decrease in size of lesion, and decrease in size of nodular enhancement along the medial aspect (*arrow*). The patient was eventually treated with liver transplan-tation. Pathology of the explanted liver showed focus of hepatocellular carcinoma associated with necrosis.

Table 2
Imaging characteristics of lesions in the cirrhotic liver

	T2-weighted	Unenhanced T1-weighted	In/Opposed Phase	Enhanced T1-weighted- Arterial Phase	Enhanced T1-weighted- PV/Delayed Phases	Other Distinguishing Feature
Regenerative nodule	Hypo- to isointense; rarely hyperintense in setting of infarction or Budd-Chiari	Variable; may be hypointense especially if siderotic	When siderotic, more hypointense on in-phase images	Typically isointense; may be hyperintense in setting of Budd-Chiari or autoimmune hepatitis	Typically isointense; may be hyperintense or hypointense in setting of Budd-Chiari or autoimmune hepatitis	Have rarely been reported to contain fat
Dysplastic nodule	Typically hypointense; may be isointense	Typically hyperintense, may be isointense or hypointense if siderotic	When siderotic, more hypointense on in-phase images	Isointense; sometimes hyperintense when higher grade	Typically isointense	Usually lack enhancing capsule/pseudocapsule
Hepatocellular carcinoma	Typically mild-moderately hyperintense; less commonly isointense or hypointense	Typically hypointense; less commonly hyperintense	May drop signal on opposed phase imaging when contain intracellular lipid or fat	Typically hyperintense; rarely isointense	Typically hypointense (washout); rarely remain hyper- or isointense; may see progressive central enhancement if peliotic change	Enhancing capsule/pseudocapsule; restricted diffusion; vascular invasion; unless well differentiated, will not accumulate hepatobiliary agent
Hemangioma (in setting of cirrhosis)	Mild to moderately hyperintense	Typically hypointense	Typically hypointense	Peripheral nodular hyperintensity that follows blood-pool; homogeneously hyperintense if flash-filling, but similar to blood-pool	Progressive centripetal hyperintensity; although in cirrhosis centrally sclerosed and may show only persistent peripheral hyperintensity	More commonly solitary; may remain stable or sclerose and decrease in size over time; rarely associated with capsular retraction

Focal hepatic fibrosis	Mildly hyperintense	Iso- to hypointense	Iso- to hypointense	Typically isointense, but rarely can be hyperintense	Typically progressive hyperintensity on delayed phases	Typical straight margins, wedge shape, location in segments 4 and 8; volume loss, capsular retraction, lack of mass effect or biliary dilatation
Intrahepatic cholangio carcinoma	Heterogeneously hyper- or hypointense	Typically hypointense	Typically hypointense	May be isointense or may demonstrate thick irregular peripheral hyperintensity that is not similar to blood-pool	Progressive or persistent hyperintensity, especially centrally	Masslike with bulging margins, associated capsular retraction, biliary dilatation, vascular compression rather than invasion/direct extension; associated with primary sclerosing cholangitis or other cholangitides
Transient hepatic intensity differences	Typically isointense; rarely hyperintense	Typically isointense	Typically isointense	Hyperintense but typically triangular shaped with straight margins, peripherally located; rarely round and mimic true lesion	Typically isointense and do not wash out; isointense on hepatobiliary phase	May wax and wane in size on follow-up, may follow segmental anatomy, may have normal vessels coursing through; must look for underlying focal lesion or vascular abnormality

Abbreviation: PV, portal vein.

rim on the T2-weighted images representing reactive change.[121] Marked T2 signal intensity may sometimes be present suggesting biloma formation or liquefactive necrosis. This is different from the less intense moderate irregular nodular focus of T2 signal intensity typically seen that would suggest tumor recurrence.[122,123] A recent study suggested that ablation should be considered incomplete when tumor is seen outside a central hyperintense zone on unenhanced T1-weighted images obtained 2 days after RFA.[124] On contrast-enhanced imaging, complete treatment response is suggested by lack of enhancement within the ablative cavity (**Fig. 12**).[121] Although focal irregular nodular enhancement at the margin of the lesion may suggest residual or recurrent tumor,[121] this must be distinguished from inflammatory reaction in tissue surrounding the lesion, which appears as a thin rim of enhancement[121,122] and can persist for several months.[28] Local tumor regrowth has been shown to typically occur at the periphery of the ablated focus as irregular thickening or may also occur adjacent to large vessels, both areas of relatively low heat accumulation potentially lacking response to therapy.[122] Wedge-shaped areas of enhancement on the arterial phase may also be seen adjacent to the treated areas and likely represent peripheral arterioportal shunts. These should also be distinguished from true tumor enhancement.[121,122] Although size of the ablation cavity should normally be larger than the actual lesion initially (see **Fig. 12**), it should also be monitored and should eventually start to regress in size.[28] Optimal time interval for initial follow-up after therapy imaging varies from 1 to 3 months with subsequent follow-up studies every 3 months.[124]

Treatment of HCC via TACE involves selective embolization with chemotherapeutic agents mixed with lipiodol. The lipiodol is radiodense on CT and its distribution indicates foci of uptake within the tumor. The radiodense lipiodol can, however, make assessment of contrast enhancement within the treated lesion difficult on CT (**Fig. 13**).[125] Lipiodol can also cause transient T1-hyperintense signal intensity within the tumor within the first 3 months after therapy.[126] Similar to other investigators,[28] we have observed loss of signal intensity on the opposed phase images in areas of lipiodol. Findings of good therapeutic response include increased T1-weighted signal intensity, decreased T2-weighted signal intensity, and negligible enhancement in the lesion on immediate gadolinium-enhanced images (see **Fig. 13**).[127] Although dynamic contrast-enhanced MRI is more accurate in predicting treatment response based on lesion enhancement,[125,128] this

evaluation is difficult in lesions that exhibit high unenhanced T1-weighted signal intensity.[128] The presence of necrosis even without decrease in size of the lesion is a good predictor of positive response. The limitations of tumor size in this regard have been reinforced subsequently. In a study by Kamel and colleagues,[66] 38 lesions treated with TACE did not respond based on size criteria, however demonstrated significant reduction in tumor enhancement and significant increase in ADC values. Diffusion-weighted imaging is another tool that can be used to predict response in patients after embolization. A significant increase in the ADC value of the treated lesions may be seen secondary to necrosis, which leads to decreased diffusion restriction of water molecules and may precede response based on size criteria.[66] At our institution, we typically perform an unenhanced CT scan on the day of therapy to check for distribution of lipiodol within the lesion. Posttreatment follow-up MRI is performed at 1 month, and then every 3 to 6 months thereafter.

Another form of transarterial embolization technique that has been developed recently is radioembolization with Y-90, a pure beta emitter that imparts local radiotherapeutic effect to the tumor. Follow-up imaging after treatment is usually performed 1 to 2 months after the procedure and every 3 months thereafter.[129] Although size has been used to assess response, as with other solid tumors using criteria from the World Health Organization (WHO) and Response Evaluation Criteria in Solid Tumors (RECIST),[13,130,131] Keppke and colleagues[13] have shown that evaluation of necrosis in combination with the RECIST criteria adds accuracy and allows for earlier assessment of response to Y-90 therapy. Although necrosis was defined as lack of enhancing tissue, thin peripheral rim enhancement only rarely suggested tumor progression[13] and has been shown to have a 93% positive predictive value for favorable response.[132] Of note, in contrast to lesions treated with RFA, tumors treated with Y-90 that show nodular enhancement after therapy do not always metastasize or grow. These nodular areas may actually represent delayed response within treated tumor or posttreatment change. When they represent delayed response, the lesions may eventually necrose and not enhance on subsequent follow-up imaging.[13] When persistent or progressive in size, these areas of enhancement may represent residual or recurrent tumor (**Fig. 14**). Similar to its utility in imaging of post-TACE lesions, functional MR imaging with DWI has been suggested as an additional tool that may be able to assess tumor response earlier based on decreased diffusion restriction of water molecules secondary to necrosis.[67,68] Increased ADC values 1 month after therapy suggesting response to therapy have been shown to precede decreased size of lesions on follow-up anatomic imaging.[67,68]

SUMMARY

When evaluating the cirrhotic liver for the presence of HCC with MRI, high field magnets with optimal imaging techniques are required. Breath-hold techniques and fat suppression are critical to eliminate artifacts from respiration and motion. The most important sequence to evaluate is the hepatic arterial phase, and hypervascular lesions on the arterial phase need to be evaluated closely to determine if they are hepatocellular carcinoma. On more delayed phases, these lesions should be closely evaluated for washout. Features that are highly suggestive for HCC include arterial hyperenhancement, washout on more delayed images, increased signal intensity on T2-weighted images, restricted diffusion, and tumor thrombus. Atypical features may be seen and not all of these features may be present. Knowledge of imaging appearance of treated HCC is important to assess treatment response and evaluation should be based not only on size, but also enhancement pattern, as well as presence or absence of restricted diffusion. A summary of typical imaging features of HCC and that of lesions that can mimic HCC in the cirrhotic liver are provided in **Table 2**.

REFERENCES

1. El-Serag HB, Rudolph KL. Hepatocellular carcinoma: epidemiology and molecular carcinogenesis. Gastroenterology 2007;132(7):2557–76.
2. Parkin DM, Bray F, Ferlay J, et al. Global cancer statistics, 2002. CA Cancer J Clin 2005;55(2): 74–108.
3. Altekruse SF, McGlynn KA, Reichman ME. Hepatocellular carcinoma incidence, mortality, and survival trends in the United States from 1975 to 2005. J Clin Oncol 2009;27:1485–91.
4. Seeff LB. Introduction: the burden of hepatocellular carcinoma. Gastroenterology 2004;127(5 Suppl 1): S1–4.
5. Ahn J, Flamm SL. Hepatocellular carcinoma. Dis Mon 2004;50:556–73.
6. Mendizabal M, Reddy KR. Current management of hepatocellular carcinoma. Med Clin North Am 2009;93:885–900.
7. Fattovich G, Stroffolini T, Zagni I, et al. Hepatocellular carcinoma in cirrhosis: incidence and risk factors. Gastroenterology 2004;127:S35–50.
8. Bruix J, Sherman M. Management of hepatocellular carcinoma. Hepatology 2005;42:1208–36.
9. Teufel A, Weinmann A, Centner A, et al. Hepatocellular carcinoma in patients with autoimmune hepatitis. World J Gastroenterol 2009;15:578–82.
10. Park SZ, Nagorney DM, Czaja AJ. Hepatocellular carcinoma in autoimmune hepatitis. Dig Dis Sci 2000;45:1944–8.
11. Yeoman AD, Al-Chalabi T, Karani JB, et al. Evaluation of risk factors in the development of hepatocellular carcinoma in autoimmune hepatitis: implications for follow-up and screening. Hepatology 2008;48:863–70.
12. Vilgrain V, Lewin M, Vons C, et al. Hepatic nodules in Budd-Chiari syndrome: imaging features. Radiology 1999;210:443–50.
13. Keppke AL, Salem R, Reddy D, et al. Imaging of hepatocellular carcinoma after treatment with yttrium-90 microspheres. Am J Roentgenol 2007; 188:768–75.
14. Yuen MF, Cheng CC, Lauder IJ, et al. Early detection of hepatocellular carcinoma increases the chance of treatment: Hong Kong experience. Hepatology 2000;31:330–5.
15. Zhang BH, Yang BH, Tang ZY. Randomized controlled trial of screening for hepatocellular carcinoma. J Cancer Res Clin Oncol 2004;130(7): 417–22.
16. Hanna RF, Aguirre DA, Kased N, et al. Cirrhosis-associated hepatocellular nodules: correlation of histopathologic and MR imaging features. Radiographics 2008;28:747–69.
17. Terminology of nodular hepatocellular lesions. International working party. Hepatology 1995; 22(3):983–93.
18. Dodd GD III, Baron RL, Oliver JH III, et al. Spectrum of imaging findings of the liver in end-stage cirrhosis: part II, focal abnormalities. Am J Roentgenol 1999;173:1185–92.
19. Brown J, Naylor MJ, Yagan N. Imaging of hepatic cirrhosis. Radiology 1997;202(1):1–16.
20. Krinsky GA, Lee VS. MR imaging of cirrhotic nodules. Abdom Imaging 2000;25(5):471–82.
21. Krinsky GA, Lee VS, Theise ND. Focal lesions in the cirrhotic liver: high resolution ex vivo MRI with pathologic correlation. J Comput Assist Tomogr 2000; 24:189–96.
22. Brancatelli G, Federle MP, Grazioli L, et al. Large regenerative nodules in Budd-Chiari syndrome and other vascular disorders of the liver: CT and MR imaging findings with clinicopathologic correlation. Am J Roentgenol 2002;178:877–83.
23. Qayyum A, Graser A, Westphalen A, et al. CT of benign hypervascular liver nodules in autoimmune hepatitis. Am J Roentgenol 2004;183:1573–6.
24. Roncalli M, Roz E, Coggi G, et al. The vascular profile of regenerative and dysplastic nodules of

the cirrhotic liver: implications for diagnosis and classification. Hepatology 1999;30(5):1174–8.

25. Krinsky GA, Israel G. Nondysplastic nodules that are hyperintense on T1-weighted gradient-echo MR imaging: frequency in cirrhotic patients undergoing transplantation. Am J Roentgenol 2003;180: 1023–7.

26. Matsui O, Kadoya M, Kameyama T, et al. Benign and malignant nodules in cirrhotic livers: distinction based on blood supply. Radiology 1991;178(2): 493–7.

27. Hussain SM, Zondervan Pe I, Jzermans JN, et al. Benign versus malignant hepatic nodules: MR imaging findings with pathologic correlation. Radiographics 2005;22:1023–36.

28. Willatt JM, Hussain HK, Adusumilli, et al. MR imaging of hepatocellular carcinoma in the cirrhotic liver: challenges and controversies. Radiology 2008;247:311–30.

29. Krinsky GA, Lee VS, Nguyen MT, et al. Siderotic nodules in the cirrhotic liver at MR imaging with explant correltaion: no increased frequency of dysplastic nodules and hepatocellular carcinoma. Radiology 2001;218:47–53.

30. Ito K, Mitchell DM, Gabata T, et al. Hepatocellular carcinoma: association with increased iron deposition in the cirrhotic liver at MR imaging. Radiology 1999;212:235–40.

31. Earls JP, Theise ND, Weinreb JC, et al. Dysplastic nodules and hepatocellular carcinoma: thin section MR imaging of explanted cirrhotic livers and pathologic correlation. Radiology 1996;201:207–14.

32. Park YN, Yang CP, Fernandez GJ, et al. Neoangiogenesis and sinusoidal "capillarization" in dysplastic nodules of the liver. Am J Surg Pathol 1998;22(6):656–62.

33. Borzio M, Fargion S, Borizo F, et al. Impact of large regenerative, low grade and high grade dysplastic nodules in hepatocellular carcinoma development. J Hepatol 2003;39(2):208–14.

34. Krinsky GA, Lee VS, Theise ND, et al. Hepatocellular carcinoma and dysplastic nodules in patients with cirrhosis: prospective diagnosis with MR imaging and explantation correlation. Radiology 2001;219(2):445–54.

35. Baron RL, Peterson MS. From the RSNA refresher courses: screening the cirrhotic liver for hepatocellular carcinoma with CT and MR imaging: opportunities and pitfalls. Radiographics 2001;21: S117–32.

36. Krinsky GA, Theise ND, Rofsky NM, et al. Dysplastic nodules in cirrhotic liver: arterial phase enhancement at CT and MR imaging—A case report. Radiology 1998;209:461–4.

37. Krinsky GA, Lee VS, Nguyen MT, et al. Siderotic nodules at MR imaging: regenerative of dysplastic? J Comput Assist Tomogr 2000;24:773–6.

38. Taouli B, Losada M, Holland A, et al. Magnetic resonance imaging of hepatocellular carcinoma. Gastroenterology 2004;127:S144–52.

39. Kobayashi M, Ikeda K, Hosaka T, et al. Dysplastic nodules frequently develop into hepatocellular carcinoma in patients with chronic viral hepatitis and cirrhosis. Cancer 2006;106(3):636–47.

40. Borzio M, Borzio F, Croce A, et al. Ultrasonography-detected macroregenerative nodules in cirrhosis: a prospective study. Gastroenterology 1997; 112(5):1617–23.

41. Bartolozzi C, Crocetti L, Lencioni R, et al. Biliary and reticuloendothelial impairment in hepatocarcinogenesis: the diagnostic role of tissue-specific MR contrast media. Eur Radiol 2007;17: 2519–30.

42. Yu JS, Cho ES, Kim KH, et al. Newly developed hepatocellular carcinoma (HCC) in chronic liver disease: MR imaging findings before the diagnosis of HCC. J Comput Assist Tomogr 2006;30:765–71.

43. Kelekis NL, Semelka RC, Worawattanakul S, et al. Hepatocellular carcinoma in North America: a multi-institutional study of appearance on T1-weighted, T2-weighted, and serial gadolinium-enhanced gradient-echo images. Am J Roentgenol 1998; 170:1005–13.

44. Hecht EM, Holland AF, Israel GM, et al. Hepatocellular carcinoma in the cirrhotic liver: gadolinium-enhanced 3D T1-weighted MR imaging as a stand-alone sequence for diagnosis. Radiology 2006;239:438–47.

45. Murakami T, Kim T, Takamura M, et al. Hypervascular hepatocellular carcinoma: detection with double arterial phase multi-detector row helical CT. Radiology 2001;218(3):763–7.

46. Honda H, Ochiai K, Adachi E, et al. Hepatocellular carcinoma: correlation of CT, angiographic, and histopathologic findings. Radiology 1993;189(3): 857–62.

47. Marrero JA, Hussain HK, Nghiem HV, et al. Improving the prediction of hepatocellular carcinoma in cirrhotic patients with an arterially-enhancing liver mass. Liver Transpl 2005;11(3): 281–9.

48. Monzawa S, Ichikawa T, Nakajima H, et al. Dynamic CT for detecting small hepatocellular carcinoma: usefulness of delayed phase imaging. AJR Am J Roentgenol 2007;188(1):147–53.

49. Lutz AM, Willmann JK, Goepfert K, et al. Hepatocellular carcinoma in cirrhosis: enhancement patterns at dynamic gadolinium- and supermagnetic iron-oxide-enhanced T1-weighted MR imaging. Radiology 2005;237(2):520–8.

50. Freeny PC, Baron RL, Teefey SA. Hepatocellular carcinoma: reduced frequency of typical findings with dynamic contrast-enhanced CT in a non-Asian population. Radiology 1992;182(1):143–8.

51. Stevens WR, Johnson CD, Stephens DH, et al. CT findings in hepatocellular carcinoma: correlation of tumor characteristics with causative factors, tumor size, and histologic tumor grade. Radiology 1994;191(2):531–7.

52. Kadoya M, Matsui O, Takashima T, et al. Hepatocellular carcinoma: correlation of MR imaging and histopathologic findings. Radiology 1992;183(3):819–25.

53. Ishigami K, Yoshimitsu K, Nishihara Y, et al. Hepatocellular carcinoma with a pseudocapsule on gadolinium enhanced MR images: correlation with histopathologic findings. Radiology 2009;250(2):435–43.

54. Graziolo L, Olivetti L, Fugazzola C, et al. The pseudocapsule in hepatocellular carcinoma: correlation between dynamic MR imaging and pathology. Eur Radiol 1999;9(1):62–7.

55. Imaeda T, Kanematsu M, Mochizuki R, et al. Extracapsular invasion of small hepatocellular carcinoma: MR and CT findings. J Comput Assist Tomogr 1994;18(5):755–60.

56. Hussain HK, Syed I, Nghiem HV, et al. T2-weighted MR imaging in the assessment of cirrhotic liver. Radiology 2004;230:637–44.

57. Pawluk RS, Tummala S, Brown JJ, et al. A retrospective analysis of the accuracy of T2-weighted images and dynamic gadolinium-enhanced sequences in the detection and characterization of focal hepatic lesions. J Magn Reson Imaging 1999;9(2):266–73.

58. Semelka RC, Shoenut JP, Kroeker MA, et al. Focal liver disease: comparison of dynamic contrast-enhanced CT and T2-weighted fat-suppressed, FLASH, and dynamic gadolinium-enhanced MR imaging at 1.5 T. Radiology 1992;184(3):687–94.

59. Bennett GL, Petersein A, Mayo-Smith WW, et al. Addition of gadolinium chelates to heavily T2-weighted MR imaging: limited role in differentiating hepatic hemangiomas from metastases. AJR Am J Roentgenol 2000;174(2):477–85.

60. Ebara M, Fukuda H, Kojima Y, et al. Small hepatocellular carcinoma: relationship of signal intensity to histopathologic findings and metal content of the tumor and surrounding hepatic parenchyma. Radiology 1999;210(1):81–8.

61. Kelekis NL, Semelka RC, Woosley JT. Malignant lesions of the liver with high signal intensity on T1-weighted MR images. J Magn Reson Imaging 1996;6(2):291–4.

62. Sandrasegaran K, Akisik FM, Lin C, et al. The value of diffusion-weighted imaging in characterizing focal liver masses. Acad Radiol 2009;16(10):1208–14.

63. Miller FH, Hammond N, Siddiqi AJ, et al. Utility of diffusion-weighted MRI in distinguishing benign and malignant hepatic lesions. J Magn Reson Imaging 2010;32(1):138–47.

64. Nasu K, Kuroki Y, Tsukamoto T, et al. Diffusion-weighted imaging of surgically resected hepatocellular carcinoma: imaging characteristics and relationship among signal intensity, apparent diffusion coefficient, and histopathologic grade. AJR Am J Roentgenol 2009;193(2):438–44.

65. Sandrasegaran K, Akisik FM, Lin C, et al. Value of diffusion-weighted MRI for assessing liver fibrosis and cirrhosis. AJR Am J Roentgenol 2009;193(6):1556–60.

66. Kamel IR, Bluemke DA, Eng J, et al. The role of functional MR imaging in the assessment of tumor response after chemoembolization in patients with hepatocellular carcinoma. J Vasc Interv Radiol 2006;17:505–12.

67. Rhee TK, Naik NK, Deng J, et al. Tumor response after yttrium-90 radioembolization for hepatocellular carcinoma: comparison of diffusion-weighted functional MR imaging with anatomic MR imaging. J Vasc Interv Radiol 2008;19:1180–6.

68. Kamel IR, Reyes DK, Liapi E, et al. Functional MR imaging assessment of tumor response after 90Y microsphere treatment in patients with unresectable hepatocellular carcinoma. J Vasc Interv Radiol 2007;18(1 Pt 1):49–56.

69. Muhi A, Ichikawa T, Motosugi U, et al. High-b-value diffusion-weighted MR imaging of hepatocellular lesions: estimation of grade of malignancy of hepatocellular carcinoma. J Magn Reson Imaging 2009;30(5):1005–11.

70. Loyer EM, Chin H, DuBrow RA, et al. Hepatocellular carcinoma and intrahepatic peripheral cholangiocarcinoma: enhancement patterns with quadruple phase helical CT—a comparative study. Radiology 1999;212(3):866–75.

71. Catalano OA, Choy G, Zhu A, et al. Differentiation of malignant thrombus from bland thrombus of the portal vein in patients with hepatocellular carcinoma: application of diffusion-weighted MR imaging. Radiology 2010;254(1):154–62.

72. Tublin ME, Dodd GD III, Baron RL. Benign and malignant portal vein thrombosis: differentiation by CT characteristics. AJR Am J Roentgenol 1997;168(3):719–23.

73. Carr BI. Hepatic arterial 90Yttrium glass microspheres (Therasphere) for unresectable hepatocellular carcinoma: interim safety and survival data on 65 patients. Liver Transpl 2004;10(2 Suppl 1):S107–10.

74. Salem R, Lewandowski R, Roberts C, et al. Use of Yttrium-90 glass microspheres (TheraSphere) for the treatment of unresectable hepatocellular carcinoma in patients with portal vein thrombosis. J Vasc Interv Radiol 2004;15(4):335–45.

75. Stevens WR, Gulino SP, Batts KP, et al. Mosaic pattern of hepatocellular carcinoma: histologic

basis for a characteristic CT appearance. J Comput Assist Tomogr 1996;20(3):337—42.

76. Asayama Y, Yoshimitsu K, Nishihara Y, et al. Arterial blood supply of hepatocellular carcinoma and histologic grading: radiologic-pathologic correlation. AJR Am J Roentgenol 2008;190(1):W28—34.

77. Kudo M. Atypical large well-differentiated hepatocellular carcinoma with benign nature: a new clinical entity. Intervirology 2004;47(3—5):227—37.

78. Kanematsu M, Semelka RC, Leonardou P, et al. Hepatocellular carcinoma of diffuse type: MR imaging findings and clinical manifestations. J Magn Reson Imaging 2003;18(2):189—95.

79. Kim YK, Han YM, Kim CS. Comparison of diffuse hepatocellular carcinoma and intrahepatic cholangiocarcinoma using sequentially acquired gadolinium-enhanced and Resovist-enhanced MRI. Eur J Radiol 2009;70(1):94—100.

80. Martin J, Sentis M, Zidan A, et al. Fatty metamorphosis of hepatocellular carcinoma: detection with chemical shift gradient-echo MR imaging. Radiology 1995;195:125—30.

81. Yoshikawa J, Matsui O, Takashima T, et al. Fatty metamorphosis in hepatocellular carcinoma: radiologic features in 10 cases. Am J Roentgenol 1988; 151:717—20.

82. Valls C, Iannacconne R, Alba E, et al. Fat in the liver: diagnosis and characterization. Eur Radiol 2006;16(10):2292—308.

83. Mitchell DG, Rubin R, Siegelman ES, et al. Hepatocellular carcinoma within siderotic regenerative nodules: appearance as a nodule within a nodule on MR images. Radiology 1991;178(1):101—3.

84. Sadek AG, Mitchell DG, Siegelman ES, et al. Early hepatocellular carcinoma that develops within macroregenerative nodules: growth rate depicted at serial MR imaging. Radiology 1995;195(3): 753—6.

85. Lupescu IG, Capsa RA, Gheorghe L, et al. Tissue specific MR contrast media role in the differential diagnosis of cirrhotic liver nodules. J Gastrointestin Liver Dis 2008;17:341—5.

86. Sun HY, Lee JM, Shin CI, et al. Gadoxetic acid-enhanced magnetic resonance imaging for differentiating small hepatocellular carcinomas ($\leq$2 cm in diameter) from arterial enhancing pseudolesions: special emphasis of hepatobiliary phase imaging. Invest Radiol 2010;45:96—103.

87. Choi SH, Lee JM, Yu NM, et al. Hepatocellular carcinoma in liver transplantation candidates: detection with gadobenate dimeglumine-enhanced MRI. Am J Roentgenol 2008;191: 529—36.

88. Ichikawa T, Saito K, Yoshioka N, et al. Detection and characterization of focal liver lesions: a Japanese phase III, multicenter comparison between gadoxetic acid disodium-enhanced magnetic resonance imaging and contrast-enhanced computed tomography predominantly in patients with hepatocellular carcinoma and chronic liver disease. Invest Radiol 2010;45:133—41.

89. Kim SH, Kim SH, Lee J, et al. Gadoxetic acid-enhanced MRI versus triple-phase MDCT for the preoperative detection of hepatocellular carcinoma. Am J Roentgenol 2009;192:1675—81.

90. Marin D, Di Martino M, Guerrisi A, et al. Hepatocellular carcinoma in patients with cirrhosis: qualitative comparison of gadobenate dimeglumine-enhanced MR imaging and multiphasic 64-section CT. Radiology 2009;251:85—95.

91. Madhoun MF, Fazili J, Bright BC, et al. Hepatitis C prevalence in patients with hepatocellular carcinoma without cirrhosis. Am J Med Sci 2010; 339(2):169—73.

92. Winston CB, Schwartz LH, Fong Y, et al. Hepatocellular carcinoma: MR imaging findings in cirrhotic livers and noncirrhotic livers. Radiology 1999; 210(1):75—9.

93. Brancatelli G, Federle MP, Grazioli L, et al. Hepatocellular carcinoma in noncirrhotic liver: CT, clinical, and pathologic findings in 39 US residents. Radiology 2002;222(1):89—94.

94. Lwakatare F, Hayashida Y, Yamashita Y. MR imaging of hepatocellular carcinoma arising in genetic hemochromatosis. Magn Reson Med Sci 2003;2:57—9.

95. Mastropasqua M, Kanematsu M, Leonardou P, et al. Cavernous hemangiomas in patients with chronic liver disease: MR imaging findings. Magn Reson Imaging 2004;22:15—8.

96. Brancatelli G, Federle MP, Blachar, et al. Hemangioma in the cirrhotic liver: diagnosis and natural history. Radiology 2001;219:69—74.

97. Heiken JP. Distinguishing benign from malignant liver tumours. Cancer Imaging 2007;7:S1—14.

98. Vilgrain V, Boulos L, Vullierme M, et al. Imaging of atypical hemangiomas of the liver with pathologic correlation. Radiographics 2000;20:379—97.

99. Blachar A, Federle MP, Brancatelli G. Hepatic capsular retraction: spectrum of benign and malignant etiologies. Abdom Imaging 2002;27(6): 690—9.

100. Yu J, Kim KW, Park M, et al. Hepatic cavernous hemangiomas in cirrhotic liver: imaging findings. Korean J Radiol 2000;1:185—90.

101. Semelka RC, Brown ED, Ascher SM, et al. Hepatic hemangiomas: a multi-institutional study of appearance on T2-weighted and serial gadolinium-enhanced gradient-echo MR images. Radiology 1994;192(2):401—6.

102. Jang HJ, Choi BI, Kim TK, et al. Atypical small hemangiomas of the liver: "bright dot" sign at two-phase spiral CT. Radiology 1998;208(2): 543—8.

103. Hoshimoto S, Morise Z, Suzuki K, et al. Hepatocellular carcinoma with extensive peliotic change. J Hepatobiliary Pancreat Surg 2009;16(4):566–70.

104. Maetani Y, Itoh K, Egawa H, et al. Benign hepatic nodules in Budd-Chiari syndrome: radiologic-pathologic correlation with emphasis on the central scar. Am J Roentgenol 2002;178:869–75.

105. Bilaj F, Hyslop WB, Rivero H, et al. MR imaging findings in autoimmune hepatitis: correlation with clinical staging. Radiology 2005;236:896–902.

106. Ohtomo K, Baron RL, Dodd GD, et al. Confluent hepatic fibrosis in advanced cirrhosis: evaluation with MR imaging. Radiology 1993;189(3):871–4.

107. Ahn IO, de Lange EE. Early hyperenhancement of confluent hepatic fibrosis on dynamic MR imaging. AJR Am J Roentgenol 1998;171(3):901–2.

108. Colagrande S, Centi N, Galdiero R, et al. Transient hepatic intensity differences: part 1, those associated with focal lesions. Am J Roentgenol 2007; 188:154–9.

109. Colagrande S, Centi N, Galdiero R, et al. Transient hepatic intensity differences: part 2, those not associated with focal lesions. Am J Roentgenol 2007;188:160–6.

110. Kim HJ, Kim AY, Kim TK, et al. Transient hepatic attenuation differences in focal hepatic lesions: dynamic CT features. AJR Am J Roentgenol 2005;184(1):83–90.

111. Holland AE, Hecht EM, Hahn WY, et al. Importance of small (≤20-mm) enhancing lesions seen only during the hepatic arterial phase at MR imaging of the cirrhotic liver: evaluation and comparison with whole explanted liver. Radiology 2005;237:938–44.

112. Tsuchiyama TS, Terasaki S, Kaneko S, et al. Tiny staining spots in liver cirrhosis associated with HCV infection observed by computed tomographic hepatic arteriography: follow-up study. J Gastroenterol 2002;37(10):807–14.

113. Shimizu A, Ito K, Koike S, et al. Cirrhosis or chronic hepatitis: evaluation of small (≤2-cm) early-enhancing hepatic lesions with serial contrast-enhanced dynamic MR imaging. Radiology 2003; 226:550–5.

114. Jeong YY, Mitchell DG, Kamishima T. Small (<20 mm) enhancing hepatic nodules seen on arterial phase MR imaging of the cirrhotic liver: clinical implications. Am J Roentgenol 2002;178:1327–34.

115. Kim YK, Lee YH, Kwak HS, et al. Clinical implication of small (<20 mm) enhancing hepatic nodules observed only during three-dimensional gadobenate dimeglumine-enhanced hepatic arterial-phase MRI of the hepatitis B virus-induced mild cirrhosis. Clin Imaging 2008;32:453–9.

116. Mazzaferro V, Regalia E, Doci R, et al. Liver transplantation for the treatment of small hepatocellular carcinomas in patients with cirrhosis. N Engl J Med 1996;334:693–9.

117. Yao FY, Ferrell L, Bass NM, et al. Liver transplantation for hepatocellular carcinoma: expansion of the tumor size limits does not adversely impact survival. Hepatology 2001;33(6):1394–403.

118. Yao FY, Xiao L, Bass NM, et al. Liver transplantation for hepatocellular carcinoma: validation of the UCSF-expanded criteria based on preoperative imaging. Am J Transplant 2007;7(11):2587–96.

119. Onaca N, Davis GL, Goldstein RM, et al. Expanded criteria for liver transplantation in patients with hepatocellular carcinoma: a report from the international registry of hepatic tumors in liver transplantation. Liver Transpl 2007;13:391–9.

120. Schwartz M. Liver transplantation for hepatocellular carcinoma. Gastroenterology 2004;127:S268–76.

121. Kim SK, Lim HK, Kim YH, et al. Hepatocellular carcinoma treated with radio-frequency ablation: spectrum of imaging findings. Radiographics 2003;23:107–21.

122. Dromain C, de Baere T, Elias D, et al. Hepatic tumors treated with percutaneous radio-frequency ablation: CT and MR imaging follow-up. Radiology 2002;223:255–62.

123. Schima W, Ba-Ssalamah A, Kurtaran A, et al. Post-treatment imaging of liver tumours. Cancer Imaging 2007;7:S28–36.

124. Khankan AA, Murakami T, Onishi H, et al. Hepatocellular carcinoma treated with radio frequency ablation: an early evaluation with magnetic resonance imaging. J Magn Reson Imaging 2008;27: 546–51.

125. Kloeckner R, Otto G, Biesterfeld S, et al. MDCT versus MRI assessment of tumor response after transarterial chemoembolization for the treatment of hepatocellular carcinoma. Cardiovasc Intervent Radiol 2009;33(3):532–40.

126. De Santis M, Alborino S, Tartoni PL, et al. Effects of lipiodol retention on MRI signal intensity from hepatocellular carcinoma and surrounding liver treated by chemoembolization. Eur Radiol 1997; 7(1):10–6.

127. Semelka RC, Worawattanakul S, Mauro MA, et al. Malignant hepatic tumors: changes on MRI after hepatic arterial chemoembolization—preliminary findings. J Magn Reson Imaging 1998;8:48–56.

128. Kubota KN, Hisa N, Nishikawa T, et al. Evaluation of hepatocellular carcinoma after treatment with transcatheter arterial chemoembolization: comparison of Lipiodol-CT, power Doppler sonography, and dynamic MRI. Abdom Imaging 2001;26(2): 184–90.

129. Atassi B, Bangash AK, Baharani A, et al. Multimodality imaging following ^{90}Y radioembolization: a comprehensive review and pictorial essay. Radiographics 2008;28:81–99.

130. Ibrahim SM, Nikolaidis P, Miller FH, et al. Radiologic findings following Y90 radioembolization for

primary liver malignancies. Abdom Imaging 2009; 34(5):566–81.

131. Therasse P, Arbuck SG, Eisenhauer EA, et al. New guidelines to evaluate the response to treatment in solid tumors. J Natl Cancer Inst 2000;92:205–16.

132. Riaz A, Kulik L, Lewandowski RJ, et al. Radiologic-pathologic correlation of hepatocellular carcinoma treated with internal radiation using Yttrium-90 microspheres. Hepatology 2009;49(4): 1185–93.

Diffusion-Weighted MRI and Liver Metastases

Hersh Chandarana, MD[a], Bachir Taouli, MD[b],*

abstract
KEYWORDS
- Liver • Metastases • MRI • Diffusion

BACKGROUND OF LIVER METASTASES

Liver metastases are the most frequently encountered malignant liver lesions in the Western countries, including the United States. In a large German autopsy series of more than 12,000 cases, liver metastases were found to represent 5.0% of cases, followed by hepatocellular carcinoma (3.1%).[1] Many primary neoplasms, including colorectal, breast, kidney, pancreas, and melanoma, can metastasize to the liver.[2,3] Accurate diagnosis of liver metastases is essential for appropriate management of these patients; patients without evidence of metastases to the liver and extrahepatic sites may benefit from definitive surgical treatment, whereas patients with liver metastases may need to be treated with systemic chemotherapy or segmental hepatectomy, or locoregional therapies such as chemoembolization and radiofrequency ablation.[4,5] Although patients with liver metastases, especially from colorectal cancer, who meet the criteria for surgical resection have significant improvement in survival, fewer than 25% of patients with disease limited to the liver are candidates for surgical resection.[6] Hence, in patients with primary extrahepatic malignancies, accurate detection of liver metastases is essential.

ROLE OF IMAGING FOR DETECTION OF LIVER METASTASES

Multiple imaging modalities, including ultrasound, CT, positron emission tomography (PET), PET-CT, and MRI are available for evaluating patients with suspected or known liver metastases. Transabdominal ultrasound has a limited sensitivity of 50% to 75% for detecting hepatic lesions, and even lower sensitivity for smaller lesions.[7] The use of contrast-enhanced ultrasound can improve lesion detection and characterization, but the ultrasound contrast is not yet approved by the US Food and Drug Administration (FDA).[7–9] Furthermore, ultrasound is user-dependent and may require another confirmatory study to characterize liver lesions in many instances.

Multidetector CT (MDCT) is routinely used for evaluating metastatic disease in patients with primary malignancies.[10] It is widely available, relatively inexpensive, and user independent. Multiphasic contrast-enhanced CT with acquisition in both the arterial (20 to 30 seconds after contrast injection) and portal venous phases (70 to 90 seconds after contrast administration) of enhancement has been shown to optimize detection of hypervascular and hypovascular liver metastases, respectively.[11–14] Limitations of multiphasic CT include exposure to ionizing radiation,[15] and the risk of contrast induced nephropathy from exposure to iodinated contrast media. Another limitation of CT is its inability to definitively characterize subcentimeter lesions. These lesions are reported as "too small to accurately characterize," even in patients with known primary malignancies.[16–18]

Fluorodeoxyglucose (FDG)-PET and PET-CT have been used increasingly in the evaluation of metastatic disease in patients with primary

---

The authors have nothing to disclose.
[a] Department of Radiology, NYU Langone Medical Center, 550 First Avenue, New York, NY 10016, USA
[b] Department of Radiology, Mount Sinai School of Medicine, One Gustave Levy Place, Box 1234, New York, NY 10029, USA
* Corresponding author.
E-mail address: bachir.taouli@mountsinai.org

Magn Reson Imaging Clin N Am 18 (2010) 451–464
doi:10.1016/j.mric.2010.07.001
1064-9689/10/$ – see front matter © 2010 Elsevier Inc. All rights reserved.

malignancies. Studies have shown high sensitivity and specificity for detection of liver metastases.[19,20] Truant and colleagues[21] reported a similar sensitivity of 76% for both CT and FDG-PET. Ogunbiyi and colleagues[20] reported that FDG-PET had a high sensitivity (95%) and specificity (100%) for detecting liver metastases, and that it was superior to that of the CT, which had sensitivity and specificity of 74% and 85%, respectively.

In a meta-analysis that reviewed 61 articles published between 1990 and 2003 to compare CT, PET-CT, and MRI in the diagnosis of colorectal liver metastases,[22] the authors concluded that PET-CT had a significantly higher sensitivity on a per-patient basis but not on a per-lesion basis.[22] PET has also been shown to be superior to CT for detecting extrahepatic metastases. Lai and colleagues[23] found previously unsuspected extrahepatic disease, predominantly involving the celiac lymph nodes, in 32% patients scheduled for hepatic metastasectomy. Sahani and colleagues[24] reported that FDG-PET identified extrahepatic disease in 9 of the 34 patients involved in their study. However, limitations of PET-CT include radiation exposure, cost, and limited availability.

CT and ultrasound allow evaluation of liver lesions based on a single physical parameter, such as attenuation and echotexture, respectively. In contrast, MRI provides an unique ability to interrogate multiple parameters like T1, T2, diffusion, and enhancement patterns of focal liver lesions, enabling accurate liver lesion detection and characterization (Table 1).[25–27] Three-dimensional T1-weighted fat-suppressed gradient-recalled echo sequence performed before and after intravenous contrast administration is the workhorse of the liver MR examination. Multiphasic acquisition after injection of extracellular gadolinium-based contrast agents during the hepatic arterial, portal venous, and equilibrium phases can be obtained without radiation exposure and has been shown to have high accuracy in the detection and characterization of liver lesions.[28,29] MRI with the use of intravenous gadolinium contrast agents was found to have higher accuracy (98% vs 86% and 66%, respectively) than contrast-enhanced PET-CT and unenhanced PET-CT for detecting colorectal metastases.[30] Liver-specific contrast agents, including hepatobiliary agents such as gadolinium-ethoxybenzyl (Gd-EOB-DTPA, Eovist or Primovist, Bayer Healthcare Pharmaceuticals, Montville, NJ, USA) and gadobenate dimeglumine (Gd-BOPTA, MultiHance, Bracco Diagnostics Inc, Princeton, NJ, USA), and reticuloendothelial agents such as superparamagnetic iron oxide particles (SPIO, Feridex, Bayer Healthcare Pharmaceuticals, Montville, NJ, USA), have shown considerable promise in further improving the sensitivity and specificity of MRI for diagnosis and characterization of focal liver lesions.[31–34] However, SPIO contrast was recently withdrawn from the market in the United States.

Drawbacks of MRI include limited availability, higher cost, and longer examination time that

Table 1
Suggested MRI protocol for liver imaging in patients with suspected liver metastases

Sequence	Acquisition Plane	TR/TE	Slice Thickness (mm)/gap (%)	Matrix
T1 GRE in and out of phase	Axial	188/2.2–4.4	8/20	178 × 256
T2 TSE fat-suppressed	Axial	~2000–4000/85	8/20	192 × 256
Single shot T2 TSE non fat suppressed	Coronal	90–infinity/65	4/20	256 × 256
Fat-suppressed SS EPI diffusion[a] (breath-hold or respiratory triggered)	Axial	1600–2000 (BH)-1 respiratory cycle (RT)/minimum	6 (RT)–7 (BH)/20	144 × 192
Three-dimensional T1 fat-suppressed GRE Pre– and 3 post–contrast acquisitions (dual arterial, portal venous [60 s], and equilibrium [180 s] phases)	Axial	3.5/1.6	2.1–2.5/NA	256 × 256 (interpolated)

Abbreviations: BH, breath-hold; GRE, gradient-recalled echo; NA, not available; RT, respiratory-triggered; SS EPI, single-shot echo planar imaging; TE, echo time; TR, repetition time; TSE, turbo spin echo.
[a] b Values: 0, 50, 500 s/mm^2 (BH) or 0, 50, 500, 1000 s/mm^2 (RT).

requires patients to hold their breath during many acquisitions. Nephrogenic systemic fibrosis is a rare and potentially life-threatening condition that has been recently reported in patients with advanced renal failure receiving gadolinium-based contrast agents.[35,36] Consequently, extreme caution is advised in administering gadolinium-based contrast material in patients with severely impaired renal function (glomerular filtration rate <30 mL/min/1.73 m²).[37] Therefore, noncontrast MR techniques, such as diffusion-weighted imaging (DWI), are attractive in this patient population.

DWI ACQUISITION, PROCESSING, AND INTERPRETATION
Principles of DWI

As a result of recent advances in MR technology, DWI is now feasible outside the brain with improved image quality and promising results. This noncontrast technique is easy to implement in clinical practice as it can be added to the existing protocols without significant time penalty.

Diffusion-weighted imaging quantifies thermally induced motion of water molecules known as *Brownian motion* in tissues.[38,39] The apparent diffusion coefficient (ADC) calculation has been used to quantify combined effects of capillary perfusion and tissue diffusion.

The ADC is calculated by performing a monoexponential fit to the relationship between the measured signal intensity (in logarithmic scale) and the b values as follows:

$$ADC = \ln(SI_0/SI)/b$$

where SI_0 is signal intensity for $b = 0$, and SI is for higher b value.

The slope of the line that describes this relationship for each voxel represents the ADC. The calculated ADCs for all voxels are usually displayed as a parametric map (automated on most clinical MR systems) and, by drawing a region of interest (ROI) onto this map, the mean or median ADC value in the region of interest can be measured.

DWI Acquisition

DWI is routinely performed before intravenous gadolinium administration, although recently published studies suggest the possibility of performing DWI after contrast administration without loss of diagnostic capability for liver lesion detection and characterization.[40,41] Ultrafast single-shot echo planar imaging (SS EPI) is the most commonly used technique in abdominal imaging. SS EPI sequences are prone to ghosting and distortion artifacts. Thus, optimal acquisition techniques are necessary to generate diagnostic quality images.

SS EPI is routinely performed with fat saturation[42,43] (spectral attenuated inversion recovery or chemical excitation with spectral suppression) to decrease ghosting artifacts. Breath-hold SS EPI is routinely used in liver imaging because the entire liver can be imaged in one to two breath-holds of approximately 20 seconds each. However, the disadvantages of breath-hold imaging include lower signal-to-noise ratio (SNR), lower resolution due to thicker slices (which helps compensate for low SNR), greater sensitivity to artifacts, and a limitation on the number of b values that can be included in the measurement.[44]

Free-breathing imaging can be performed with either multiple signal-averaging to reduce the effects of motion or with respiratory or cardiac triggering.[45,46] Most major vendors now propose routinely respiratory-triggered SS EPI sequences, using bellows or navigators. Although respiratory-triggered diffusion imaging of the liver may take longer (3–6 minutes of acquisition time), the use of multiple signal averages results in images with higher SNR. Consequently, thinner image sections (5 mm or less) can be obtained, and more b values can be accommodated within the longer measurement.

A prior study showed improved liver lesion detection with respiratory-triggered sequence when compared with breath-hold DWI (sensitivity for lesion detection, 93.7% vs 84.3%),[47] likely due to improved image quality and higher SNR (**Fig. 1**). In addition, the authors have shown that respiratory-triggered DWI using navigator echo improves ADC quantification over breath-hold DWI[45] because of lower noise contamination. The noise contamination in liver ADC as measured using the coefficient of variability (CV) was 33% lower with the navigator triggered sequence than with the breath-hold DWI. However, a recent study in volunteers showed that the ADC values obtained using the free-breathing technique were more reproducible compared with breath-hold or navigator-triggered images.[48] Clearly more work needs to be done to determine the value of breath-hold versus free-breathing versus navigator-triggered DWI schemes.

In addition, in the left hepatic lobe, cardiac motion results in spin-dephasing, which causes artifacts, especially at higher b values, and can result in decreased lesion conspicuity[49] and spuriously high ADC values.

Diffusion in the liver shows lack of significant anisotropy or directionality to water diffusion,[50] and therefore DWI in the liver is routinely performed by applying gradients in one to three directions (along each of the three directions: x, y, z,

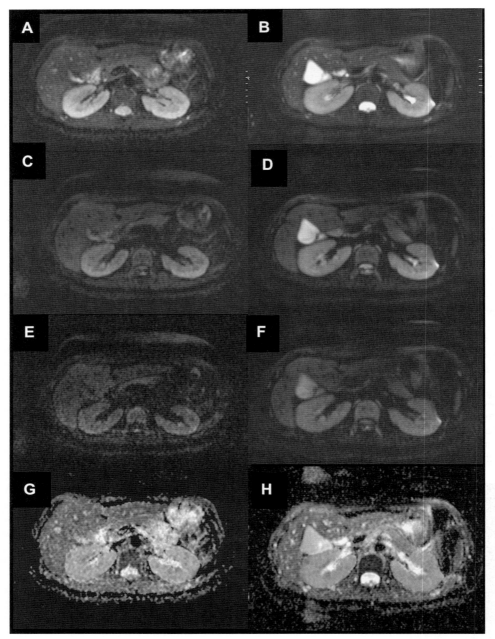

Fig. 1. Axial fat-suppressed breath-hold (left column, *A*, *C*, *E*, *G*) versus respiratory-triggered (right column, *B*, *D*, *F*, *H*) abdominal single-shot echo-planar imaging diffusion images in a 46-year-old woman with normal liver. Respiratory-triggered acquisition (using navigator echo) shows better image quality and signal-to-noise ratio with better organ edge delineation for all *b* values (in s/mm^2) (*B*, *b* = 0; *D*, *b* = 50; *F*, *b* = 500) and more homogeneous apparent diffusion coefficient (ADC) map (*H*) compared with breath-hold acquisition (*A*, *b* = 0; *C*, *b* = 50; *E*, *b* = 500; *G*, ADC map). A strong signal drop of the gallbladder is present with high ADC value, as seen on respiratory-triggered images (only a small portion of the gallbladder is seen on breath-hold images because of slice acquisition differences).

which serves to improve SNR). The authors use tri-directional gradients, and assess the trace (average) image for clinical interpretation.

Diffusion Weighting (b value)

The strength of diffusion weighting can be altered through changing the b value or b factor. The b value increases with the square of the gradient amplitude, the square of the gradient diffusion length, and approximately with the time between the two diffusion gradient pulses. Hence, diffusion weighting increases with higher b values. No consensus exists among studies about the appropriate b values to use for liver imaging. Recently published guidelines have suggested using b values between 100 and 750 s/mm² for liver DWI.[51] At the authors' institution, DWI is performed with at least three b values (see **Table 1**), including both lower and higher values (eg, using $b = 0$, $b \leq 100$, and $b \geq 500$ s/mm²).[44] Additional b values can be considered when the primary goal is to obtain an accurate ADC measurement (eg, to assess tumor response or liver fibrosis), because increasing the number of data points can reduce the error in the ADC estimation. However, this increases the acquisition time.

Image Interpretation

The images acquired from each individual b value can be assessed qualitatively, and this is routinely used in clinical practice for liver lesion detection and characterization.[47,52] Highly cellular tissues, such as tumors, will show restricted diffusion (high signal intensity) on the higher b-value (≥ 400–500 s/mm²) images and correspondingly lower ADC values, whereas less cellular benign lesions tend to have a relatively lower signal intensity on the high b-value images with corresponding high ADC values (**Figs. 2** and **3**). However, the signal intensity observed on the diffusion image depends on diffusivity, tissue T2-relaxation time, and microcapillary perfusion. A lesion may seem to show high signal intensity on a high b-value image, because of incomplete suppression of T2 effect from long T2-relaxation time rather than the true restriction to diffusion (T2 shine-through). The presence of a T2 shine-through effect should be recognized by noting higher lesion ADC rather than low ADC (dark on ADC map), which should be seen with true restriction to diffusion. Therefore, diffusion images should always be interpreted concurrently with the ADC map.

Quantitative ADC values are less routinely used in clinical practice but are being investigated with considerable promise, especially for diagnosis of liver fibrosis and cirrhosis[53,54] and characterization of focal liver lesions.[47] ADC value can be obtained by placing an ROI on the ADC map and the ADC values are usually expressed in "$\times 10^{-3}$ mm²/s."

ROLE OF DWI IN DETECTING LIVER METASTASES

Qualitative evaluation of low and high b value images with corresponding ADC maps can be

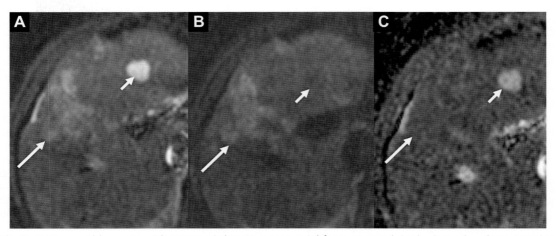

Fig. 2. A 55-year-old woman with metastatic breast cancer. Axial fat-suppressed single-shot echo planar imaging diffusion-weighted images at $b = 0$ s/mm² (A), $b = 500$ s/mm² (B), and ADC map (C) show a metastatic lesion in the right hepatic lobe (*long arrow*) and a cyst in the medial left lobe (*short arrow*). The metastatic lesion shows restricted diffusion: it is mildly hyperintense at $b = 0$ s/mm², remaining hyperintense at $b = 500$ s/mm², with low ADC. The cyst shows free diffusion: it is hyperintense at $b = 0$ s/mm² and hypointense at $b = 500$ s/mm², with high ADC. (*Reproduced from* Parikh T, Drew SJ, Lee VS, et al. Focal liver lesion detection and characterization with diffusion-weighted MR imaging: comparison with standard breath-hold T2-weighted imaging. Radiology 2008;246(3):812–22; with permission.)

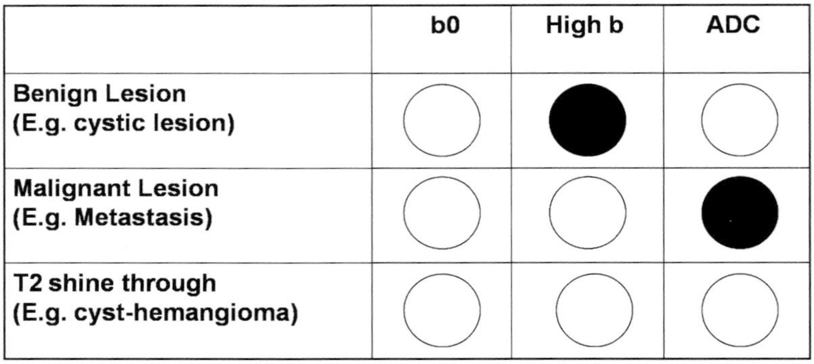

	b0	High b	ADC
Benign Lesion (E.g. cystic lesion)	○	●	○
Malignant Lesion (E.g. Metastasis)	○	○	●
T2 shine through (E.g. cyst-hemangioma)	○	○	○

Fig. 3. Visual liver lesion characterization with DWI. This figure gives a simplified approach to lesion characterization using visual assessment of $b = 0$ s/mm^2, higher b value, and ADC maps. A benign fluid-containing lesion shows strong signal drop with high ADC, whereas a cellular malignant lesion shows no or minimal signal drop, with low ADC compared with surrounding liver parenchyma. A lesion with long T2 can sometimes show a T2 shine-through effect. (*Reproduced from* Taouli B, Koh DM. Diffusion-weighted MR imaging of the liver. Radiology 2010;254:47–66; with permission.)

used to detect focal liver lesions. Several studies have shown higher sensitivity of DWI for detecting lesions compared with T2-weighted imaging (T2WI),[47,55,56] and comparable accuracy of DWI to contrast-enhanced T1W acquisitions.[57]

Low b value acquisition (<100 s/mm^2) provides background vascular signal suppression equivalent to black-blood images, which increases the conspicuity of liver lesions and improves sensitivity for lesion detection.[52,58,59] In a study comparing black-blood DWI (using $b = 50$ s/mm^2) with fat-suppressed T2WI at 1.5T, Zech and colleagues[58] showed better image quality, fewer artifacts, and better sensitivity for lesion detection with DWI than with T2WI (83% vs 61%). Similar findings were reported at 3T by van den Bos and colleagues,[59] who reported that DWI was comparable to T2WI in terms of image quality, with improved suppression of fat and blood signals, and high contrast-to-noise ratio and SNR in a single breath-hold acquisition. In 53 patients with 211 lesions, the authors found that DWI performs better than standard breath-hold T2WI for lesion detection and characterization using b values of 50 and 500 s/mm^2, with a sensitivity for detection of 87.7% versus 70.1% for all lesions, and 86.4% versus 62.9% for malignant lesions (P<.001), respectively (**Figs. 4** and **5**).[47,48] In addition, DWI significantly improved detection of small malignant lesions (<2 cm) compared with breath-hold T2WI (78.5% vs 45.8%; P<.001).[47]

Bruegel and colleagues[55] compared respiratory-triggered DWI with five different T2WI sequences (breath-hold fat-suppressed- single shot (HASTE), breath-hold fat-suppressed turbo spin-echo (TSE), breath-hold STIR, respiration-triggered fat-suppressed TSE, and respiration-triggered STIR) for diagnosing liver metastases. DWI showed higher accuracy (area under the curve [AUC], 0.91–0.92) compared with T2WI turbo spin echo (TSE) sequences (AUC, 0.47–0.67). These differences were even more pronounced for small metastatic lesions (≤1 cm).

The use of DWI in place of gadolinium chelates is very attractive in patients with severe renal dysfunction who are at increased risk of nephrogenic systemic fibrosis. In addition, the combination of DWI with contrast-enhanced T1WI may improve accuracy compared to either sequence alone. However, there is limited data directly comparing DWI with contrast-enhanced studies (see **Fig. 5**). Nasu and colleagues[49] found that DWI was more sensitive than SPIO-enhanced MRI (82% vs 66%) for detecting colorectal hepatic metastases, except in the left hepatic lobe. In their study, SPIO-enhanced MRI was 2.3 times less sensitive for detecting metastases smaller than 1 cm than for those larger than 1 cm in diameter. However, DWI was more robust in detecting smaller lesions and showed no significant difference in sensitivity for detecting metastases larger or smaller than 1 cm in diameter.

Koh and colleagues[60] compared DWI with mangafodipir trisodium (MnDPDP)—enhanced MRI for detecting colorectal liver metastases, and found that DWI had a lower diagnostic accuracy compared with MnDPDP for observer 1 (AUC, 0.83 vs 0.92), and no significant difference between DWI and MnDPDP for observer 2 (AUC, 0.90 vs 0.88). More importantly, the addition of DWI significantly improved the diagnostic accuracy for detecting colorectal liver metastases compared

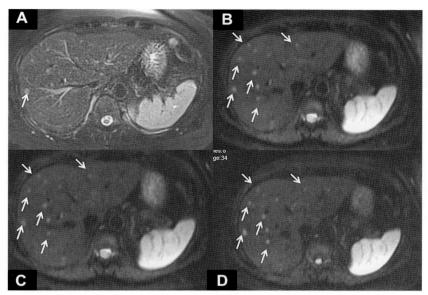

Fig. 4. Liver metastases from breast cancer better detected with DWI than with T2WI. Axial fat-suppressed fast spin echo T2WI (*A*, slice thickness 8 mm) shows a small metastatic lesion (*arrow*). However, many more metastatic lesions (*arrows*) are identified on axial fat-suppressed single-shot echo planar imaging diffusion images (*B*, $b = 50$ s/mm^2; *C*, $b = 500$ s/mm^2; *D*, $b = 1000$ s/mm^2; slice thickness 7 mm) in a 42-year-old woman with breast cancer. The lesions are more easily detected on diffusion images, and remain bright on high b value, consistent with malignant lesions. (*Reproduced from* Taouli B, Koh DM. Diffusion-weighted MR imaging of the liver. In: Taouli B, editor. Extracranial applications of diffusion-weighted MR imaging. Cambridge (UK): Cambridge University Press; 2001; with permission.)

with either technique alone for both readers (AUC, 0.94 for observer 1 and 0.96 for observer 2).

Other studies have postulated the advantages of performing DWI after SPIO-enhanced imaging. Naganawa and colleagues[61] showed that the addition of SPIO contrast medium to DWI improved detection of focal lesions in all patients for both $b = 600$ s/mm^2 and $b = 1000$ s/mm^2 acquisition. Low and Gurney[62] compared DWI with Gadopentetate Dimeglumine (Gd-DTPA; extracellular gadolinium chelates)—enhanced MRI for tumor detection and showed additional tumor detection with DWI compared with contrast-enhanced MRI; however, the study was not specifically focused on liver lesions.

A recent study by Hardie and colleagues[57] compared DWI with Gd-DTPA—enhanced T1WI for detecting liver metastases. In this study, two observers retrospectively assessed 51 patients with extrahepatic malignancies. Neither observer saw a difference in diagnostic performance between the DWI and Gd-DTPA—enhanced T1WI in diagnosing metastatic lesions per-patient. For per-lesion analysis, sensitivity of DWI was equivalent to contrast-enhanced T1WI for observer 1 (67.3% vs 63.3%; $P = .67$), and lower for observer

2 (65.3% vs 83.7%; $P = .007$). When pooling data from both observers, the sensitivity of DWI and contrast-enhanced MRI was 66.3% and 73.5%, respectively, and the difference was not statistically significantly ($P = .171$).

This study suggested that DWI can be a reasonable alternative to gadolinium-enhanced T1WI for detecting liver metastases. Although not assessed in this study, an integrated approach using both DWI and contrast-enhanced MRI must be explored to improve accuracy for liver lesion detection, especially for lesions smaller than 1 cm.

Some studies[47,50,55,63—68] have suggested that ADC maps and mean ADC values may be helpful in discriminating benign from malignant lesions (see **Fig. 2**, **Figs. 5** and **6**), and may help segment out lesions through discriminating cellular from necrotic components without the use of intravenous contrast (**Fig. 7**). Measuring ADC on necrotic portions of the tumors is generally not recommended.

ADC cutoffs between 1.4 and 1.6 $\times 10^{-3}$ mm^2/s have been described in the literature for diagnosing malignant liver lesions, with reported sensitivity of 74% to 100% and specificity of 77% to 100% (**Table 2**).[47,50,55,63—68] These cutoffs vary

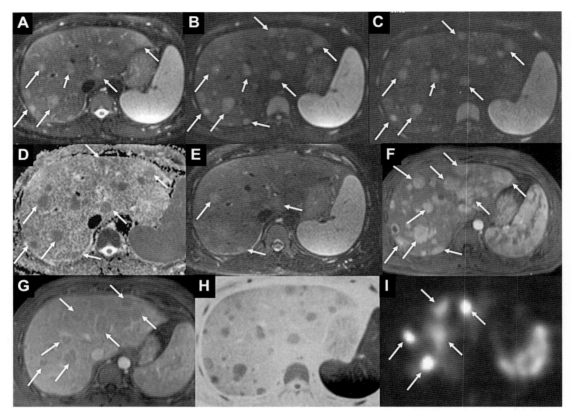

Fig. 5. Neuroendocrine liver metastases in a 65-year-old man. Axial fat-suppressed single-shot echo planar imaging diffusion images (*A, b* = 0 s/mm^2; *B, b* = 500 s/mm^2; *C, b* = 1000 s/mm^2; slice thickness 7 mm), and ADC map (*D*, using 0-50-500-1000) show multiple metastatic liver lesions (*arrows*) with restricted diffusion (hyperintense on high *b* values with decreased ADC). The lesions are not as conspicuous on axial fat-suppressed breath-hold T2WI (*E*, slice thickness 8 mm). Postcontrast T1WI at the arterial (*F*) and portal venous (*G*) phases show hypervascular lesions with washout. A diffusion image (*b* = 1000) with inverted contrast (*H*, positron emission tomography—like image) is shown next to octreotide scan image (*I*) showing multiple areas of hepatic uptake compatible with neuroendocrine metastases.

depending on the patient population included and sequence parameters. The study by Parikh and colleagues[47] showed AUC, sensitivity, and specificity of 0.839, 74%, and 77%, respectively, through using a threshold ADC cutoff of 1.6 × 10^{-3} mm^2/s (for *b* values 0, 50, and 500 s/mm^2, respectively).

Some potential pitfalls of DWI must be kept in mind when using it for liver lesion characterization. Some overlap exists among cellular benign hepatic lesions (eg, focal nodular hyperplasia and adenoma), metastases, and hepatocellular carcinomas. Moreover, mucinous or necrotic malignant tumors may have no diffusion restriction with correspondingly high ADC, and can be falsely misinterpreted as benign lesions (**Fig. 8**). Therefore, diffusion images should always be interpreted in conjunction with all available conventional

sequences including post—contrast imaging and clinical history.

Assessment of Treatment Response

Considerable interest in advanced MRI techniques such as DWI is because of their potential not only in improving lesion characterization beyond existing conventional techniques, such as T2WI and contrast-enhanced T1WI, but also in providing additional functional information that cannot be obtained using these routine sequences. One potential advantage of DWI is its ability to provide information about the tumor environment, and hence its ability to diagnose and predict treatment response to various systemic and locoregional therapies in patients with liver metastases.[69–71]

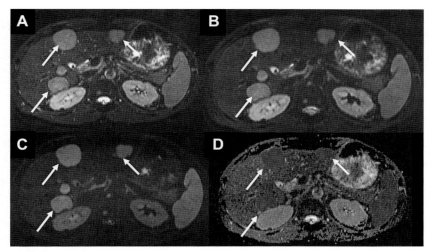

Fig. 6. Neuroendocrine liver metastases in a 51-year-old man. Axial fat-suppressed single-shot echo planar imaging diffusion images (A, $b = 0$ s/mm^2; B, $b = 500$ s/mm^2; C, $b = 1000$ s/mm^2), and ADC map (D, using 0-50-500-1000) show multiple metastatic liver lesions (*arrows*) with restricted diffusion (remaining hyperintense on high b values, with low ADC) in relation with high tumor cellularity.

Koh and colleagues[72] showed an increase in colorectal metastasis ADC in lesions that showed at least a partial response to chemotherapy according to the response evaluation criteria in solid tumors (RECIST). This rise in ADC was not observed in the lesions that showed either no change or disease progression according to conventional RECIST criteria. In another study, an increase in ADC was noted as early as 3 to 7 days after initiation of chemotherapy in responders but not in nonresponders.[73] Another interesting finding was that the colorectal metastases with a high pretreatment ADC responded poorly to chemotherapy, suggesting that tumors that were more necrotic before treatment were more likely to be chemoresistant.[72]

Although these series are small, these findings illustrate the potential value of quantitative ADC measurements in diagnosing and predicting treatment response. However, larger prospective studies are needed to validate these promising results.

LIMITATIONS AND FUTURE DIRECTIONS

DWI is an imaging technique that still often requires varying degrees of optimization to ensure consistent high-quality performance. Some of the limitations of the DWI include poor SNR, limited spatial resolution, susceptibility to motion artifact, and other artifacts, including ghosting, distortion, and blurring. The readers can refer to a recently

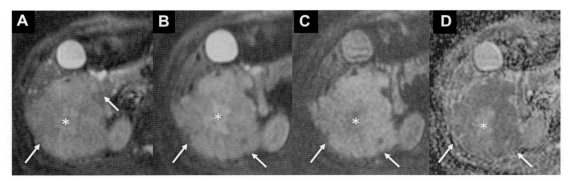

Fig. 7. Partially necrotic liver metastasis from gastrinoma in a 38-year-old man. Axial fat-suppressed single-shot echo planar imaging diffusion images (A, $b = 0$ s/mm^2; B, $b = 50$ s/mm^2; C, $b = 500$ s/mm^2) and ADC map (D, using 0-50-500) show a large metastatic liver lesion (*arrows*) with restricted diffusion (hyperintense on high b values with decreased ADC), except for a small central area of necrosis (*) showing signal drop and higher ADC.

Table 2
Mean ADC of focal liver lesions and cutoff values for diagnosing malignancy

	Kim et al[66,a]	Taouli et al[50,b]	Bruegel et al[67]	Gourtsoyianni et al[68]	Parikh et al[47]
Number of patients/ lesions	126/79	66/52	102/204	38/37	53/211
b values (s/mm^2)	$\leq$846	$\leq$500	50 to 300–600	0–50 to 500–1000	0–50 to 500
ADC values					
Metastases	1.06–1.11	0.94	1.22	0.99	1.50
Hemangiomas	2.04–2.10	2.95	1.92	1.90	2.04
Cysts	2.91–3.03	3.63	3.02	2.55	2.54
ADC cutoff for diagnosis of malignant liver lesions[c]	1.60	1.50	1.63	1.47	1.60
Sensitivity (%)	98	84	90	100	74
Specificity (%)	80	89	86	100	77

[a] ADCs for $b<850$ s/mm^2 are given.
[b] ADCs for $b = 0$ to 500 s/mm^2 are given.
[c] Lesions with apparent diffusion coefficients (ADCs) below the cutoff value are considered malignant, whereas those with ADCs above are considered benign. Malignant lesions include metastases and hepatocellular carcinomas.
Adapted from Taouli B, Koh DM. Diffusion-weighted MR imaging of the liver. Radiology 2010;254:47–66; with permission.

published review article discussing diffusion image optimization.[44] ADC can vary as a result of hardware, human, or biologic factors. Even when using the same MR system, because single-shot echo-planar imaging is prone to inherent low SNR and multiple artifacts, variability in ADC values is possible, as shown in a recent brain diffusion study.[74] Few studies have assessed ADC reproducibility in liver parenchyma,[75,76] but data on liver lesions are limited,[77] and further work

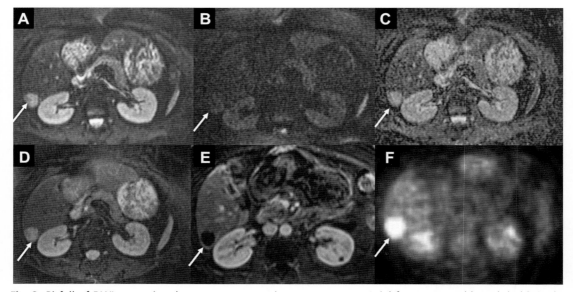

Fig. 8. Pitfall of DWI: necrotic colon cancer metastasis post treatment. Axial fat-suppressed breath-hold single-shot echo planar imaging diffusion images in a 50-year-old man with metastatic colon cancer treated with systemic chemotherapy, obtained using b values of 0 (*A*) and 500 s/mm^2 (*B*) with corresponding ADC map (*C*), T2WI (*D*), and postcontrast image (*E*). The metastatic lesion is hyperintense at $b = 0$ s/mm^2, but shows no diffusion restriction with corresponding high ADC, in relation with its necrotic content, as shown on the postcontrast image. FDG-PET image (*F*) acquired before chemotherapy showed lesion uptake.

evaluating the precision and accuracy of ADC values obtained with different MRI systems will allow studies to be compared reliably and DWI to be applied in clinical practice.

A debate remains about the optimal selection of *b* values for liver imaging. Selection of *b* values affects the ADC measurement, making results from different institutions and studies difficult to compare. A more standardized approach to DWI may help overcome the variability in ADC quantification.[51] Recent studies are evaluating possibility of performing DWI using both low and high *b* values as per the principle of intravoxel incoherent motion DWI to generate perfusion and tissue diffusion information simultaneously.[78,79] Studies are needed to validate these measures in the evaluation of focal liver lesions and treatment response.

SUMMARY

DWI is now available on most commercial scanners, and clinical experience with DWI in evaluating liver disease is expanding. DWI can be used for liver lesion detection and lesion characterization, with better results than with T2WI and potential additional value to contrast-enhanced T1WI sequences, especially in detecting small lesions. Furthermore, in patients who cannot receive gadolinium contrast agents, DWI is a reasonable alternative to contrast-enhanced imaging. However radiologists should be aware of potential pitfalls and limitations of the technique, and the authors suggest that diffusion images should always be interpreted in conjunction with conventional sequences and clinical history. In the authors' opinion, DWI should be a routine component of liver MRI protocols for evaluating metastatic disease to the liver in patients with primary malignancy. The role of DWI for tumor treatment response assessment is promising and should be further investigated.

REFERENCES

1. Kasper HU, Drebber U, Dries V, et al. Liver metastases: incidence and histogenesis. Z Gastroenterol 2005;43(10):1149−57 [in German].
2. Baker ME, Pelley R. Hepatic metastases: basic principles and implications for radiologists. Radiology 1995;197(2):329−37.
3. Martinez L, Puig I, Valls C. Colorectal liver metastases: radiological diagnosis and staging. Eur J Surg Oncol 2007;33(Suppl 2):S5−16.
4. Sharma S, Camci C, Jabbour N. Management of hepatic metastasis from colorectal cancers: an update. J Hepatobiliary Pancreat Surg 2008;15(6):570−80.
5. Ruers T, Bleichrodt RP. Treatment of liver metastases, an update on the possibilities and results. Eur J Cancer 2002;38(7):1023−33.
6. Ravikumar TS, Steele GD Jr. Hepatic cryosurgery. Surg Clin North Am 1989;69(2):433−40.
7. Konopke R, Kersting S, Bergert H, et al. Contrast-enhanced ultrasonography to detect liver metastases: a prospective trial to compare transcutaneous unenhanced and contrast-enhanced ultrasonography in patients undergoing laparotomy. Int J Colorectal Dis 2007;22(2):201−7.
8. Bartolotta TV, Taibbi A, Midiri M, et al. Focal liver lesions: contrast-enhanced ultrasound. Abdom Imaging 2009;34(2):193−209.
9. Quaia E, Bartolotta TV, Midiri M, et al. Analysis of different contrast enhancement patterns after microbubble-based contrast agent injection in liver hemangiomas with atypical appearance on baseline scan. Abdom Imaging 2006;31(1):59−64.
10. Kamel IR, Fishman EK. Recent advances in CT imaging of liver metastases. Cancer J 2004;10(2):104−20.
11. Bonaldi VM, Bret PM, Reinhold C, et al. Helical CT of the liver: value of an early hepatic arterial phase. Radiology 1995;197(2):357−63.
12. Francis IR, Cohan RH, McNulty NJ, et al. Multidetector CT of the liver and hepatic neoplasms: effect of multiphasic imaging on tumor conspicuity and vascular enhancement. AJR Am J Roentgenol 2003;180(5):1217−24.
13. Kanematsu M, Kondo H, Goshima S, et al. Imaging liver metastases: review and update. Eur J Radiol 2006;58(2):217−28.
14. Soyer P, Poccard M, Boudiaf M, et al. Detection of hypovascular hepatic metastases at triple-phase helical CT: sensitivity of phases and comparison with surgical and histopathologic findings. Radiology 2004;231(2):413−20.
15. Fazel R, Krumholz HM, Wang Y, et al. Exposure to low-dose ionizing radiation from medical imaging procedures. N Engl J Med 2009;361(9):849−57.
16. Khalil HI, Patterson SA, Panicek DM. Hepatic lesions deemed too small to characterize at CT: prevalence and importance in women with breast cancer. Radiology 2005;235(3):872−8.
17. Schwartz LH, Gandras EJ, Colangelo SM, et al. Prevalence and importance of small hepatic lesions found at CT in patients with cancer. Radiology 1999;210(1):71−4.
18. Krakora GA, Coakley FV, Williams G, et al. Small hypoattenuating hepatic lesions at contrast-enhanced CT: prognostic importance in patients with breast cancer. Radiology 2004;233(3):667−73.

19. Erturk SM, Ichikawa T, Fujii H, et al. PET imaging for evaluation of metastatic colorectal cancer of the liver. Eur J Radiol 2006;58(2):229–35.

20. Ogunbiyi OA, Flanagan FL, Dehdashti F, et al. Detection of recurrent and metastatic colorectal cancer: comparison of positron emission tomography and computed tomography. Ann Surg Oncol 1997;4(8):613–20.

21. Truant S, Huglo D, Hebbar M, et al. Prospective evaluation of the impact of [18F]fluoro-2-deoxy-D-glucose positron emission tomography of resectable colorectal liver metastases. Br J Surg 2005;92(3): 362–9.

22. Bipat S, van Leeuwen MS, Comans EF, et al. Colo-rectal liver metastases: CT, MR imaging, and PET for diagnosis—meta-analysis. Radiology 2005; 237(1):123–31.

23. Lai DT, Fulham M, Stephen MS, et al. The role of whole-body positron emission tomography with [18F]fluorodeoxyglucose in identifying operable colorectal cancer metastases to the liver. Arch Surg 1996;131(7):703–7.

24. Sahani DV, Kalva SP, Fischman AJ, et al. Detection of liver metastases from adenocarcinoma of the colon and pancreas: comparison of mangafodipir trisodium-enhanced liver MRI and whole-body FDG PET. AJR Am J Roentgenol 2005;185(1):239–46.

25. McFarland EG, Mayo-Smith WW, Saini S, et al. Hepatic hemangiomas and malignant tumors: improved differentiation with heavily T2-weighted conventional spin-echo MR imaging. Radiology 1994;193(1):43–7.

26. Kelekis NL, Semelka RC, Woosley JT. Malignant lesions of the liver with high signal intensity on T1-weighted MR images. J Magn Reson Imaging 1996;6(2):291–4.

27. de Lange EE, Mugler JPIII, Bosworth JE, et al. MR imaging of the liver: breath-hold T1-weighted MP-GRE compared with conventional T2-weighted SE imaging—lesion detection, localization, and charac-terization. Radiology 1994;190(3):727–36.

28. Elsayes KM, Narra VR, Yin Y, et al. Focal hepatic lesions: diagnostic value of enhancement pattern approach with contrast-enhanced 3D gradient-echo MR imaging. Radiographics 2005;25(5):1299–320.

29. Quillin SP, Atilla S, Brown JJ, et al. Characterization of focal hepatic masses by dynamic contrast-enhanced MR imaging: findings in 311 lesions. Magn Reson Imaging 1997;15(3):275–85.

30. Cantwell CP, Setty BN, Holalkere N, et al. Liver lesion detection and characterization in patients with colo-rectal cancer: a comparison of low radiation dose non-enhanced PET/CT, contrast-enhanced PET/CT, and liver MRI. J Comput Assist Tomogr 2008;32(5): 738–44.

31. Reimer P, Rummeny EJ, Daldrup HE, et al. Enhancement characteristics of liver metastases, hepatocellular carcinomas, and hemangiomas with Gd-EOB-DTPA: preliminary results with dynamic MR imaging. Eur Radiol 1997;7(2):275–80.

32. Vogl TJ, Schwarz W, Blume S, et al. Preoperative evaluation of malignant liver tumors: comparison of unenhanced and SPIO (Resovist)-enhanced MR imaging with biphasic CTAP and intraoperative US. Eur Radiol 2003;13(2):262–72.

33. Hammerstingl R, Huppertz A, Breuer J, et al. Diag-nostic efficacy of gadoxetic acid (Primovist)-enhanced MRI and spiral CT for a therapeutic strategy: comparison with intraoperative and histo-pathologic findings in focal liver lesions. Eur Radiol 2008;18(3):457–67.

34. Ward J, Robinson PJ, Guthrie JA, et al. Liver metas-tases in candidates for hepatic resection: comparison of helical CT and gadolinium- and SPIO-enhanced MR imaging. Radiology 2005;237(1):170–80.

35. Grobner T. Gadolinium—a specific trigger for the development of nephrogenic fibrosing dermopathy and nephrogenic systemic fibrosis? Nephrol Dial Transplant 2006;21(4):1104–8.

36. Sadowski EA, Bennett LK, Chan MR, et al. Nephro-genic systemic fibrosis: risk factors and incidence estimation. Radiology 2007;243(1):148–57.

37. Thomsen HS. How to avoid nephrogenic systemic fibrosis: current guidelines in Europe and the United States. Radiol Clin North Am 2009;47(5): 871–5, vii.

38. Le Bihan D. Molecular diffusion nuclear magnetic resonance imaging. Magn Reson Q 1991;7(1):1–30.

39. Bammer R. Basic principles of diffusion-weighted imaging. Eur J Radiol 2003;45(3):169–84.

40. Chiu FY, Jao JC, Chen CY, et al. Effect of intravenous gadolinium-DTPA on diffusion-weighted magnetic resonance images for evaluation of focal hepatic lesions. J Comput Assist Tomogr 2005;29(2): 176–80.

41. Choi JS, Kim MJ, Choi JY, et al. Diffusion-weighted MR imaging of liver on 3.0-Tesla system: effect of intravenous administration of gadoxetic acid disodium. Eur Radiol 2009;20(5): 1052–60.

42. Butts K, Riederer SJ, Ehman RL, et al. Echo-planar imaging of the liver with a standard MR imaging system. Radiology 1993;189(1):259–64.

43. Turner R, Le Bihan D, Chesnick AS. Echo-planar imaging of diffusion and perfusion. Magn Reson Med 1991;19(2):247–53.

44. Taouli B, Koh DM. Diffusion-weighted MR imaging of the liver. Radiology 2010;254(1):47–66.

45. Taouli B, Sandberg A, Stemmer A, et al. Diffusion-weighted imaging of the liver: comparison of navi-gator triggered and breathhold acquisitions. J Magn Reson Imaging 2009;30(3):561–8.

46. Koh DM, Takahara T, Imai Y, et al. Practical aspects of assessing tumors using clinical diffusion-weighted

imaging in the body. Magn Reson Med Sci 2007;6(4):211–24.

47. Parikh T, Drew SJ, Lee VS, et al. Focal liver lesion detection and characterization with diffusion-weighted MR imaging: comparison with standard breath-hold T2-weighted imaging. Radiology 2008;246(3):812–22.

48. Kwee TC, Takahara T, Koh DM, et al. Comparison and reproducibility of ADC measurements in breath-hold, respiratory triggered, and free-breathing diffusion-weighted MR imaging of the liver. J Magn Reson Imaging 2008;28(5):1141–8.

49. Nasu K, Kuroki Y, Nawano S, et al. Hepatic metastases: diffusion-weighted sensitivity-encoding versus SPIO-enhanced MR imaging. Radiology 2006;239(1):122–30.

50. Taouli B, Vilgrain V, Dumont E, et al. Evaluation of liver diffusion isotropy and characterization of focal hepatic lesions with two single-shot echo-planar MR imaging sequences: prospective study in 66 patients. Radiology 2003;226(1):71–8.

51. Padhani AR, Liu G, Koh DM, et al. Diffusion-weighted magnetic resonance imaging as a cancer biomarker: consensus and recommendations. Neoplasia 2009;11(2):102–25.

52. Hussain SM, De Becker J, Hop WC, et al. Can a single-shot black-blood T2-weighted spin-echo echo-planar imaging sequence with sensitivity encoding replace the respiratory-triggered turbo spin-echo sequence for the liver? An optimization and feasibility study. J Magn Reson Imaging 2005;21(3):219–29.

53. Lewin M, Poujol-Robert A, Boelle PY, et al. Diffusion-weighted magnetic resonance imaging for the assessment of fibrosis in chronic hepatitis C. Hepatology 2007;46(3):658–65.

54. Taouli B, Tolia AJ, Losada M, et al. Diffusion-weighted MRI for quantification of liver fibrosis: preliminary experience. AJR Am J Roentgenol 2007;189(4):799–806.

55. Bruegel M, Gaa J, Waldt S, et al. Diagnosis of hepatic metastasis: comparison of respiration-triggered diffusion-weighted echo-planar MRI and five t2-weighted turbo spin-echo sequences. AJR Am J Roentgenol 2008;191(5):1421–9.

56. Coenegrachts K, Delanote J, Ter Beek L, et al. Improved focal liver lesion detection: comparison of single-shot diffusion-weighted echoplanar and single-shot T2 weighted turbo spin echo techniques. Br J Radiol 2007;80(955):524–31.

57. Hardie AD, Naik M, Hecht EM, et al. Diagnosis of liver metastases: value of diffusion-weighted MRI compared with gadolinium-enhanced MRI. Eur Radiol 2010;20(6):1431–41.

58. Zech CJ, Herrmann KA, Dietrich O, et al. Black-blood diffusion-weighted EPI acquisition of the liver with parallel imaging: comparison with a standard T2-weighted sequence for detection of focal liver lesions. Invest Radiol 2008;43(4):261–6.

59. van den Bos IC, Hussain SM, Krestin GP, et al. Liver imaging at 3.0 T: diffusion-induced black-blood echo-planar imaging with large anatomic volumetric coverage as an alternative for specific absorption rate-intensive echo-train spin-echo sequences: feasibility study. Radiology 2008;248(1):264–71.

60. Koh DM, Brown G, Riddell AM, et al. Detection of colorectal hepatic metastases using MnDPDP MR imaging and diffusion-weighted imaging (DWI) alone and in combination. Eur Radiol 2008;18(5):903–10.

61. Naganawa S, Sato C, Nakamura T, et al. Diffusion-weighted images of the liver: comparison of tumor detection before and after contrast enhancement with superparamagnetic iron oxide. J Magn Reson Imaging 2005;21(6):836–40.

62. Low RN, Gurney J. Diffusion-weighted MRI (DWI) in the oncology patient: value of breathhold DWI compared to unenhanced and gadolinium-enhanced MRI. J Magn Reson Imaging 2007;25(4):848–58.

63. Ichikawa T, Haradome H, Hachiya J, et al. Characterization of hepatic lesions by perfusion-weighted MR imaging with an echoplanar sequence. AJR Am J Roentgenol 1998;170(4):1029–34.

64. Namimoto T, Yamashita Y, Sumi S, et al. Focal liver masses: characterization with diffusion-weighted echo-planar MR imaging. Radiology 1997;204(3):739–44.

65. Yamada I, Aung W, Himeno Y, et al. Diffusion coefficients in abdominal organs and hepatic lesions: evaluation with intravoxel incoherent motion echo-planar MR imaging. Radiology 1999;210(3):617–23.

66. Kim T, Murakami T, Takahashi S, et al. Diffusion-weighted single-shot echoplanar MR imaging for liver disease. AJR Am J Roentgenol 1999;173(2):393–8.

67. Bruegel M, Holzapfel K, Gaa J, et al. Characterization of focal liver lesions by ADC measurements using a respiratory triggered diffusion-weighted single-shot echo-planar MR imaging technique. Eur Radiol 2008;18(3):477–85.

68. Gourtsoyianni S, Papanikolaou N, Yarmenitis S, et al. Respiratory gated diffusion-weighted imaging of the liver: value of apparent diffusion coefficient measurements in the differentiation between most commonly encountered benign and malignant focal liver lesions. Eur Radiol 2008;18(3):486–92.

69. Liapi E, Geschwind JF, Vossen JA, et al. Functional MRI evaluation of tumor response in patients with neuroendocrine hepatic metastasis treated with transcatheter arterial chemoembolization. AJR Am J Roentgenol 2008;190(1):67–73.

70. Buijs M, Kamel IR, Vossen JA, et al. Assessment of metastatic breast cancer response to chemoembolization with contrast agent enhanced and diffusion-weighted MR imaging. J Vasc Interv Radiol 2007; 18(8):957–63.

71. Buijs M, Vossen JA, Hong K, et al. Chemoembolization of hepatic metastases from ocular melanoma: assessment of response with contrast-enhanced and diffusion-weighted MRI. AJR Am J Roentgenol 2008;191(1):285–9.

72. Koh DM, Scurr E, Collins D, et al. Predicting response of colorectal hepatic metastasis: value of pretreatment apparent diffusion coefficients. AJR Am J Roentgenol 2007;188(4):1001–8.

73. Cui Y, Zhang XP, Sun YS, et al. Apparent diffusion coefficient: potential imaging biomarker for prediction and early detection of response to chemotherapy in hepatic metastases. Radiology 2008; 248(3):894–900.

74. Sasaki M, Yamada K, Watanabe Y, et al. Variability in absolute apparent diffusion coefficient values across different platforms may be substantial: a multivendor, multi-institutional comparison study. Radiology 2008;249(2):624–30.

75. Braithwaite AC, Dale BM, Boll DT, et al. Short- and midterm reproducibility of apparent diffusion coefficient measurements at 3.0-T diffusion-weighted imaging of the abdomen. Radiology 2009;250(2): 459–65.

76. Dale BM, Braithwaite AC, Boll DT, et al. Field strength and diffusion encoding technique affect the apparent diffusion coefficient measurements in diffusion-weighted imaging of the abdomen. Invest Radiol 2010;45(2):104–8.

77. Koh DM, Blackledge M, Collins DJ, et al. Reproducibility and changes in the apparent diffusion coefficients of solid tumours treated with combretastatin A4 phosphate and bevacizumab in a two-centre phase I clinical trial. Eur Radiol 2009;19(11): 2728–38.

78. Luciani A, Vignaud A, Cavet M, et al. Liver cirrhosis: intravoxel incoherent motion MR imaging—pilot study. Radiology 2008;249(3):891–9.

79. Patel J, Sigmund EE, Rusinek H, et al. Diagnosis of cirrhosis with intravoxel incoherent motion diffusion MRI and dynamic contrast-enhanced MRI alone and in combination: preliminary experience. J Magn Reson Imaging 2010;31(3):589–600.

Hepatic Perfusion Imaging: Concepts and Application

Masoom A. Haider, MD[a,b,]*, Farzin A. Farhadi, MD[a],
Laurent Milot, MD[b]

KEYWORDS

- Liver • MR imaging • Perfusion
- Dynamic contrast enhancement • Cirrhosis
- Hepatocellular carcinoma • Metastases

PERFUSION IMAGING OF THE LIVER

Perfusion imaging of the liver can be described as a quantitative imaging method reflective of hepatic parenchymal and hepatic lesion blood flow. In the realm of magnetic resonance (MR) imaging, perfusion imaging has become synonymous with dynamic contrast-enhanced (DCE) MR imaging. There are other MR imaging methods such as arterial spin labeling (ASL)[1] that can reflect hepatic blood flow but a discussion of this technique is beyond the scope of this review. DCE MR imaging differs from the standard dynamic MR imaging performed in clinical practice in that it involves quantification of enhancement as opposed to qualitative assessment. A key requirement of perfusion imaging is a high temporal resolution (much greater than in routine DCE MR imaging), which is acquired in selected regions.

The diagnostic value of the dynamic enhancement characteristics of the background liver and liver tumor has been well recognized. Terms such as hypervascular, hypovascular, and washout are an important part of the descriptive lexicon of radiologists and play an important role in the differential diagnosis of disease.[2] These terms reflect observations related to altered perfusion states within hepatic tumors and alterations in the balance of hepatic portal and arterial flow. Many studies have been devoted to determining the optimal timing for assessment of lesion vascularity within the constraints of imaging within a breath-hold and the typical qualitative nature of enhancement assessment remains.[3] The lure of quantitative perfusion assessment lies in the ability to improve lesion assessment through objective measures that may be used for characterization of hepatic tumors, assessment of biologic aggressiveness, and of therapeutic response. Perfusion MR imaging indices may also represent a potential biomarker for a variety of diffuse liver diseases through detection of changes in the complex balance of arterial and venous blood flow fractions that may facilitate prognostication and timing of therapeutic intervention.

The increased interest in hepatic perfusion imaging is catalyzed by technologic improvements in MR imaging. Fast gradients have resulted in reduced scan times, and parallel imaging and partial k-space filling methods have further enabled high temporal resolution imaging. Such technological advances permit coverage of much of the liver in scan times of less than 10 seconds using two-dimensional (2D) and three-dimensional (3D) gradient echo sequences thus opening the door for pharmacokinetic analysis based on DCE MR imaging as part of a future clinical routine.

In this review, the methodologies and potential clinical applications of hepatic perfusion with MR imaging are discussed (a glossary of abbreviations is available in **Table 1**).

[a] Joint Department of Medical Imaging, University Health Network and Mount Sinai Hospital, University of Toronto, 610 University Avenue, Toronto, ON M5G 2M9, Canada
[b] Department of Medical Imaging, Sunnybrook Health Sciences Center, University of Toronto, 2075 Bayview Avenue, Toronto, ON M4N 3M5, Canada
* Corresponding author.
E-mail address: m.haider@utoronto.ca

Magn Reson Imaging Clin N Am 18 (2010) 465–475
doi:10.1016/j.mric.2010.07.009

Table 1
Glossary of abbreviations

DCE	Dynamic contrast enhanced
ASL	Arterial spin labeling
DWI	Diffusion-weighted imaging
AIF	Arterial input function
BV	Blood volume
BF	Blood flow
PS, K^{trans}	Permeability surface area product
MTT	Mean transit time
HAF	Hepatic arterial fraction
HPI	Hepatic perfusion index
IAUCC	Initial area under the Gd concentration curve
v_e	Extravascular extracellular volume fraction
$k_{ep}=K^{trans}/v_e$	Efflux rate from extracellular extravascular space to plasma
R2*	Decay constant (1/T2*) related to magnetic susceptibility
TACE	Transarterial chemoembolization

LIVER BLOOD SUPPLY

The liver is uniquely supported by a dual blood supply contributed from the hepatic artery (25%) and the portal vein (75%).[4] The arterial and venous supplies to the liver are not independent systems. There can be several communications between vessels, including trans-sinusoidal, vasal, tumoral, and plexal-peribiliary routes. Decreases in portal blood flow can be compensated for by an increase in arterial flow, thus the arterial perfusion fraction may be an important indicator of underlying hepatic pathology.[5,6] Relative changes in arterial and portal blood supply combined with arterial neoangiogenesis are also important features of primary hepatic tumors such as hepatocellular carcinoma (HCC).[7] Thus, in evaluating the liver parenchyma or primary hepatic tumors, this dual blood supply must be considered. In-flowing blood eventually reaches liver sinusoids and is separated from hepatocytes by fenestrated endothelial cells and the space of Disse. The permeability of the sinusoidal vascular space can be affected in cirrhosis as a result of deposition of collagen in the space of Disse and loss of endothelial fenestration.[8] Such changes may be reflected in the hepatic enhancement kinetics of low-molecular-weight contrast agents used in imaging.

The relative arterial and portal blood supply may be less critical in the assessment of liver metastases, which are considered to be supplied predominantly by the arterial circulation. As such, simpler models based on pure arterial circulation may be sufficient for assessment of tumor perfusion.

METHODOLOGY

In this article the discussion of perfusion MR imaging is limited to T1-weighted DCE MR imaging. This is only one of many techniques available for evaluating hepatic perfusion. Much work in hepatic perfusion has been done with DCE computed tomography (CT) and this work is referenced throughout this review. Both DCE CT and MR imaging use low-molecular-weight chelates, which diffuse rapidly from the vascular space into the interstitial space. In addition, contrast-enhanced ultrasound (CEUS), which unlike CT or MR imaging evaluates the intravascular compartment exclusively, is being investigated for hepatic tumor evaluation and may provide valuable ancillary information.[9,10] Particular advantages of MR imaging include better contrast sensitivity than CT, the lack of ionizing radiation, an increased sensitivity for tumor detection, and the potential to combine perfusion indices with other quantitative MR imaging techniques in the same examination such as diffusion-weighted imaging. There is no current consensus on a standard methodology for perfusion MR imaging of the liver and this is a major issue for broad acceptance and evaluation. Efforts are being made to develop industry-wide standards by the radiology community such as the Quantitative Imaging Biomarkers Alliance (http://qibawiki.rsna.org/).[11]

Analytical approaches can be divided into semi-quantitative methods that characterize enhancement patterns or curves and quantitative methods that typically use pharmacokinetic models of tissue enhancement. For many applications semi-quantitative methods may be sufficient and there is debate regarding the need for complex modeling. A representative scheme for quantitative DCE MR imaging perfusion imaging is presented in **Table 2**. The core components are steps 2, 5, 6, and 7.

Converting MR Imaging Signal to Gadolinium Concentration

To achieve measurements of tumor or liver perfusion in meaningful units (ie, mL/min/100 g) arbitrary image signal intensities on MR images must be converted into concentration of gadolinium. It is assumed that [Gd] is directly proportional to

Table 2
Summary of steps for hepatic perfusion imaging with MR imaging

	Step	Details	Example
1.	Convert MR imaging signal to gadolinium concentration	Requires T1 mapping precontrast and/or phantom for calibration of signal intensity to concentration	Acquire multiflip angle gradient echo images through the liver to calculate baseline T1 of tissue
2.	Acquire rapid DCE image for 120 s or longer after injection of a bolus of contrast agent using an automated injector	Usually a T1 gradient echo image with a temporal resolution of <10 s covering as much of the tumor or liver as possible. Fat suppression is usually avoided	Volume interpolated 3D spoiled gradient echo with 2 direction parallel imaging for a combined reduction factor of 4. Typical injection of Gd-DTPA with automated injector 0.1 mmol/kg at 2 mL/s with 30 mL saline flush at 2 mL/s. Patient instructed to hold breath for arterial run and images acquired during quiet breathing for remainder of acquisition time. Coverage should include aorta and portal vein
3.	Motion correction	Patients cannot hold their breath for the entire length of the DCE acquisition. Motion correction algorithm applied for images acquired during quiet breathing	Proprietary workstation for postacquisition correction. Methods that use breathing information acquired during acquisition may be used such as navigator echoes or respiratory bellows
4.	Arterial input function defined	Operator draws ROI over aorta ± (portal vein)	Proprietary workstation or in-house software used for analysis
5.	Pixelwise- or ROI-based analysis of enhancement curve	Typical end points are either based on pharmacokinetic analysis or more basic enhancement curve properties	Proprietary workstation used for analysis. Pharmacokinetic end points used include total hepatic blood flow, permeability surface area product, hepatic arterial fraction, mean transit time. More basic curve properties include IAUCC contrast arrival time, time to peak, washin rate, washout rate
6.	Segmentation	Define ROI of tumor or lobes of liver	This can be done manually or in an automated or semi-automated fashion from the source data or parametric maps. An example would be to define a liver metastases boundary by looking at the hypervascular rim on an IAUCC map
7.	Summary end point calculated	A summary of the quantitative end point derived as a single number is usually required for clinical application	Median of ROI for each of the parametric maps

Abbreviations: DTPA, diethylene triamine pentaacetic acid; ROI, region of interest.

relaxivity. By measuring baseline tissue T1 before contrast injection and knowing the contrast agents relaxivity it is possible to perform such a conversion (Eq. 1).

$$C_t \sim \frac{1}{r_1 T_{10}} \left(\frac{S(t) - S(0)}{S(0)} \right) \qquad (1)$$

where C_t is the concentration of contrast at time t, r_1 is the relaxivity of contrast agent, T_{10} is the baseline T1 of tissue (precontrast), $S(t)$ is the signal intensity at time t, and $S(0)$ is the signal intensity at $t = 0$.

One common method of measuring T1 is to perform multiple gradient echo images with varying flip angles before contrast injection.[12] This technique is affected by poor B1 homogeneity and although most modern MR imaging scanners have good B1 homogeneity such that determination of B1 homogeneity is not routinely performed, this step does improve the accuracy of DCE MR imaging end point calculation, especially if 3-T systems are being used.[13] Despite these limitations the multi flip angle approach is one of the most commonly used; M_0 and T1 are the unknowns in Eq. 2 and can be solved by curve fitting or analytically.

$$S(\alpha) = M_0 \sin\alpha \frac{1 - e^{-TR/T1}}{1 - \cos\alpha e^{-TR/T1}} \qquad (2)$$

where $S(\alpha)$ is the signal intensity at flip angle α, M_0 is the longitudinal magnetization, and TR is the repetition time.

Other methods such as single breath-hold, segmented, inversion recovery prepared, true fast imaging with steady-state precession (sIR-TrueFISP) have been proposed for optimal T1 mapping, which may be more robust but are not as widely available.[14] One may forego T1 mapping and assume a linear relationship between signal intensity change and change in [Gd] although this may affect the range of results.[15] The optimal approach is highly dependent on the pulse sequences, MR imaging platform, and range of Gd concentrations expected.

The DCE Series

Once the series to calculate a T1 map has been acquired, a DCE series is obtained. A standard low-molecular-weight contrast agent such as Gd-diethylene triamine pentaacetic acid (DTPA) (Magnevist, Bayer-Schering, Germany) is injected into an antecubital vein using an automated injector at a dose of 0.1 mmol/kg at 2 mL/s with a flush of 30 mL of saline. Capturing the peak enhancement time point in the aorta is of importance, thus injection rates that are too rapid may result in missing the arterial peak with acquisition temporal resolutions from 3 to 5 seconds. Typically injection rates of 2 to 4 mL/s are used with Gd-DTPA. The DCE series is typically a T1-weighted spoiled gradient echo sequence (**Table 3**). Sagittal or coronal oblique acquisition planes are typically chosen to facilitate motion correction. The aorta, target lesion (if applicable) and portal vein should be covered in each series. 3D sequences are favored because of their higher signal-to-noise ratio (SNR) and fewer issues with slice excitation profile. For reproducible quantification of DCE MR imaging, higher temporal resolutions in the 1- to 5-second range compared with 15 to 30 seconds for standard dynamic liver MR imaging are necessary. For semi-quantitative approaches (such as often used for focal lesion characterization rather than for determination of therapeutic response), the lower temporal resolutions may be adequate (ie, 10–30 seconds). Images are acquired over the same region repeatedly for 2 to 5 minutes during the injection of the contrast bolus. Several baseline images (2–10 phases) are acquired before injection to ensure stable and high SNR images for baseline signal intensity (S[0]) measurement. The patient is usually instructed to breath quietly during this series. Although breath-hold approaches can be applied, the patient often needs to breath during the critical time when contrast is arriving in the portal vein and arterial washout may be occurring in the tumors, and the resultant poor quality images can negatively affect the analysis. Single breath-hold approaches rely on first-pass perfusion analysis and have the advantage of reducing the need for motion correction.[16] Serial breath-hold approaches improve precision and accuracy compared with single breath-hold approaches but require more patient cooperation.[17]

Motion Correction

If motion correction is not applied the resulting analysis of perfusion can be adversely affected, particularly at the margin of tumors. Various transforms can be applied to register the dynamic series. The simplest approaches involve 2D rigid transforms and help improve precision.[18–20] Inclusion of the right hemidiaphragm in the dynamic series can help to provide a contrast-invariant boundary to further improve motion compensation.

Analysis

The method of image analysis is dependent on several factors including the purpose for which the perfusion parameters will be used and the pulse sequences. Tracer kinetic modeling has the advantage of providing measures that can be

Table 3
An example of MR imaging parameters for a DCE scan of the liver

Pulse Sequence	3D FLASH or 2D FLASH with Non—slice-selective Inversion or Saturation 3D Preferred
TR	Minimum
TE	Minimum
Plane	Oblique coronal or sagittal to include aorta, portal vein and tumor. Tumor and vessels preferably near center slice. Include diaphragm to help with motion correction
Phase encoding	Anterior-posterior or left-right
Reduction factor	2 or more
Flip angles for T1 mapping	$2-14°$
Flip angle for DCE	$14-20°$
Temporal resolution	3 s or less preferred to minimize breathing motion artifact
Respiration	Quiet breathing or serial breath-hold
Matrix	128—256 (frequency) × 128 (phase)
Gadolinium	0.2 mmol/kg at 2 mL/s and 30 mL saline flush at 2 mL/s using automated injector. Start injection after a few phases (ie, 5) of multiphase DCE scan have been acquired
Total scan time for DCE series	2—5 min
Fat suppression	Off
Slice thickness	8—10 mm

Abbreviations: FLASH, fast low-angle shot; TE, echo time.

related to microvasculature. Model-free approaches have the advantage of being simple to perform.

For model-free approaches, the spleen has been used as a control tissue to help define the enhancement kinetics of the hepatic arterial circulation. The hepatic perfusion index (HPI) was proposed by Miles and colleagues[21] (Eq. 3):

$$HPI = AP/(AP+PP) \times 100\% \qquad (3)$$

where arterial perfusion (AP) = maximum slope of liver enhancement ($S_{maxliver}$) before time to peak spleen enhancement (T_{sp})/peak aortic enhancement (Ao_p), portal perfusion (PP) = $S_{maxliver}$ after T_{sp}/Ao.

Tracer kinetic modeling involves fitting the [Gd] versus time curve within a region of interest (ROI) or on a voxel by voxel basis. A detailed review of models is beyond the scope of this article. The parameters derived from the model are dependent on the type of model and assumptions that are made. Models typically require measurement of an arterial input function (AIF) and may require definition of a portal venous function as well. Historically measurement of the AIF has been technically difficult with MR imaging for a variety of reasons including time of flight effects, rapid change of signal resulting in difficulty measuring

true peak enhancement, and loss of linearity between signal intensity and [Gd] at high concentrations. Errors in AIF measurement are propagated through the model and this has been a continuing problem in blood flow parameter estimates in liver and other organs.[22] Optimal solutions to the AIF measurement problem with MR imaging are still needed.

The best model for assessing perfusion in the liver remains undefined. Current approaches make many assumptions. The most common models include an AIF or a portal venous input function, use single- or dual-compartment models and may or may not include assumptions about instantaneous mixing of contrast between compartments. Model complexity may not necessarily lead to better clinically applicable results. Typical parameters derived from these models include one or more of the following: blood flow (BF), blood volume (BV, v_b), permeability surface area product (PS, K^{trans}), mean transit time (MTT), hepatic arterial fraction (HAF), and extravascular extracellular space (v_e).

A model commonly used for metastatic disease where the dominant supply is assumed to be arterial is the Toft model (**Figs. 1** and **2**), which is a bidirectional, dual-compartment, single-input model.[23] The second term in Eq. (4) is often dropped with

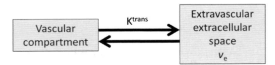

Fig. 1. Toft model.

the assumption that the plasma volume fraction in tissue is small.

$$C_t = DK^{trans} \sum_{i=1}^{2} \frac{e^{-(K^{trans}/v_e)t} - e^{-m_i t}}{m_i - K^{trans}/v_e}$$

$$+ v_p D \sum_{i=1}^{2} a_i e^{-m_i t} \qquad (4)$$

where a_i and m_i are related to the biexponential fit of the AIF, v_e is the extravascular extracellular volume fraction, K^{trans} is the permeability constant, D is the dose of contrast agent, v_p is the plasma volume fraction, k_{ep} is the K^{trans}/v_e efflux rate from extracellular extravascular space to plasma.

The assumption of a dominant arterial supply to metastases may not be true[24,25] and in the surrounding liver is certainly not true. The clinical usefulness of more complex models remains to be seen, however the need for more accurate modeling to reflect true hepatic pathophysiology is recognized[25] Other confounding factors also limit accurate evaluation of perfusion. For example, the very rapid movement of Gd-DTPA, and other low-molecular-weight chelates used in clinical practice, from the vascular space into the interstitium makes it difficult to accurately calculate intravascular compartment parameters such as blood volume with the temporal resolutions of current scanners.

Defining a Summary End Point

For quantitative assessment a summary value must be derived. This can be derived by drawing an ROI on the parametric maps of perfusion parameters generated from semi-quantitative or quantitative modeling and taking a mean or median. Alternatively the ROI can be drawn first on the DCE MR image and then a mean or median can be taken; with this summary curve, a pharmacokinetic model can be fitted or semi-quantitative analysis done to derive a summary value. This latter approach has the advantage of having good SNR, however information regarding tissue heterogeneity is lost. In addition, if there are areas of necrosis within the ROI that do not enhance, these violate the model assumptions and can affect the final result. Alternatively the ROI can be drawn on the parametric map itself. A mean or median value can be used. Within tumors the distribution of values may not be normal and thus a median would be a better summary value (**Fig 3**). ROI placement on a parametric map also permits the assessment of the relative proportion of voxel subgroups within a tumor, and allows estimation of the percentage of nonenhancing tumor; such subgroup analysis may contribute further value to the quantitative tumor evaluation. Variability

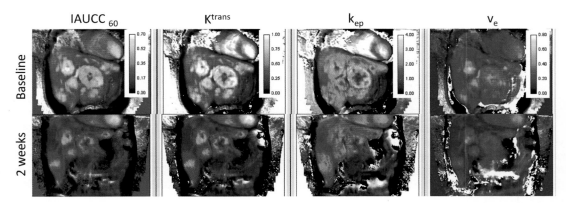

Fig. 2. Toft model parametric maps of renal cell carcinoma metastases treated with a tyrosine kinase inhibitor. Coronal perfusion images were obtained at baseline and 2 weeks after therapy with an antiangiogenic drug in a patient with metastatic renal cell carcinoma to the liver. Parametric maps are displayed on a color scale from black to yellow (see **Fig 3** for scales). IAUCC$_{60}$ is an example of a semi-quantitative parameter; the others are derived from a Tofts model. This model has a single vascular input function and thus is not descriptive of the hepatic parenchyma but is often used for metastases where the dominant supply is assumed to be arterial. There is a clear change in parametric maps at 2 weeks after treatment with a decrease in all parameters within the tumors.

ROI from IAUC map

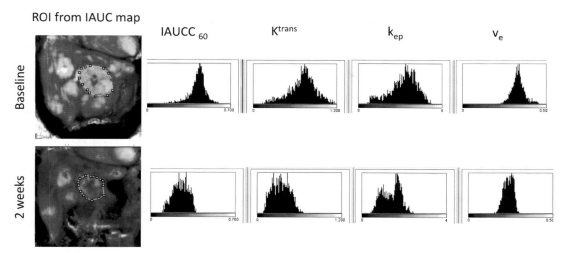

Fig. 3. Summary of response parameters. $IAUCC_{60}$ maps are derived from coronal DCE MR imaging data from the same patient as in see **Fig 2**, which have been motion corrected (*left*). ROIs are manually drawn on the $IAUCC_{60}$ maps around a target lesion. From this ROI the distribution of each of the pharmacokinetic parameters is displayed as a histogram in the 4 graphs (*horizontal*) before and after therapy (*vertical*). This can be done as a 2D or 3D ROI. Histograms show a decrease in the mean and median of all distributions. Note that the distributions are not normal and important information regarding response behavior may reside in other end points derived from these distributions.

in definition of ROI boundaries can introduce variability in end points as much of the dynamic vascular changes occur at the margin of tumors. Our approach has been to use the initial area under the Gd concentration curve (IAUCC) maps for visual assessment of ROI boundaries. The optimal approach may be to use semi-automated segmentation to help reduce interobserver variability.

CLINICAL APPLICATIONS
Therapeutic Response Assessment

The interest in using MR liver perfusion imaging for therapy response assessment is based on the introduction of antiangiogenic therapies in clinical practice for cancers including HCC[26] and renal cell carcinoma.[27] These therapies curb new vessel formation and thus tumor growth. Such antiangiogenic drugs are costly and often tumor size as

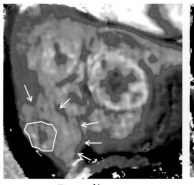

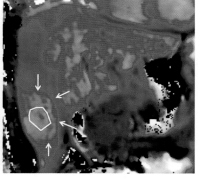

Baseline   2 weeks

Fig. 4. Changes in liver parenchyma (k_{ep} maps). k_{ep} maps derived from coronal DCE MR imaging data from the same patient as in **Fig 2** are shown with a color scale with yellow indicating a higher value and black a lower value. In the same patient there are peritumoral changes occurring (*white arrows*), particularly in the hepatic parenchyma surrounding the metastases (*white ROI*). The Toft model is probably not the best for characterization of the liver parenchyma, because it does not reflect the dual vascular supply. Changes in parenchyma have been quantified using HPI which is increased in metastatic disease[21] and further work in assessment of these changes using 2-compartment dual-input models is also being pursued in the hopes that this may provide prognostic information.

Table 4
Summary table of techniques for DCE

DCE Technique	(Promising) Indications	Advantage(s)	Limitation(s)
MR imaging model-based with dual-input function	Therapy response assessment Determine degree of cirrhosis or severity of diffuse liver disease Characterization of hepatic arterial fraction in disease that affects the balance of portal and arterial perfusion such as HCC and cirrhosis	Extraction of quantitative data is based on physiologic parameters	Analysis is time intensive Requires expertise knowledge in personnel and specialized propriety hardware and software No consensus/standardized model because based on differing physiologic assumptions No standard operating procedure for image acquisition Experience with MR imaging setting is limited and optimized pulse sequences to give good input function measures are needed
MR imaging model-based with single AIF	Therapy response assessment with assumption of dominant arterial supply to hepatic tumor	Extraction of quantitative data is based on physiologic parameters	Analysis is time and cost intensive although less complex than dual-input function model Limitations are similar to dual-input function model approaches
HPI	May be a predictor of metastatic disease to the liver (CT) Determining severity of cirrhosis (Child-Pugh class)	Simple to derive, calculate and compare across time and institutions Takes into account the dual blood supply of the liver	Relies on the spleen as a control tissue, which may lead to problems if spleen is affected by the pathophysiologic process Parameter is not directly quantifiable as a blood flow measurement (ie, mL/min/100 g of tissue)
IAUCC	Measure of early therapeutic response to therapies for metastatic disease such as antiangiogenic drugs	Relatively robust and insensitive to noise Correlated with PS Easy to calculate	Parameter is not directly quantifiable as a blood flow measurement (ie, mL/min/100 g of tissue)
CT	All the same indications as MR imaging	Readily available Linear relationship of signal to iodine concentration	Sensitivity to small concentrations of contrast is limited Large radiation doses limit repeated application Limited coverage of tissues (this is improving with newer multidetector scanners)

measured using Response Evaluation Criteria in Solid Tumors (RECIST) criteria[28] reflects poorly on drug activity, particularly in the early stages of treatment. As the variety of drugs increases it may be of value to determine those responding best to the treatment by using parameters derived from DCE MR imaging as early biomarkers of therapeutic response. Approaches to evaluation have ranged from simply assessing percent enhancement of tumors from standard pre- and postcontrast CT to determining changes in HPI and data from pharmacokinetic modeling. Simple enhancement assessment is showing promise in CT trials. The best known simple criteria is the Choi criteria defined as a 10% decrease in tumor size or a 15% decrease in tumor density on contrast-enhanced CT.[29] Such enhancement criteria have been shown to predict outcome in renal cell carcinoma being treated with tyrosine kinase inhibitors. In a recent CT study of 53 patients, Smith and colleagues[30,31] showed a favorable response based on the modified Choi criteria, at a median of 61 days after therapy, had a sensitivity of 75% and specificity of 100% for identifying patients with progression-free survival of more than 250 days, versus 16% and 100% for RECIST criteria. Other studies performed to date have involved small groups of patients using HPI with MR imaging or CT.[32,33] HPI has been shown to be increased in patients with cirrhosis (median 0.65, range 0.3–1) and metastatic disease (median 0.65, range 0.4–1).[21] Transarterial chemoembolization and radiofrequency ablation response and recurrence may benefit form liver perfusion assessment.[34,35] The precise clinical role of hepatic perfusion MR imaging in therapeutic response assessment has yet to be established and its advantage over CT for this application remains uncertain. The commonest end points used for assessment of therapy response in liver and other metastases are IAUCC$_{60}$ (initial area under the Gd concentration versus time curve at 60 seconds from contrast arrival) and K^{trans} (Figs. 2–4).

Cirrhosis and HCC

Much of the work related to cirrhosis perfusion assessment has been done with DCE CT. In cirrhosis, an increase in hepatic arterial perfusion and decrease in portal vein perfusion has been described.[21,36,37] DCE-related parameters have been shown to correlate with the severity of cirrhosis.[38] Hepatic perfusion changes reported in cirrhosis include portal perfusion decrease but MTT and arterial fraction increase.[39,40] In a DCE MR imaging study using a dual-input

single-compartment model, Hagiwara and colleagues[41] have shown that MTT, distribution volume, and arterial flow are good predictors of liver fibrosis with a sensitivity of 76.9% to 82.4% and a specificity of 76.9% to 84.6%. As hepatic perfusion MR imaging is refined it is possible that these parameters may help predict advancing cirrhosis but further study is required.

It is possible that characterization of relative arterial versus portal circulation in HCC may have benefit in improving diagnosis and characterizing nodules in cirrhosis. This is done in a qualitative sense when arterial versus portal venous enhancement patterns are assessed. MR imaging is the best modality for assessment of small nodules in cirrhosis but the overall performance of imaging in this setting is still in need of improvement. Sahani and colleagues[42] have shown BF, BV, and PS are decreased in poorly differentiated HCC.[42] A biomarker of aggressiveness of small nodules in cirrhosis would be of great value in triaging patients for therapy.

SUMMARY

Noninvasive assessment of hepatic perfusion with MR imaging is a complex task because of a variety of factors ranging from the difficulties with MR imaging quantification to modeling the complex nature of hepatic diseases. For DCE MR imaging of the liver to become part of clinical practice, standardized operating procedures are needed that will allow further evaluation. The combined used of simple perfusion MR imaging methods with other methods of tissue characterization such as DWI, ASL, R2* mapping, and fat quantification may allow for improved characterization and prognostication in liver disease and focal hepatic lesion assessment. A summary of DCE MR imaging techniques is shown in **Table 4**.

ACKNOWLEDGMENTS

The authors would like to thank Professor Gregory Stanisz, Dr Georg Bjarnason and Colleen Bailey from Sunnybrook Health Sciences Center in Toronto for contributing source data and Alastair J. Martin, PhD, for his editorial comments on this manuscript.

REFERENCES

1. De Bazelaire C, Rofsky NM, Duhamel G, et al. Arterial spin labeling blood flow magnetic resonance imaging for the characterization of metastatic renal cell carcinoma (1). Acad Radiol 2005;12(3):347–57.
2. Elsayes KM, Narra VR, Yin Y, et al. Focal hepatic lesions: diagnostic value of enhancement pattern

approach with contrast-enhanced 3D gradient-echo MR imaging. Radiographics 2005;25(5):1299–320.

3. Hussain HK, Londy FJ, Francis IR, et al. Hepatic arterial phase MR imaging with automated bolus-detection three-dimensional fast gradient-recalled-echo sequence: comparison with test-bolus method. Radiology 2003;226(2):558–66.

4. Chiandussi L, Greco F, Sardi G, et al. Estimation of hepatic arterial and portal venous blood flow by direct catheterization of the vena porta through the umbilical cord in man. Preliminary results. Acta Hepatosplenol 1968;15(3):166–71.

5. Richter S, Mucke I, Menger MD, et al. Impact of intrinsic blood flow regulation in cirrhosis: maintenance of hepatic arterial buffer response. Am J Physiol Gastrointest Liver Physiol 2000;279(2): G454–62.

6. Gulberg V, Haag K, Rossle M, et al. Hepatic arterial buffer response in patients with advanced cirrhosis. Hepatology 2002;35(3):630–4.

7. Matsui O. Imaging of multistep human hepatocarcinogenesis by CT during intra-arterial contrast injection. Intervirology 2004;47(3-5):271–6.

8. Martinez-Hernandez A. The hepatic extracellular matrix. II. Electron immunohistochemical studies in rats with CCl4-induced cirrhosis. Lab Invest 1985; 53(2):166–86.

9. Brannigan M, Burns PN, Wilson SR. Blood flow patterns in focal liver lesions at microbubble-enhanced US. Radiographics 2004;24(4):921–35.

10. Qi XL, Burns P, Hong J, et al. Characterizing blood volume fraction (BVF) in a VX2 tumor. Magn Reson Imaging 2008;26(2):206–14.

11. Quantitative Imaging Biomarkers Alliance (QIBA). RSNA. Available at: http://qibawiki.rsna.org/index.php?title=MR_Acquisition_Protocols. Accessed July 27, 2010.

12. Wang HZ, Riederer SJ, Lee JN. Optimizing the precision in T1 relaxation estimation using limited flip angles. Magn Reson Med 1987;5(5):399–416.

13. Treier R, Steingoetter A, Fried M, et al. Optimized and combined T1 and B1 mapping technique for fast and accurate T1 quantification in contrast-enhanced abdominal MRI. Magn Reson Med 2007; 57(3):568–76.

14. Bokacheva L, Huang AJ, Chen Q, et al. Single breath-hold T1 measurement using low flip angle TrueFISP. Magn Reson Med 2006;55(5):1186–90.

15. Bokacheva L, Rusinek H, Chen Q, et al. Quantitative determination of Gd-DTPA concentration in T1-weighted MR renography studies. Magn Reson Med 2007;57(6):1012–8.

16. Jackson A, Haroon H, Zhu XP, et al. Breath-hold perfusion and permeability mapping of hepatic malignancies using magnetic resonance imaging and a first-pass leakage profile model. NMR Biomed 2002;15(2):164–73.

17. Orton MR, Miyazaki K, Koh DM, et al. Optimizing functional parameter accuracy for breath-hold DCE-MRI of liver tumours. Phys Med Biol 2009; 54(7):2197–215.

18. Melbourne A, Atkinson D, White MJ, et al. Registration of dynamic contrast-enhanced MRI using a progressive principal component registration (PPCR). Phys Med Biol 2007;52(17):5147–56.

19. Noseworthy MD, Haider MA, Sussman MS, et al. Free-breathing motion compensation using template matching: a technique allowing for tracer kinetic modeling of liver metastases. J Comput Assist Tomogr 2007;31(2):193–7.

20. Buonaccorsi GA, Roberts C, Cheung S, et al. Tracer kinetic model-driven registration for dynamic contrast enhanced MRI time series. Med Image Comput Comput Assist Interv 2005;8(Pt 1):91–8.

21. Miles KA, Hayball MP, Dixon AK. Functional images of hepatic perfusion obtained with dynamic CT. Radiology 1993;188(2):405–11.

22. Roberts C, Buckley DL, Parker GJ. Comparison of errors associated with single- and multi-bolus injection protocols in low-temporal-resolution dynamic contrast-enhanced tracer kinetic analysis. Magn Reson Med 2006;56(3):611–9.

23. Tofts PS. Modeling tracer kinetics in dynamic Gd-DTPA MR imaging. J Magn Reson Imaging 1997; 7(1):91–101.

24. Liu Y, Matsui O. Changes of intratumoral microvessels and blood perfusion during establishment of hepatic metastases in mice. Radiology 2007;243(2):386–95.

25. Koh TS, Thng CH, Lee PS, et al. Hepatic metastases: in vivo assessment of perfusion parameters at dynamic contrast-enhanced MR imaging with dual-input two-compartment tracer kinetics model. Radiology 2008;249(1):307–20.

26. Llovet JM, Ricci S, Mazzaferro V, et al. Sorafenib in advanced hepatocellular carcinoma. N Engl J Med 2008;359(4):378–90.

27. Escudier B, Eisen T, Stadler WM, et al. Sorafenib in advanced clear-cell renal-cell carcinoma. N Engl J Med 2007;356(2):125–34.

28. Eisenhauer EA, Therasse P, Bogaerts J, et al. New response evaluation criteria in solid tumours: revised RECIST guideline (version 1.1). Eur J Cancer 2009; 45(2):228–47.

29. Benjamin RS, Choi H, Macapinlac HA, et al. We should desist using RECIST, at least in GIST. J Clin Oncol 2007;25(13):1760–4.

30. van der Veldt AA, Meijerink MR, van den Eertwegh AJ, et al. Choi response criteria for early prediction of clinical outcome in patients with metastatic renal cell cancer treated with sunitinib. Br J Cancer 2010;102(5):803–9.

31. Smith AD, Lieber ML, Shah SN. Assessing tumor response and detecting recurrence in metastatic renal cell carcinoma on targeted therapy: importance of size

and attenuation on contrast-enhanced CT. AJR Am J Roentgenol 2010;194(1):157—65.

32. Meijerink MR, van Cruijsen H, Hoekman K, et al. The use of perfusion CT for the evaluation of therapy combining AZD2171 with gefitinib in cancer patients. Eur Radiol 2007;17(7):1700—13.

33. Miyazaki K, Collins DJ, Walker-Samuel S, et al. Quantitative mapping of hepatic perfusion index using MR imaging: a potential reproducible tool for assessing tumour response to treatment with the antiangiogenic compound BIBF 1120, a potent triple angiokinase inhibitor. Eur Radiol 2008;18(7):1414—21.

34. Chen G, Ma DQ, He W, et al. Computed tomography perfusion in evaluating the therapeutic effect of transarterial chemoembolization for hepatocellular carcinoma. World J Gastroenterol 2008;14(37):5738—43.

35. Meijerink MR, van Waesberghe JH, van der Weide L, et al. Early detection of local RFA site recurrence using total liver volume perfusion CT initial experience. Acad Radiol 2009;16(10):1215—22.

36. Bolton RP, Mairiang EO, Parkin A, et al. Dynamic liver scanning in cirrhosis. Nucl Med Commun 1988;9(3):235—47.

37. Blomley MJ, Coulden R, Dawson P, et al. Liver perfusion studied with ultrafast CT. J Comput Assist Tomogr 1995;19(3):424—33.

38. Hashimoto K, Murakami T, Dono K, et al. Assessment of the severity of liver disease and fibrotic change: the usefulness of hepatic CT perfusion imaging. Oncol Rep 2006;16(4):677—83.

39. Annet L, Materne R, Danse E, et al. Hepatic flow parameters measured with MR imaging and Doppler US: correlations with degree of cirrhosis and portal hypertension. Radiology 2003;229(2):409—14.

40. Van Beers BE, Leconte I, Materne R, et al. Hepatic perfusion parameters in chronic liver disease: dynamic CT measurements correlated with disease severity. AJR Am J Roentgenol 2001;176(3):667—73.

41. Hagiwara M, Rusinek H, Lee VS, et al. Advanced liver fibrosis: diagnosis with 3D whole-liver perfusion MR imaging—initial experience. Radiology 2008;246(3):926—34.

42. Sahani DV, Holalkere NS, Mueller PR, et al. Advanced hepatocellular carcinoma: CT perfusion of liver and tumor tissue—initial experience. Radiology 2007;243(3):736—43.

Magnetic Resonance Imaging of Biliary Tumors

Celso Matos, MD*, Eva Serrao, MD, Maria Antonieta Bali, MD

KEYWORDS
- Biliary system • Biliary malignancies • Gallbladder cancer
- Cholangiocarcinoma • Magnetic resonance imaging

BILE DUCT IMAGING

Magnetic resonance (MR) imaging has been accepted as a major noninvasive diagnostic modality for investigating the bile ducts. MR imaging with MR cholangiopancreatography (MRCP) may be used as a replacement for diagnostic endoscopic retrograde cholangiopancreatography (ERCP) in many indications and has gained acceptance by gastroenterologists, surgeons, and general practitioners because of its high success rate, and because of the ability to project a virtual cholangiogram image display.

MR imaging assessment of bile duct morphology may be combined with evaluation of the liver parenchyma, adjacent soft tissues, and vascular network for biliary tumor detection, staging, and surgical planning. Rapid T1- and T2-weighted sequences with high spatial resolution are commonly available as a result of the technological advances in MR imaging. Furthermore, the detection of hepatobiliary malignancy through the use of nonconventional MR imaging techniques has become more readily accessible because of the advances in functional MR techniques in the abdomen, such as diffusion-weighted imaging (DWI) with high b values and acceptable signal-to-noise ratio. This article discusses the current MR imaging techniques for the diagnosis of biliary tumors. Emphasis is placed on the importance of a comprehensive protocol that includes: T2-weighted imaging and MRCP, gadolinium-enhanced T1-weighted imaging, and DWI. Imaging characteristics that may indicate a specific diagnosis of biliary tumor are described.

MR IMAGING TECHNIQUE
General Considerations

Comprehensive MR imaging of biliary tumors should:

1. Show the size and location of a primary lesion and assess the longitudinal and radial extent of bile duct involvement
2. Enable the characterization of a biliary stenosis
3. Show involvement of the hepatic artery (main and lobar branches) and portal vein (main and lobar branches) with the tumor, for the purpose of surgical planning
4. Depict the presence and extent of liver invasion and lobar atrophy or hypertrophy
5. Enable the detection of regional lymph nodes and metastases.

To achieve such a level of assessment, MR imaging should be performed at high field strength using multichannel, phased-array coils, parallel imaging technology, and ideally before any biliary drainage procedure. Such an approach allows high-resolution images to be obtained with substantially reduced acquisition times.

The major advantage of parallel imaging is a reduction in acquisition time. Parallel imaging in conjunction with turbo spin-echo (TSE) T2-weighted sequences, allows shortening of the

MR Imaging Division, Department of Radiology, Cliniques Universitaires de Bruxelles, Hôpital Erasme, Université Libre de Bruxelles, Route de Lennik 808, B-1070, Belgium
* Corresponding author.
E-mail address: cmatos@ulb.ac.be

Magn Reson Imaging Clin N Am 18 (2010) 477–496
doi:10.1016/j.mric.2010.08.004

mri.theclinics.com

echo train length without loss of spatial resolution, and consequently decreases signal decay and reduces image blurring. The use of parallel imaging to shortening the acquisition time is also beneficial in gradient-echo (GRE) T1-weighted imaging, because it permits image acquisition within a breath hold. A further advantage of parallel imaging is the reduction in geometric distortion and image ghosting when it is used in combination with modern fat suppression schemes, which is particularly helpful for DWI.

DWI of the liver is of particular interest as a means of exploring new contrast mechanisms in which signal intensity reflects the degree of restriction of microscopic water movements in tissues and is correlated to tissue cellularity, the integrity of cell membranes, and the amount of tissue fibrosis. DWI is therefore a sensitive sequence for the detection of tumors and inflammation and may be beneficial in the assessment of patients with contraindications for gadolinium administration.[1] In addition, DWI has the potential advantage of performing quantitative data analysis through the generation of apparent diffusion coefficient (ADC) maps, which could contribute to objective disease assessment and monitoring of response to therapy. With modern MR scanners a complete assessment of the biliary system and its surrounding tissues can be performed in approximately 30 minutes.

Practical Setup

Patients are required to fast for 4 to 6 hours before the examination, to permit gallbladder distension and promote gastric emptying. The presence of a large amount of fluid in the bowel may interfere with image interpretation because of the visualization of overlapping bowel loops. Strategies to overcome the potential obscuring of biliary structures by fluid in bowel include the administration of a T2-negative oral contrast agent (iron oxide particles, or pineapple juice or 1 mL of gadolinium mixed with 50 mL of water).[2,3] However, duodenal distension may be desirable when detailed visualization of the duodenal papilla and the confluence of bile and pancreatic ducts is required. In such selected patients duodenal distension may be achieved with administration of secretin, which stimulates pancreatic exocrine fluid and to a lesser extent secretion of bile duct fluid.[4]

The 4 principle sequences used for imaging the hepatobiliary system are:

1. TSE T2-weighted imaging
2. Thick-slab MRCP cholangiogram
3. DWI

4. Pre- and postgadolinium-enhanced volumetric fat-suppressed GRE T1-weighted imaging.

Sequences

1. *T2-weighted sequence:* Thin section T2-weighted images are acquired in the axial and coronal planes using a single-shot TSE sequence during free breathing with respiratory triggering or a navigator echo, to minimize the need for patient cooperation. The field of view should include the whole liver, the pancreas, and the duodenum, with a typical section thickness of 4 to 5 mm. To preserve the delineation of surrounding anatomy, fat suppression is not routinely applied. The T2-weighted images provide good contrast between lesions with high water content and the adjacent liver and soft tissues and depict the bile ducts and the pancreatic ducts in cross section. The T2-weighted images are also used as a guide for thick-slab MRCP acquisition (**Table 1** and **Fig. 1**).

2. *Single-shot TSE T2-weighted sequence:* Imaging of the bile ducts is obtained with a single-shot TSE T2-weighted sequence using a long echo time (about 1 second) to selectively display fluid-containing bile ducts with high signal intensity and reduce visualization of background soft tissues through a reduction in signal intensity. Our routinely adopted sequence uses a single, 20- to 50-mm-thick section that can be obtained in any desired plane during a single short breath hold (<3 seconds). This approach does not require post-processing and offers high-signal ERCP-like views. At least 2 different planes (coronal and transversal) are acquired, providing selectively display of bile ducts with no respiratory artifact and a good in-plane resolution. The transverse plane is particularly useful when assessing proximal biliary obstruction associated with intrahepatic bile duct dilatation. It allows better evaluation of ductal involvement in tumors of the porta hepatis and better differentiation of the involved liver segments. Alternatively a navigator-based respiratory-triggered three-dimensional (3D) acquisition scheme with longer acquisition time may be implemented, which provides better signal intensity and contrast and better delineation of biliary anatomy and requires less medical interaction. However, in the setting of malignant bile duct obstruction, no statistically significant difference in accuracy between the single thick section and navigator-based respiratory-triggered 3D acquisition has been reported for

Table 1
Suggested MR imaging protocol

Sequence	Parameters
Axial and coronal single-shot TSE T2-weighted	Motion correction: respiratory triggering Echo time: 80 ms; echo train length: 72 Parallel imaging: sense factor 2 in the phase-encoding direction Slice thickness: 4–5 mm Field of view: 400 × 450 Matrix size: 226 × 400
Axial and coronal thick-slab single-shot TSE T2-weighted	Selective fat saturation Echo time: 1000 ms; echo train length: 256 Slice thickness: 20–50 mm Field of view: 250 × 250 Matrix size: 256 × 256
Axial diffusion-weighted SE-EPI	Short inversion time inversion recovery fat suppression (inversion time: 180 ms at 1.5 T) Motion correction: respiratory triggering Repetition time/echo time: 2000 ms/70 ms Parallel imaging: acceleration factor 2 in the phase-encoding direction b values: 0, 150, 1000 s/mm^2 Slice thickness: 5 mm Field of view: 400 × 450 Matrix size: 272 × 189
Axial 3D GRE T1-weighted	Selective fat saturation Motion correction: breath hold (18s) Repetition time/echo time: 3.9 ms/1.9 ms Parallel imaging: sense factor 2 in the phase-encoding direction Slice thickness: 2 mm Field of view: 400 × 400 Matrix size: 192 × 256

evaluating disease extent.[5] Therefore, we prefer the single thick section acquisition scheme to the 3D sequence because it has the advantage of a faster acquisition time and the ability to assess common bile duct physiologic changes with dynamic image acquisition.

3. *DWI*: DWI images are obtained in the axial plane using a respiratory-triggered fat-saturated spin-echo echo planar sequence (SE-EPI) with b values of 0, 150, and 1000 s/mm^2 and the same geometry parameters (number of slices, slice thickness, and field of view) as the TSE T2-weighted acquisition. Although the acquisition time is longer compared with breath-hold techniques such strategy allows acquiring more slices and permits combining both datasets (T2-weighted and diffusion-weighted) in a fused image to increase the conspicuity of diffusion-positive lesions.[6]

4. *T1-weighted sequence*: T1-weighted images may be acquired with two-dimensional GRE (using both in- and out-of-phase echo times) or with 3D GRE sequences. The latter are specifically designed to be used along with intravenous gadolinium administration. A volumetric acquisition is obtained with a breath-hold fat-suppressed technique generally in the axial plane with nearly isotropic voxels. This sequence allows improved spatial resolution and multiplanar reformatting. However, patient cooperation is required. The sequence is repeated at least 3 times to obtain the information in the arterial, portal venous, and delayed phases. To optimize the arterial phase, fluoroscopic triggering of the contrast bolus may be used. Subsequent multiphase angiographic renderings may be reconstructed from the source images using maximum intensity projection (MIP) algorithms.

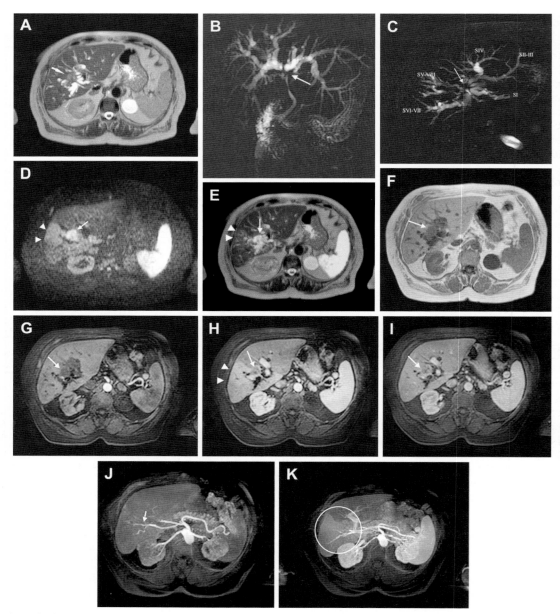

Fig. 1. Hilar cholangiocarcinoma: contribution of different MR sequences routinely used. (*A*) Respiratory-triggered TSE T2-weighted section shows a moderately hyperintense lesion (*arrow*) associated with bile duct dilation in both liver lobes. (*B*) Coronal thick-slab MRCP shows complete narrowing of the bile duct at the porta hepatis (*white arrow*) and associated intrahepatic bile duct dilation. (*C*) Axial thick-slab MRCP (view from below) better shows the multiple strictures involving the different liver segments; the tumor is seen as a signal void (*arrow*). (*D*) b = 1000 s/mm² axial diffusion-weighted SE-EPI confirms and highlights the obstructing hilar mass (*arrow*) consistent with cholangiocarcinoma. An area of decreased perfusion caused by tumor infiltration (*arrowheads*) is better depicted compared with (*A*). (*E*) Fusion imaging displaying both T2-weighted and diffusion-weighted information. (*F*) In-phase GRE T1-weighted section showing a moderately hypointense lesion at the level of the porta hepatis (*arrow*). (*G*, *H*, *I*) Arterial phase (*G*), portal venous phase (*H*) and delayed phase (*I*) fat-suppressed 3D GRE T1-weighted sections show progressive and delayed enhancement of the lesion (*long arrows*) and associated perfusion defect (*arrowheads*). (*J*, *K*) Arterial (*J*) and portal venous (*K*) angiographic renderings display narrowing of segmental hepatic artery (*arrow*) and of corresponding portal vein (*circle*).

BILIARY TUMORS

Most biliary tract tumors are malignant and have traditionally been divided into cancers of the gallbladder, the extrahepatic bile ducts, and the ampulla of Vater, whereas intrahepatic bile duct cancers have been classified as primary liver cancers. More recently cholangiocarcinoma has been used to describe all cancers arising from the epithelial cells of the bile ducts regardless of their location. The most common presenting symptoms of biliary tract cancer are caused by bile duct obstruction and include jaundice, pruritus and weight loss. When bile duct obstruction is distally located (common bile duct and ampulla of Vater) symptoms may occur early. A more insidious course with late symptoms and advanced disease at presentation is associated with proximal bile duct obstruction (intrahepatic and perihilar cholangiocarcinoma, gallbladder carcinoma). Abdominal pain in the right upper quadrant is the most frequent symptom in gallbladder cancer but is not typically associated with cholangiocarcinoma.[7]

Gallbladder Carcinoma

Primary carcinoma of the gallbladder is the most common malignancy of the biliary tract. Most often it occurs in women and the incidence increases steadily with age. Postmenopausal status and cigarette smoking are risk factors.[8] It has been postulated that the most important risk factor is the presence of long-standing gallbladder inflammation, usually related to stones. Although the exact pathogenesis remains unclear there seems to be a metaplasia-dysplasia-carcinoma sequence in the development of most invasive carcinomas of the gallbladder.[9] Nearly 70% of gallbladder carcinomas are diffusely infiltrative lesions, and the remainder show intraluminal polypoid growth.[10] Infiltrative forms are associated with gallstones and are more prone to invade adjacent organs (liver, colon, duodenum, and pancreas) and metastasize to lymph nodes. The spread of gallbladder carcinoma to the liver is common (65% of cases)[10] and is facilitated by the thinness of the muscular layer and the continuity of the connective tissue of the gallbladder wall with the interlobular connective tissue of the liver, facilitating its direct venous drainage to the hepatic veins and spread to lymphatic channels. At diagnosis lymphatic spread is present in more than 50% of patients with gallbladder cancer and usually involves the cystic and pericholedochal nodes initially and subsequently extends into the posterior pancreaticoduodenal, retroportal and celiac nodes; involvement of intercaval nodes occurs later. Because of the late stage of the disease at presentation in most cases,

the therapeutic options are limited (surgery vs palliative therapy). Recent reports suggest that highly selected patients who undergo extended and complete surgical resection have a 5-year survival of 31% compared with an overall survival of 13%.[11] Therefore imaging studies play a major role in optimizing patient selection to appropriate treatment.

MR Imaging Findings

Gallbladder cancer has 3 major patterns of presentation: focal or diffuse mural thickening, a soft-tissue mass occupying or replacing the gallbladder lumen, and an intraluminal polypoid mass.

Mural thickening Focal or diffuse mural thickening of more than 10 mm with marked asymmetry is highly suggestive of the diagnosis.[12] Gallbladder cancer usually shows low- to intermediate signal intensity on T1-weighted sequences and heterogeneous hyperintensity on T2-weighted sequences with a characteristically ill-defined tumor-liver interface. After the administration of gadolinium marked nodular or asymmetric enhancement of the wall is observed during the arterial phase that persists during the venous phases on T1-weighted imaging. When tumor is diffuse or localized in the neck of the gallbladder, bile duct dilatation may be present as a result of associated cystic duct and common hepatic duct involvement (**Fig. 2**). In such circumstances the features may overlap with chronic cholecystitis. Diffuse symmetric mural thickening and smooth contrast enhancement in the early phase and delayed contrast enhancement are suggestive of a benign lesion (**Fig. 3**). Although no reported data are available, in our experience contribution of DWI is limited in this setting, because restricted diffusion is observed with malignant and benign gallbladder disease.

Soft-tissue mass replacement of gallbladder Gallbladder cancer manifesting as a large solid mass replacing the gallbladder may be associated with nonvisualization of the gallbladder and the presence of stones within the mass, which can be helpful in making the diagnosis.[12]

Intraluminal polypoid mass Approximately 25% of gallbladder carcinomas present as an intraluminal polypoid mass. Malignant polypoid lesions are usually larger than 10 mm and may have a thickened implantation base. Lesions exhibit low signal intensity relative to bile on T2-weighted imaging and are therefore easily detected (**Fig. 4**). In contrast to benign lesions that show early enhancement with subsequent washout, malignant lesions show early and prolonged

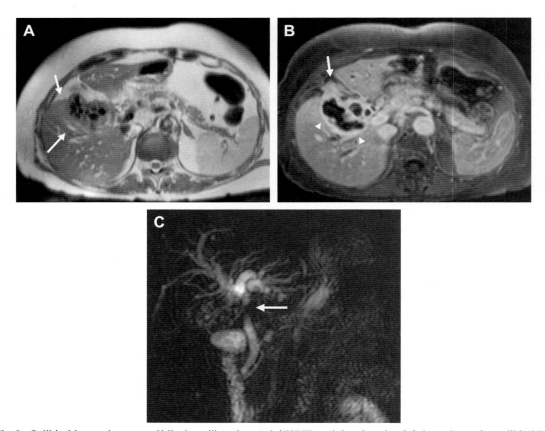

Fig. 2. Gallbladder carcinoma and bile duct dilatation. Axial TSE T2-weighted section (*A*) shows irregular gallbladder wall thickening with ill-defined liver interface (*arrows*). Delayed phase fat-suppressed gadolinium-enhanced T1-weighted section (*B*) shows marked gallbladder wall enhancement (*arrowheads*) and tumor infiltration of the liver (*long arrow*). Corresponding MRCP (*C*) shows invasion of the common hepatic duct and intrahepatic bile duct dilation.

enhancement after contrast administration.[12] The combined use of MR imaging, MRCP, and contrast-enhanced MR angiography has a high sensitivity for detecting direct liver invasion (100%) and lymphadenopathy (nearly 92%) and for identifying the level and the cause of bile duct obstruction (direct tumor invasion or extrinsic compression by the tumor or lymph nodes).[12,13] When bile duct invasion is suspected and conventional MR imaging is not diagnostic, the display of diffusion images fused to conventional MR images may help in identifying the cause without the need for gadolinium administration (see **Fig. 4**).

Cholangiocarcinoma

Cholangiocarcinoma is a malignant epithelial tumor of the biliary tree. It is the second most prevalent primary liver cancer after hepatocellular carcinoma and the incidence is rising in most countries; however, it remains a rare disease comprising less than 2% of malignancies. Only a few patients presenting with cholangiocarcinoma have known risk factors. Recognized risk factors are liver flukes (14% prevalence) and hepatolithiasis (20% prevalence) in endemic areas of southeast Asia, choledochal cyst (10%–20% incidence of malignant degeneration if the cyst is not excised by the age of 20 years), alcohol consumption, diabetes, cirrhosis (10-fold higher risk of developing cholangiocarcinoma than the general population), and primary sclerosing cholangitis (PSC), which is the most important predisposing factor in Western countries (1.5%/y cumulative risk after the development of jaundice).[14–16] Cholangiocarcinomas may develop within the liver parenchyma (intrahepatic form) or involve the biliary tree within the hepatoduodenal ligament and gallbladder (extrahepatic form). Extrahepatic cholangiocarcinomas are divided into hilar, also called Klatskin tumors,[17] or distal. Hilar lesions have been classified by Bismuth and Corlette

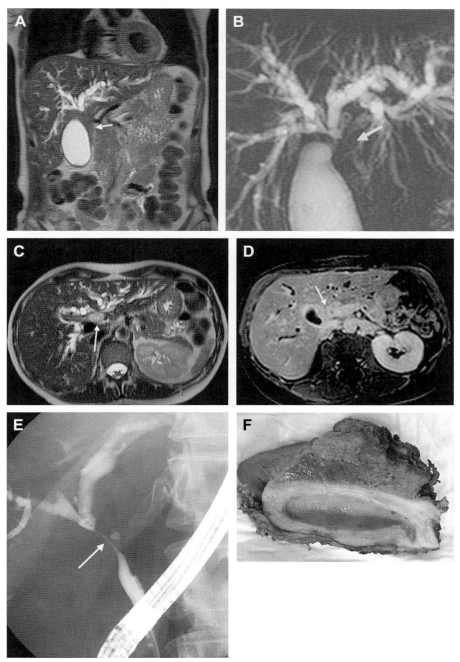

Fig. 3. Chronic cholecystitis and bile duct dilation. Coronal TSE T2-weighted section (*A*) shows homogeneous hy-pointense gallbladder wall thickening (*arrow*), and intrahepatic bile duct dilation. Corresponding MRCP (*B*) shows narrowing of the common hepatic duct (*arrow*). Axial TSE T2-weighted section (*C*) at the level of the porta hepatis shows thickening of the common bile duct wall (*long arrow*). Delayed phase fat-suppressed gadolinium-enhanced T1-weighted section (*D*) shows mild and relatively homogeneous enhancement of the gallbladder wall and of the bile duct wall (*arrow*). ERCP (*E*) more clearly shows the extrinsic compression and associated bile duct stricture (*arrow*). No filling of the cystic duct and of the gallbladder is depicted. Macroscopic pathology of the gallbladder (*F*) displays homogeneous fibrotic thickening of the different layers of the wall including the neck and proximal cystic duct.

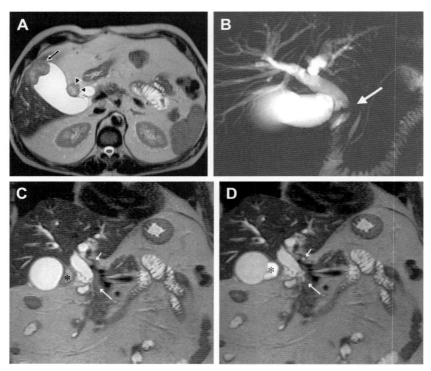

Fig. 4. Gallbladder cancer and bile duct obstruction. Axial TSE T2-weighted section (*A*) shows a polypoid lesion in the gallbladder invading the adjacent liver parenchyma (*black arrow*) and an extraluminal node adjacent to the cystic duct (*arrowheads*). Coronal MRCP projection (*B*) shows short narrowing of the suprapancreatic segment of the common bile duct (*white arrow*) and upstream bile duct dilation. Coronal TSE T2-weighted section (*C*) shows a lesion in the gallbladder neck (*black asterisk*) and lymph nodes adjacent to the hepatic artery (*short white arrow*). The lesion responsible of bile duct narrowing is not well delineated (*long white arrow*). Corresponding fusion imaging (*D*) more clearly shows the lesion causing the bile duct narrowing (*long white arrow*).

into 4 types according to the extent of ductal involvement, from the common hepatic duct (type 1) up to the second-order proximal intrahepatic bile ducts (type 4) (**Table 2**).[18] Hilar tumors represent approximately 60% to 70%, of cholangiocarcinomas. Other extrahepatic cholangiocarcinomas account for 20% to 30%, and intrahepatic cholangiocarcinomas account for 5% to 15% of this tumor type.[19] More than 90% of cholangiocarcinomas are well to moderately differentiated adenocarcinomas with a tendency to develop variable degrees of desmoplastic reaction and early perineural invasion.[20] Most hilar cholangiocarcinomas are associated with a poor prognosis, with an overall 5-year survival of only 1%. Intrahepatic cholangiocarcinoma may present as solid masses (20% to 30%), infiltrate periductal tissues, intraductal-growing, or have mixed characteristics. Extrahepatic cholangiocarcinoma may present as nodular lesions, sclerosing strictures (the most common), or as a papillary-growing lesion (rare and associated with more favorable prognosis).[14]

MR imaging findings

Intrahepatic cholangiocarcinoma: mass-forming type Mass-forming type is usually large, up to 21 cm in diameter, with irregular or lobulated

Table 2 Hilar cholangiocarcinoma Bismuth-Corlette classification	
Type I	Involves the common hepatic duct, distal to the bifurcation of the biliary tree
Type II	Affects the bifurcation
Type IIIa	Affects the right hepatic duct in addition to the bifurcation
Type IIIb	Affects the left hepatic duct in addition to the bifurcation
Type IV	Involves the bifurcation and both right and left hepatic ducts or indicates multifocal cholangiocarcinoma

margins. The MR imaging appearance depends on the degree of fibrosis or coagulative necrosis, cell debris, and mucin production.[21] Most often the lesion is hyperintense and heterogeneous on T2-weighted images and homogeneously hypointense on T1-weighted images. Central areas of low signal or high signal intensity relative to the edge of the tumor may be observed on T2-weighted images. Although the relationship is not linear, in the study by Maetani and colleagues,[21] these features correlated well with the fibrotic ratio difference between the 2 areas. At dynamic MR imaging after gadolinium administration, mass-forming cholangiocarcinoma classically shows moderate peripheral enhancement and progressive pooling of the contrast within the central portion. The area of the tumor with early enhancement and rapid washout indicates active growth, whereas the central area is composed mainly of loose connective tissue with an abundant intercellular matrix.[16] However, delayed enhancement may be variable. In the same study by Maetani and colleagues,[21] regions showing homogeneous delayed enhancement were found to have predominant fibrosis, whereas regions revealing little and delayed enhancement were found to predominantly represent coagulative necrosis. Additional features of cholangiocarcinoma commonly include capsular retraction and occasionally dilatation of the peripheral bile ducts. The presence of ancillary features with cholangiocarcinoma such as capsular retraction, satellite nodules, vascular encasement without tumor thrombus formation, hepatolithiasis, and intrahepatic bile duct dilatation favors an intrahepatic tumor.[16,21] Fig. 5 shows a case of mass-forming cholangiocarcinoma with central coagulative necrosis (hyperintense central area on T2-weighted images and on DWI with mild enhancement on delayed images including images obtained in the hepatospecific phase after intravenous gadolinium ethoxybenzyl diethylenetriamine pentaacetic acid [Gd-EOB-DTPA] administration). As with other lesions atypical patterns of enhancement may be observed. Homogeneous hypervascular enhancement may be seen in well-differentiated cholangiocarcinoma with abundant vasculature in the fibrotic stroma[22] and may therefore simulate a hepatocellular carcinoma, especially in patients with chronic liver disease.[23] Other major differential diagnosis includes metastasis, especially from colorectal origin, which may show retraction of the liver capsule. However, metastatic disease of the liver is uncommon with the background of cirrhosis.

Intrahepatic cholangiocarcinoma: periductal infiltrating type This type of cholangiocarcinoma is characterized by longitudinal growth along a dilated or narrowed bile duct and is radiologically and pathologically identical to infiltrating hilar cholangiocarcinoma (Klatskin tumor). However, the tumor location is different because it is peripheral to the secondary bile ducts. Furthermore, the tumor tends to involve one segment or lobe of the liver. The key diagnostic features include[16]:

- Long-segment stricture with an irregular margin
- Asymmetric narrowing and peripheral ductal dilatation
- Ductal enhancement
- Lymph node enlargement
- Periductal soft-tissue lesion.

In the periphery of the liver a mixed pattern (mass-forming and periductal infiltrative) is more common than a purely periductal infiltrating lesion. The early diagnosis may be difficult before significant narrowing of the bile duct occurs (**Fig. 6**).

Intrahepatic cholangiocarcinoma: intraductal-growing type Macroscopically intraductal-growing type lesions are confined to the bile duct wall and may present as either papillary or polypoid lesions, often spreading along the mucosal surface. In advanced stages the tumor may invade the ductal wall. Microscopic lesions manifest with flat or micropapillary dysplastic epithelium (BilIN1), atypical biliary epithelium (BilIN2), carcinoma in situ (BilIN3), or may coexist.[24,25] Characteristic imaging features include diffuse or focal dilatation of the bile ducts with or without a visible mass. Small lesions along the mucosal surface are difficult or impossible to visualize. Visible lesions are reported to enhance after contrast administration.[16] Variable degrees of bile duct dilatation may be observed. When bile duct dilatation is prominent and associated aneurismal dilatation occurs, mucin production and consequent bile flow obstruction should be suspected.[25] At MR imaging, mucin may have the same signal intensity as bile or manifest as multiple, cordlike filling defects that are better depicted and diagnosed at ERCP (**Fig. 7**). This pattern of intraductal-growing type tumor can be easily differentiated from other cholangiocarcinomas, which are more commonly associated with a space-occupying lesion and segmental stenoses. However, intraductal cholangiocarcinoma may also present as focal narrowing with mild upstream dilatation and no visible mass. If the tumor is not visible by cross-sectional imaging or more invasive

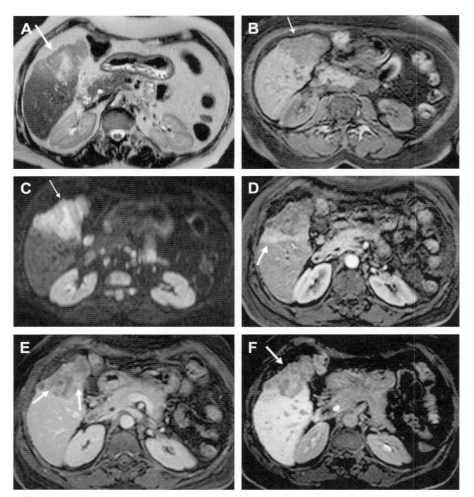

Fig. 5. Mass-forming cholangiocarcinoma. Axial TSE T2-weighted section (*A*) shows a large heterogeneous, hyperintense right liver lobe lesion with capsular retraction (*arrow*). Axial fat-suppressed T1-weighted section (*B*) shows a more homogeneous lesion hypointense relative to adjacent liver. DWI (*C*) shows a cellular malignant-appearing lesion with high water restriction; a central hyperintense area related to central necrosis is depicted. Gd-EOB-DTPA-enhanced T1-weighted sections in the arterial phase (*D*) show irregular peripheral enhancement (*arrow*). Portal venous phase (*E*) illustrates heterogeneous central enhancement of the lesion (*arrows*). On delayed phase (*F*) at 40 minutes no additional contrast enhancement is depicted.

techniques (ERCP, cholangioscopy) the involved hepatic segment may be resected if the patient is considered to be clinically at risk for malignancy.

Intrahepatic cholangiocarcinoma staging

The most important prognostic factors for intrahepatic cholangiocarcinoma are tumor size 3 cm or larger, lymph node metastasis, and vascular invasion.[26–28] Multivariate analysis showed that lymph node metastasis, multiple tumors at presentation, symptomatic tumors, and vascular invasion are independent factors associated with poor postoperative outcome.[26,27]

Cholangiocarcinoma may be difficult to stage accurately with preoperative imaging. According to Okabayashi and colleagues' study,[28] up to 37% of satellite nodules may be missed preoperatively. Assessment of vascular involvement is important and mainly concerns the portal vein. Tumor encasement of the ipsilateral portal vein should be suspected in the presence of segmental or lobar atrophy. The most important limitation of preoperative imaging concerns lymph node involvement because size criteria are predominantly used to predict nodal disease. However, functional MR imaging techniques such as high b value DWI could potentially improve MR imaging

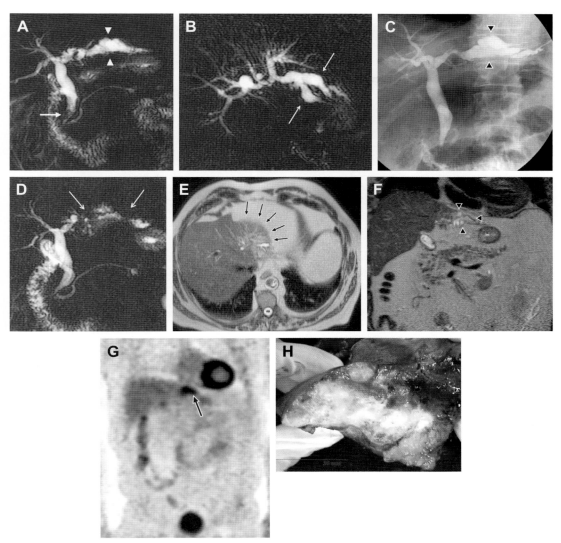

Fig. 6. Intrahepatic cholangiocarcinoma with periductal infiltration. Coronal (*A*) and axial (*B*) MRCP projections show saccular enlargement of the left intrahepatic bile ducts (*arrowheads*) and a distal common bile duct stone. ERCP (*C*) obtained after stone extraction confirms the saccular enlargement (*arrowheads*) and no significant narrowing of the bile ducts. Coronal MRCP projection obtained 1 year later as a result of a high level of CA19.9 (*D*) shows multiple strictures involving the left intrahepatic bile duct (*arrows*). Axial TSE T2-weighted section (*E*) shows a hyperintense lesion (*black arrows*) with irregular margins in the left liver lobe with associated bile duct dilation and parenchymal atrophy. Coronal fusion imaging (*F*) highlights the left liver lobe lesion (*black arrowheads*). Corresponding positron emission tomography scan (*G*) displays an area of hypermetabolic activity matching MR imaging findings. Macroscopic pathology specimen (*H*) shows a white and dense fibrotic tumor with capsular retraction.

detection and characterization of nodal involvement. ADC measurements may be helpful in discriminating between malignant and nonmalignant lymph nodes in the future.[29]

Hilar Cholangiocarcinoma

Klatskin tumors originate from the right and left hepatic ducts and from the common hepatic duct. At these locations lesions are most commonly of the infiltrating type (>70%) and less frequently they manifest as exophytic or polypoid lesions. Infiltrative growth by a scirrhous adenocarcinoma is usually observed at histologic examination.[26] The role of MR imaging is to detect and characterize the tumor, and determine resectability. On cross-sectional MR imaging the lesion

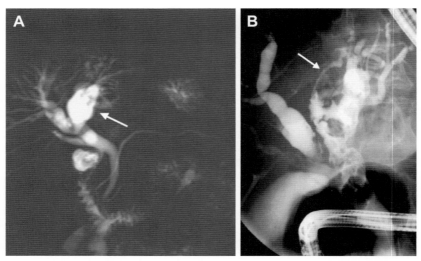

Fig. 7. Intraductal papillary mucinous tumor. MRCP (*A*) shows aneurysmal dilation of the left intrahepatic bile ducts (*arrow*). Corresponding ERCP (*B*) shows multiple filling defects related to mucin production (*arrow*).

appears most often as ill-defined, moderately hypointense or isointense on T1-weighted images and mildly hyperintense or isointense on T2-weighted images relative to adjacent liver parenchyma.[30–33] Although it is not a sensitive feature, thickening of the ductal wall more than 5 mm is suggestive of cholangiocarcinoma.[31] In our experience, adding DWI to conventional cross-sectional T2-weighted, T1-weighted, and MRCP sequences is helpful in the detection of obstructive lesions (**Fig. 8**). Therefore we include DWI as part of our routine protocol when assessing the cause of bile duct obstruction.

In the setting of hilar cholangiocarcinoma, the principle role of MRCP is to determine the level of biliary obstruction, to evaluate the morphology of the corresponding stricture, and to assess the longitudinal and the radial extent of bile ducts involvement according to the classification of Bismuth-Corlette.[18] Benign stenoses usually appear as regular, symmetric, and smooth-shaped narrowing of the lumen, whereas an abrupt, irregular, and asymmetric luminal narrowing is suggestive of malignant obstruction. The accuracy of characterization of stenoses with MRCP and ERCP has been shown to be comparable.[34] In a series of 99 patients with hilar cholangiocarcinoma, MRCP accurately determined the longitudinal extension of the tumor in 88% of the patients.[35] In another comparative study with ERCP, MRCP enabled the correct diagnosis of ductal involvement in 31 of 33 patients.[32]

Hilar cholangiocarcinoma staging
The staging of hilar or Klatskin cholangiocarcinomas is described in **Table 3**. Understaging of

cholangiocarcinoma may occur if there is lack of recognition of submucosal spread in involved bile ducts. At MRCP signal void between the right and left hepatic ducts is a typical finding of infiltrating hilar cholangiocarcinoma, which may or may not be associated with a visibly thickened wall. To avoid this pitfall, it is important to carefully evaluate signal voids along to determine the radial extent of the tumor. The axial thick-slab TSE T2-weighted cholangiographic views obtained at the hilum are the most informative about the number of strictures and the involvement of the different liver segments, including caudate lobe (see **Fig. 8; Figs. 9** and **10**). Dilatation of the intrahepatic bile ducts in a single and small hepatic lobe with hypertrophy of the contralateral lobe suggests the atrophy-hypertrophy complex, as seen with tumors chronically obstructing a single lobe and invading the ipsilateral portal vein (see **Fig. 8**).[36] Hilar cholangiocarcinomas have a variable pattern of enhancement after intravenous gadolinium chelates administration. Heterogeneous and delayed enhancement may be observed in those lesions with significant fibrosis.[30] In the study by Vogl and colleagues[32] improved visualization of the tumor was observed in the arterial-dominant phase because of corresponding enhancement of the bile duct walls. Enhancement of involved bile ducts during the arterial-dominant phase was marked (observed in 84.5% of their patients) compared with enhancement of noninvolved bile ducts and it persisted in the portal venous phase in all but 2 patients. It has been reported that adding contrast-enhanced dynamic images to

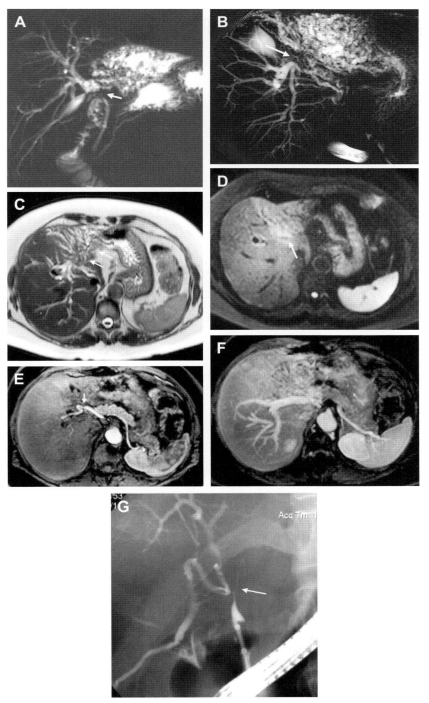

Fig. 8. Periductal infiltrating cholangiocarcinoma pT2N0Mx. Coronal MRCP projection (*A*) shows narrowing of the common hepatic duct (*short arrow*) and dilatation of the left intrahepatic bile ducts. Corresponding axial MRCP projection (*B*) better displays left and right intrahepatic bile ducts and caudate lobe involvement. The signal void area (*long arrow*) corresponds to the tumor. Axial TSE T2-weighted section (*C*) at the level of the porta hepatis shows an infiltrative, ill-defined lesion (*white arrows*) associated with lobar atrophy. Corresponding b = 1000 s/mm² diffusion-weighted image (*D*) better highlights the tumor (*white arrow*). Arterial phase (*E*) and portal venous phase (*F*) gadolinium-enhanced axial MIPs show narrowing of the hepatic artery (*arrow*) and occlusion of the left intrahepatic portal vein. ERCP (*G*) confirms the involvement of the common hepatic duct and of the left intrahepatic duct and also shows a short narrowing of the right intrahepatic duct (Bismuth type 3B lesion).

Table 3
American Joint Committee on Cancer staging of Klatskin tumors

Stage	Tumor	Node	Metastasis
0	Tis	N0	M0
I	T1	N0	M0
II	T2a–b	N0	M0
IIIA	T3	N0	M0
IIIB	T1–3	N1	M0
IVA	T4	N0–1	M0
IVB	Any T	N2	M0
	Any T	Any N	M1

Tis: carcinoma in situ.
    T1: tumor confined to the bile duct, with extension up to the muscle layer or fibrous tissue.
    T2a: tumor invades beyond the wall of the bile duct to surrounding adipose tissue.
    T2b: tumor invades adjacent hepatic parenchyma.
    T3: tumor invades unilateral branches of the portal vein or hepatic artery.
    T4: tumor invades main portal vein or its branches bilaterally; or the common hepatic artery; or the second-order biliary radicals bilaterally; or unilateral second-order biliary radicals with contralateral portal vein or hepatic artery involvement.
    N0: no regional lymph node metastasis.
    N1: regional lymph node metastasis (including nodes along the cystic duct, common bile duct, hepatic artery, and portal vein).
    N2: metastasis to periaortic, pericaval, superior mesenteric artery, and/or celiac artery lymph nodes.
    M0: no metastasis.
    M1: distant metastasis.
    From Edge SB, Byrd DR, Compton CC, et al. AJCC (American Joint Committee on Cancer) cancer staging manual. 7th edition. New York: Springer-Verlag; 2010. p. 219; with permission.

MRCP allows better diagnostic performance and interobserver agreement for assessment of the longitudinal extent of the tumor.[37]

The infiltrative growth pattern and the close proximity to the portal vein and the hepatic artery of hilar cholangiocarcinoma results in a low resectability rate, ranging between 20% and 40%.[38] The major determinants of resectability are the extent of tumor within the biliary tree, the amount of hepatic parenchyma involved, vascular invasion, hepatic lobar atrophy, and metastatic disease.[39] In the study by Park and colleagues,[40] overall accuracy rates for predicting involvement of the bilateral secondary biliary confluences were 90.7% and 85.1%, respectively, for MR imaging with MRCP and multidetector computed tomography (MDCT) compared with direct cholangiography. In the assessment of vascular involvement, lymph node metastasis, and tumor resectability diagnostic performance of both techniques (MR imaging with MRCP and MDCT) was similar. In our experience, when evaluating intrahepatic bile ducts extension axial views diagnose caudate lobe involvement better. Caudate lobe infiltration has been documented in 30% to 95% of patients with tumors at the bifurcation and above. Moreover, significantly improved 5-year survival has been reported by Sugiura and colleagues[41] in patients treated with caudate lobe resection when compared with patients treated with bile duct resection alone (46% vs 12%). The importance of caudate lobe resection was later shown by several other studies.[42–44] For detection and assessment of invasion into the liver parenchyma, not only dynamic gadolinium-enhanced MR imaging is helpful but also DWI because it improves the detection of small malignant (<2cm) lesions compared with TSE T2-weighted imaging (see **Fig. 10**) and is a reasonable alternative to gadolinium-enhanced MR imaging.[45]

Distal Extrahepatic Cholangiocarcinoma

Distal extrahepatic cholangiocarcinomas are most commonly of the infiltrative type and grow intramurally, beneath the bile duct epithelium. Depending on the extent of intramural growth the associated stricture may involve a short or long ductal segment and present gradual tapering. The accuracy of MRCP is reported to be comparable with that of ERCP for differentiating extrahepatic bile duct carcinoma from benign cause of stricture.[34] Although some overlap exists, in general the presence of a long segment of extrahepatic bile duct stricture with irregular margins and asymmetric narrowing is suggestive of cholangiocarcinoma,

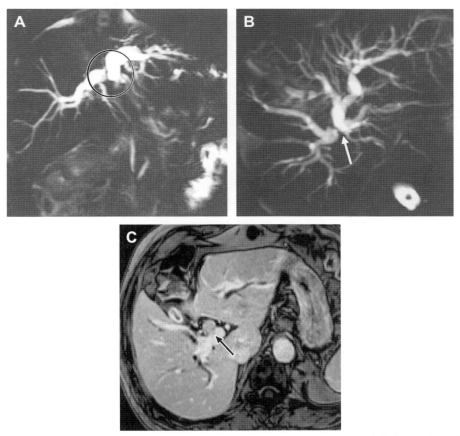

Fig. 9. Cholangiocarcinoma and portal venous invasion. Coronal MRCP projection (*A*) shows dilatation of the right and left intrahepatic bile ducts. Corresponding axial MRCP projection (*B*) shows narrowing involving the confluence of intrahepatic bile ducts (*arrow*). Gadolinium-enhanced out-of-phase GRE T1-weighted section (*C*) at the level of bile duct narrowing depicts a tumor nodule infiltrating the portal vein (*black arrow*).

whereas a short segment with regular margins and symmetric narrowing favors a benign cause.[34] The classic features of extrahepatic cholangiocarcinoma are a nodular mass with delayed enhancement after gadolinium chelate administration (**Fig. 11**) at the site of bile duct narrowing, and concentric or asymmetric thickening of the bile duct wall at the transition zone where the dilated extrahepatic duct suddenly disappears (**Fig. 12**). Although no data are available concerning DWI, it may help to visualize the cause of bile duct narrowing and identify adjacent periductal and lymph node metastasis commonly seen in the subperitoneal space of the hepatoduodenal ligament, as well as detecting subtle peritoneal seeding (see **Fig. 12**). The differential diagnosis includes several benign and malignant conditions. Common benign conditions that may mimic extrahepatic cholangiocarcinoma include PSC, AIDS

cholangiopathy, autoimmune pancreatitis, and acute and chronic pancreatitis. The most important malignant differential of extrahepatic cholangiocarcinoma that arises in the intrapancreatic portion of the common bile duct is pancreatic adenocarcinoma. An important differentiating feature is the lack of main pancreatic duct and accessory pancreatic duct involvement, which favors the diagnosis of cholangiocarcinoma (see **Fig. 12**). Although rare, intrabiliary metastasis (lung, breast, colon, testicle, prostate, pancreas, melanoma, and lymphoma) should also be considered (**Fig. 13**).[46]

Periampullary Tumors

Tumors that arise within 2 cm of the major duodenal papilla are considered periampullary carcinomas and include ampullary, bile duct, pancreatic, and

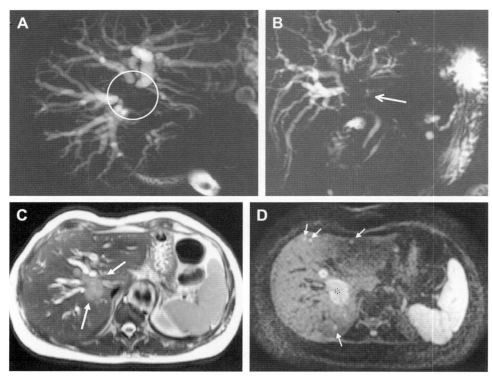

Fig. 10. Klatskin tumor and liver metastases. Axial (*A*) and coronal (*B*) MRCP projections show dilatation of the intrahepatic bile ducts and a huge defect at the liver hilum (*white circle* and *arrow*) caused by Klastkin tumor. TSE T2-weighted section (*C*) shows an infiltrating hyperintense tumor (*arrows*). Corresponding b = 1000 mm/s^2 DWI (*D*) shows additional small liver metastases (*short arrows*).

duodenal malignancies. The exact origin of the periampullary group of tumors is often difficult to determine by imaging methods and at pathology.[47] At MR imaging, the periampullary area is difficult to evaluate because of the small amount of fluid distributed in this region and the potential pitfall of pseudostricture caused by physiologic contraction of the sphincter of Oddi. In this setting serial thick-slab MRCP projections should be obtained to differentiate pathologic stenosis and physiologic

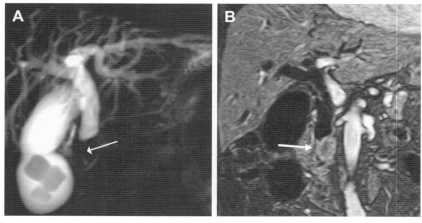

Fig. 11. Distal cholangiocarcinoma. Coronal MRCP projection (*A*) shows asymmetric narrowing of distal common bile duct (*arrow*). Main pancreatic duct is normal. Corresponding coronal gadolinium-enhanced T1-weighted section (*B*) shows a hypovascular lesion with enhancing peripheral rim (*arrow*).

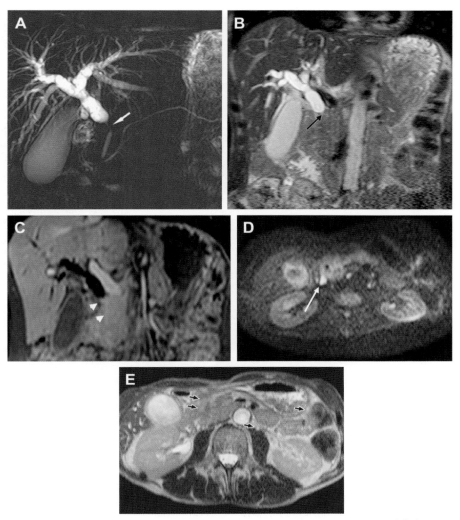

Fig. 12. Distal cholangiocarcinoma and peritoneal metastases. Coronal MRCP projection (*A*) shows a short stricture of the suprapancreatic segment of the common bile duct (*arrow*) and associated upstream dilation of the bile ducts. Pancreatic ducts are normal. Coronal TSE T2-weighted section (*B*) and coronal gadolinium-enhanced T1-weighted section (*C*) at the level of the head of the pancreas depict the dilation of the bile ducts; cause of obstruction is not depicted. Corresponding b = 1000 mm/s² axial DWI (*D*) at the level of the bile duct narrowing shows a small area of restricted diffusion (*long white arrow*) representing the tumor. Fusion imaging section (*E*) shows multiple and small peritoneal implants (*black arrows*).

narrowing of the sphincter segment.[48] In addition periampullary tumor characterization may be improved through the use of secretin to achieve good duodenal distension and increase the contrast between the intermediate signal of the tumor and the bright fluid in the duodenum on T2-weighted images. This strategy allows better assessment of the intraduodenal and the intraductal extension of the tumor (**Fig. 14**). Usually periampullary tumors present with biliary dilatation extending to the level of the duodenum. Distal bile

duct carcinomas manifest as luminal obliteration and wall thickening or as an intraductal polypoid mass without complete obliteration of the lumen (**Fig. 15**). According to a study by Kim and colleagues,[47] the distal segment of the bile duct below the obstruction is reportedly seen in more than 50% of the patients and the pancreatic duct is often normal (3-segment sign) until the tumor infiltrates the ampullary segment of both common bile duct and pancreatic duct, or directly invades the pancreas.

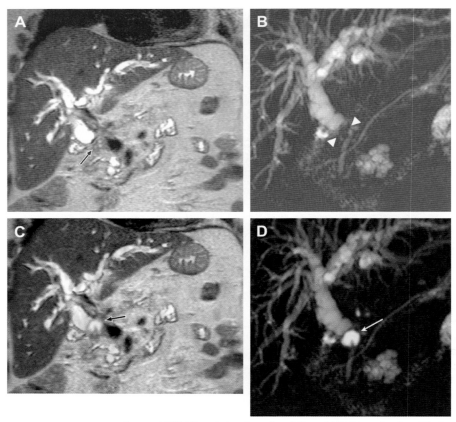

Fig. 13. Breast cancer metastases. Coronal TSE T2-weighted section (*A*) and MRCP projection (*B*) show extrahepatic bile duct obstruction (*black arrow* and *white arrowheads*). Fusion images (*C, D*) clearly depict a mass at the site of bile duct obstruction (*black* and *white arrows*).

MR imaging challenges

Despite continual advances in MR imaging technology, diagnostic and staging challenges of bile duct tumors persist. Such challenges include difficulty in detection of cholangiocarcinoma in the setting of PSC, precise evaluation of extension along intrahepatic bile ducts in hilar cholangiocarcinoma, difficulty in detection of early peritoneal spread, and detection of nodal metastasis. Strategies that may be helpful in addressing these

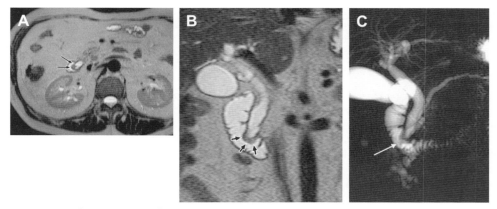

Fig. 14. Carcinoma of the ampulla of Vater. Axial (*A*) and coronal (*B*) TSE T2-weighted sections show nodular thickening of the duodenal papilla that protrudes into the lumen (*black arrows*), causing distal obstruction and dilation of both the common bile duct and the pancreatic duct, as shown on MRCP projection (*C*).

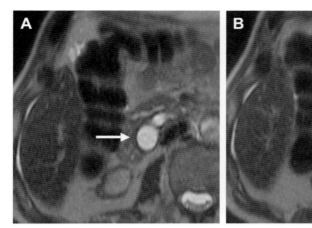

Fig. 15. Distal common bile duct carcinoma. Two contiguous axial TSE T2-weighted sections showing (*A*) common bile duct dilation (*arrow*) and a polypoid lesion (*B*) with irregular margins partially filling the lumen of the common bile duct (*arrow*).

limitations include high field imaging at 3 T to improve spatial resolution and potentially enable the detection of small intrahepatic bile ducts tumors, and DWI to potentially improve detection of metastatic disease in unenlarged lymph nodes and early peritoneal implants. Further studies concerning the role of DWI in the diagnosis and staging of biliary tumors are required.

REFERENCES

1. Koh DM, Collins DJ. Diffusion-weighted MRI in the body: application and challenges in oncology. AJR Am J Roentgenol 2007;188:1622–35.
2. Coppens E, Metens T, Winant C, et al. Pineapple juice labeled with gadolinium: a convenient oral contrast for magnetic resonance cholangiopancreatography. Eur Radiol 2005;15(10):2122–9.
3. Chan JHM, Tsui EYK, Yuen MK, et al. Gadopentate dimeglumine as an oral negative gastrointestinal contrast agent for MRCP. Abdom Imaging 2000;25:405–8.
4. Matos C, Metens T, Devière J, et al. Pancreatic duct: morphology and functional evaluation with dynamic MR pancreatography after secretin stimulation. Radiology 1997;203:435–41.
5. Choi JY, Kim MJ, Lee JM, et al. Magnetic resonance cholangiography: comparison of two- and three-dimensional sequences for assessment of malignant biliary obstruction. Eur Radiol 2008;18(1):78–86.
6. Tsushima Y, Takano A, Taketomi-Takahashi, et al. Body diffusion-weighted MR imaging using high b-value for malignant tumor screening: usefulness and necessity of referring to T2-weighted images and creating fusion images. Acad Radiol 2007;14:643–50.
7. De Groen PC, Gores GJ, LaRusso AF, et al. Biliary tract cancers. N Engl J Med 1999;341(18):1368–78.
8. Khan ZR, Neugut AI, Ahsan H, et al. Risk factors for biliary tract cancers. Am J Gastroenterol 1999;94:149–52.
9. Bartlett DL. Gallbladder cancer. Semin Surg Oncol 2000;19:145–55.
10. Levy AD, Murakata LA, Rohrmann CA. Gallbladder carcinoma: radiologic-pathologic correlation. Radiographics 2001;21:295–314.
11. Ito H, Matros E, Brooks DC, et al. Treatment outcomes associated with surgery for gallbladder cancer: a 20-year experience. J Gastrointest Surg 2004;8:183–90.
12. Catalano OA, Sahani DV, Kalva SP, et al. MR imaging of the gallbladder: a pictorial essay. Radiographics 2008;28:135–55.
13. Kim JH, Kim TK, Eun HW, et al. Preoperative evaluation of gallbladder carcinoma: efficacy of combined use of MR imaging, MR cholangiography, and contrast-enhanced dual-phase three-dimensional MR angiography. J Magn Reson Imaging 2002;16:676–84.
14. Aljiffry M, Walsh MJ, Molinari M. Advances in diagnosis, treatment and palliation of cholangiocarcinoma: 1990–2009. World J Gastroenterol 2009;15(34):4240–62.
15. Sherlock S, Dooley J. Disease of the liver and biliary system. 10th edition. London: Blackwell; 1997. p. 642–49.
16. Chung YE, Kim MJ, Park YN, et al. Varying appearances of cholangiocarcinoma: radiologic-pathologic correlation. Radiographics 2009;29:683–700.
17. Klatskin G. Adenocarcinoma of the hepatic duct at its bifurcation within the porta hepatis. An unusual tumor with distinctive clinical and pathologic features. Am J Med 1965;38:241–56.

18. Bismuth H, Corlette MB. Intrahepatic cholangioen-teric anastomosis in carcinoma of the hilus of the liver. Surg Gynecol Obstet 1975;140:170–8.

19. Patel T. Cholangiocarcinoma. Nat Clin Pract Gastro-enterol Hepatol 2006;3:33–42.

20. Lim JH, Park CK. Pathology of cholangiocarcinoma. Abdom Imaging 2004;29:540–7.

21. Maetani Y, Itoh K, Watanabe C, et al. MR imaging of intrahepatic cholangiocarcinoma with pathologic correlation. AJR Am J Roentgenol 2001;176: 1499–507.

22. Yoshida Y, Imai Y, Murakami T, et al. Intrahepatic cholangiocarcinoma with marked hypervascularity. Abdom Imaging 1999;24(1):66–8.

23. Adjei ON, Tamura S, Sugimara H, et al. Contrast-enhanced MR imaging of intrahepatic cholangiocar-cinoma. Clin Radiol 1995;50:6–10.

24. Zen Y, Adsay NV, Bardadin K, et al. Biliary intraepi-thelial neoplasia: an international interobserver agreement study and proposal for diagnostic criteria. Mod Pathol 2007;20(6):701–9.

25. Lim JH, Yoon KH, Kim SH, et al. Intraductal papillary mucinous tumor of the bile ducts. Radiographics 2004;24:53–67.

26. Yamasaki S. Intrahepatic cholangiocarcinoma: macroscopic type and stage classification. J Hepatobiliary Pancreat Surg 2003;10:288–91.

27. Uenishi T, Yamazaki O, Yamamoto T, et al. Serosal invasion in TNM staging of mass-forming intrahe-patic cholangiocarcinoma. J Hepatobiliary Pancreat Surg 2005;12:479–83.

28. Okabayashi T, Yamamoto J, Kosuge T, et al. A new staging system for mass-forming intrahepatic chol-angiocarcinoma: analysis of preoperative and post-operative variables. Cancer 2001;92:2374–83.

29. Akduman EI, Momtahen AJ, Balci NC, et al. Compar-ison between malignant and benign abdominal lymph nodes on diffusion-weighted imaging. Acad Radiol 2008;15:641–6.

30. Lee WJ, Lim HK, Jang KM, et al. Radiologic spec-trum of cholangiocarcinoma: emphasis on unusual manifestations and differential diagnosis. Radio-graphics 2001;21:S97–116.

31. Manfredi R, Barbaro B, Masselli G, et al. Magnetic resonance imaging of cholangiocarcinoma. Semin Liver Dis 2004;24:155–64.

32. Vogl TJ, Schwarz WO, Heller M, et al. Staging of Klatskin tumours (hilar cholangiocarcinomas): comparison of MR cholangiography, MR imaging, and endoscopic retrograde cholangiography. Eur Radiol 2006;16:2317–25.

33. Masselli G, Gualdi G. Hilar cholangiocarcinoma: MRI/MRCP in staging and treatment planning. Abdom Imaging 2008;33:444–51.

34. Park MS, Kim TK, Kim KW, et al. Differentiation of extrahepatic bile duct cholangiocarcinoma from benign stricture: findings at MRCP versus ERCP. Radiology 2004;233:234–40.

35. Lee SS, Kim MH, Lee SK, et al. MR cholangiography versus cholangioscopy for evaluation of longitudinal extension of hilar cholangiocarcinoma. Gastrointest Endosc 2002;56:25–32.

36. Hann LE, Gettrajdman GI, Brown KT, et al. Hepatic lobar atrophy: association with ipsilateral portal vein obstruction. AJR Am J Roentgenol 1996;167: 1017–21.

37. Kim HJ, Lee JM, Kim SH, et al. Evaluation of the longitudinal tumor extent of bile duct cancer: value of adding gadolinium-enhanced dynamic imaging to unenhanced images and magnetic resonance cholangiography. J Comput Assist Tomogr 2007; 31:469–74.

38. Gores GJ. Cholangiocarcinoma: current concepts and insights. Hepatology 2003;37:961–9.

39. Jarnagin WR, Fong Y, DeMatteo RP, et al. Staging, resectability, and outcome in 225 patients with hilar cholangiocarcinoma. Ann Surg 2001;234: 507–17.

40. Park HS, Lee JM, Choi JY, et al. Preoperative evalu-ation of bile duct cancer: MRI combined with MRCP versus MDCT with direct cholangiography. AJR Am J Roentgenol 2008;190:396–405.

41. Sugiura Y, Nakamura S, Iida S, et al. Extensive resection of the bile ducts combined with liver resec-tion for cancer of the main hepatic duct junction: a cooperative study of the Keio Bile Duct Cancer Study Group. Surgery 1994;115:445–51.

42. Lee S, Lee Y, Park K, et al. One hundred and eleven liver resections for hilar bile duct cancer. J Hepatobiliary Pancreat Surg 2000;7:135–41.

43. Tabata M, Kawarada Y, Yokoi H, et al. Surgical treat-ment for hilar cholangiocarcinoma. J Hepatobiliary Pancreat Surg 2000;7:148–54.

44. Nimura Y, Kamiya J, Kondo S, et al. Aggres-sive preoperative management and extended surgery for hilar cholangiocarcinoma: Nagoya experience. J Hepatobiliary Pancreat Surg 2000;7:155–62.

45. Hardie AD, Naik M, Hecht EM, et al. Diagnosis of liver metastases: value of diffusion-weighted MRI compared with gadolinium-enhanced MRI. Eur Radiol 2010. [Epub ahead of print]. DOI:10.1007/ s00330-009-1695-9.

46. Menias CO, Surabhi VR, Prasad SR, et al. Mimics of cholangiocarcinoma: spectrum of disease. Radio-graphics 2008;28:1115–29.

47. Kim JH, Kim MJ, Chung JJ, et al. Differential diag-nosis of periampullary carcinomas at MR imaging. Radiographics 2002;22:1335–52.

48. Kim JH, Kim MJ, Park SI, et al. Kinematic MR chol-angiopancreatography to evaluate biliary dilatation. AJR Am J Roentgenol 2002;178:909–14.

Magnetic Resonance Cholangiopancreatography of Benign Disorders of the Biliary System

Priya D. Prabhakar, MD, MPH[a], Anand M. Prabhakar, MD[b],
Hima B. Prabhakar, MD[c], Duyshant Sahani, MD[b],*

KEYWORDS

• MRCP • Benign liver disorders • Biliary • Imaging

NORMAL ANATOMY AND CONGENITAL VARIATIONS

Knowledge of biliary anatomy is often needed to plan surgical intervention.

Bile duct anatomy and variants can be well evaluated using a standard two-dimensional (2D) magnetic resonance cholangiopancreatography (MRCP) technique. Obscuration of duct anatomy caused by overlap from adjacent fluid-filled ducts and bowel was once a limitation inherent to the standard 2D technique. However, with the routine use of three-dimensional (3D) MRCP sequences and processed maximum intensity projection (MIP) images, this problem is less often encountered.[1,2]

The classically described normal anatomic configuration of the bile duct, consisting of 2 right segmental hepatic ducts (anterior and posterior) joining to form the main right hepatic duct and 2 major segmental branches of the left hepatic duct (medial and lateral) joining to form the main left hepatic duct, is present in only 50% to 60% of the population.[3] The main right and left hepatic ducts typically fuse to form the common hepatic duct 1 cm beyond the liver margin. The common hepatic duct extends from the confluence of the right and left main ducts and becomes the common bile duct (CBD) at the point where the cystic duct inserts.[4] The sphincter of Oddi consists of smooth muscle surrounding the common channel of the distal CBD and pancreatic duct as they insert into the duodenal papilla. The average CBD diameter is reported as 5 mm in individuals less than 50 year old; it can increase by 1 mm per decade after age 50 years.[5] However, after cholecystectomy, the CBD is often capacious and can measure up to 13 mm, but it shows lack of intrahepatic biliary ductal dilation—a finding useful in discrimination of CBD obstruction from normal expected dilation in these patients.

Because variant biliary duct anatomy is common, it is important to identify such variants for surgical planning before major hepatectomy, liver transplantation, and laparoscopic cholecystectomy to facilitate planned liver resection and ductal anastamosis as well as to minimize inadvertent biliary injuries during surgery.

A crossover anomaly is characterized by drainage of the right posterior segmental hepatic duct into the left main hepatic duct (**Fig. 1**). The crossover anomaly is found in 13% to 19% of the population, and is similar in prevalence to trifurcation of the biliary confluence that drains into the common hepatic duct. An accessory or aberrant right hepatic biliary duct draining into

[a] Wilmington Veterans Administration Hospital, Wilmington, DE, USA
[b] Department of Radiology, Division of Abdominal Imaging & Intervention, Massachusetts General Hospital, 55 Fruit Street, White 270, Boston, MA 02114, USA
[c] South Texas Radiology, San Antonio, TX, USA
* Corresponding author.
E-mail address: DSAHANI@partners.org

Magn Reson Imaging Clin N Am 18 (2010) 497–514
doi:10.1016/j.mric.2010.08.007
1064-9689/10/$ — see front matter © 2010 Elsevier Inc. All rights reserved.

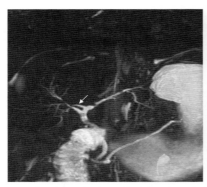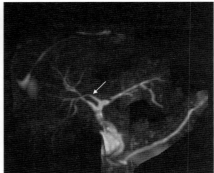

Fig. 1. Right posterior hepatic duct draining into left hepatic duct (crossover anomaly). Coronal MIP images demonstrate the right posterior segmental hepatic branch draining in the left hepatic duct (*arrows*).

the common hepatic or cystic duct can be seen in 7.4% of the population.[4,6,7]

The biliary ductal variants of surgical interest (**Tables 1** and **2**) involve those that affect the outflow, length, and course of the intra- and extrahepatic biliary ducts. A crossover anomaly and trifurcation of the biliary confluence are of surgical importance when planning a left hepatectomy, because the inadvertent surgical ligation of these variant ducts leads to atrophy and cirrhosis of liver segments VI to VII or V to VIII.[6] In addition, inadvertent resection or ligation of these anomalous ducts can lead to biliary leaks and strictures, especially in laparoscopic cholecystectomy or living donor right-lobe liver transplantation.[8]

Cystic duct anomalies are correctly identified with preoperative imaging in about 18% to 23% of cases, but such identification is important to reduce risk of major injury to the biliary tree during laparoscopic cholecystectomy. For example, in patients with a low cystic duct insertion (**Fig. 2**), the cystic duct has a long parallel course before inserting into the distal one-third of the CBD. Failure to recognize a low cystic duct insertion may lead to injury to the common duct during laparoscopic cholecystectomy. An aberrant right hepatic duct joining the common hepatic duct or cystic duct can also be inadvertently injured or ligated during laparoscopic cholecystectomy, leading to atrophy of segments VI and VII of the right hepatic lobe.[7,9] Similarly, failure to recognize

a proximal cystic duct insertion may lead to inadvertent ligation of the cystic duct and subsequent development of a stricture in the common hepatic duct. Long-term complications associated with low insertion of the cystic duct include postcholecystectomy syndrome, which is caused by development of calculi and inflammatory changes of a long cystic duct remnant, and instrumentation injury during endoscopic retrograde cholangiopancreatography (ERCP).[9]

Congenital Abnormalities of the Biliary Duct

Bile duct cysts (or choledochal cysts) are rare cystic dilations of the biliary tree. There are 5 types of biliary cysts according to the Todani classification system:

1. Type I choledochal cysts are the most common, comprising 80% to 90% of bile duct cysts, and are defined as fusiform dilatation of the extrahepatic CBD.
2. A type II cyst is a true saccular diverticulum from the extrahepatic bile duct or an intrahepatic bile duct.
3. A type III cyst, or choledochocele, represents a focal protrusion of a dilated segment of the distal CBD into the duodenum. An individual with a type III cyst may present with abdominal pain, jaundice, and vomiting, but many are incidentally detected.

Table 1 Biliary ductal variants of surgical significance	
Variant	**Prevalence (%)**
Trifurcation of the biliary duct	19
Right posterior segmental hepatic duct draining into the left hepatic duct (crossover anomaly)	13–19
Right hepatic duct emptying into the common hepatic or cystic duct	7.4

Table 2	
Cystic duct variants of surgical significance	
Variant	**Prevalence (%)**
Low medial insertion of the cystic duct into the distal CBD	9
Long parallel course of the cystic duct	10

4. Type IV cysts are subdivided into 2 subtypes: IVa, which shows fusiform dilation of the entire extrahepatic bile duct with extension into the intrahepatic ducts (**Fig. 3**), and IVb, which are characterized by multiple cystic dilatations of only the extrahepatic bile duct.

5. Type V or Caroli disease is a rare cyst disease that manifests as cystic dilatations of only the intrahepatic bile ducts and is associated with cystic renal disease and renal tubular ectasia. The key imaging feature of Caroli disease is that the cystic dilations communicate with the biliary tree.[4,10,11]

Choledochal cysts should be surgically corrected because of the risk of associated complications such as cystolithiasis, recurrent cholangitis, and subsequent biliary peritonitis, pancreatitis, and malignant transformation to cholangiocarcinoma. The correct identification of bile duct cyst distribution is therefore important for preoperative planning. The standard T2-weighted MRCP, single-shot rapid acquisition with refocused echoes (SS-RARE) or fast recovery 3D RARE serves as an excellent method to delineate the bile duct cysts and the extent of their involvement of the biliary system (**Fig. 4**). The inclusion of axial

T1-weighted gadolinium (Gd)-enhanced images also enables visualization of the pathognomonic dot sign in Caroli disease, which represents a portal or arterial branch at the periphery of or within a pseudoseptation running through a cyst.[4,10,12]

An anomalous pancreaticobiliary junction represents union of the pancreatic duct and CBD into a long common channel (more than 15 mm) outside the duodenal wall. Sphincter of Oddi dysfunction is associated with reflux of pancreatic secretions into the CBD and pancreatic duct and manifests as ductal inflammation. An anomalous pancreaticobiliary junction is often associated with choledochal cysts, biliary carcinoma, and pancreatitis. MRCP has an accuracy of 75% for diagnosis of an anomalous pancreaticobiliary junction.[13] MRCP is able to show the anomalous union of the ducts as well as the common channel; however, the length of the common channel tends to measure less on MRCP compared with ERCP because of factors such as spasm of the sphincter muscle. If needed, the delineation of the pancreatic duct at MRCP can be improved with secretin administration, which stimulates the pancreas to secrete fluid and bicarbonate, causing increased fullness and conspicuity of the duct.[14] An anomalous pancreaticobiliary junction should be treated with endoscopic sphincterotomy to prevent the onset of complications such as pancreatitis, biliary ductal distortion, or the development of cholangiocarcinoma.[7]

Biliary atresia is another congenital entity that can be evaluated with MRCP. Extrahepatic biliary atresia should be suspected if there is nonvisualization of the entire length of the extrahepatic biliary tree. Intrahepatic biliary atresia can also occur. Because normal pediatric intrahepatic bile ducts are poorly visualized on MRCP, establishing the diagnosis of intrahepatic biliary atresia on MRCP can be difficult. Features suggestive of biliary

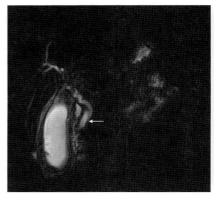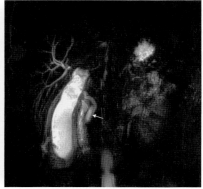

Fig. 2. Low medial insertion cystic duct into CBD. A common cystic duct variant, low medial insertion of the cystic duct into the distal common bile is shown on this coronal MIP image (*arrows*).

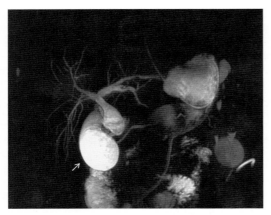

Fig. 3. Type 4A choledochal cyst. A type 4A choledochal cyst (*arrow*), which represents fusiform dilation of the entire extrahepatic bile duct with extension into the intrahepatic ducts, is seen on this coronal MIP image from MRCP.

atresia in pediatric patients include structural abnormalities of the bile ducts, liver atrophy, and masslike nodules centered near a hypertrophic portal vessel. However, MRCP is not the technique of choice to evaluate biliary atresia, because other modalities such as nuclear scintigraphy and ultrasound (US) can help make the diagnosis without the need for pediatric sedation or difficulty in visualization of small pediatric biliary.[15,16] Extrahepatic biliary atresia can be surgically corrected with hepaticojejunostomy, whereas intrahepatic biliary atresia is not amenable to surgical correction and therefore may require liver transplantation.[7]

GALLBLADDER DISEASE

Nonmalignant disease of the gallbladder is typically evaluated with US. The normal T2

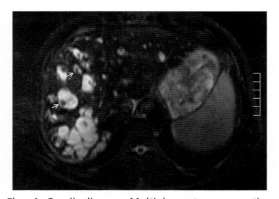

Fig. 4. Caroli disease. Multiple cysts representing cystic dilation of the intrahepatic ducts are present on this axial T2-weighted image with fat saturation. Several of these cysts show a central dot sign, consistent with an arterial or portal branch within a pseudoseptation running through the cyst (*arrows*).

appearance of the gallbladder on MRCP (T2-weighted images) is a thin low-signal intensity wall with high-signal intensity bile. However, the signal intensity of the gallbladder contents can vary depending on the concentration of water, cholesterol, and bile salts. In the fasting state, there is reabsorption of water and subsequent increased cholesterol and bile salt concentration, which results in a decreased T1 relaxation time, or bright signal on T1-weighted imaging and higher signal intensity of the gallbladder contents on T1- or T2-weighted imaging with prolongation in the fasting state.[11] Normal variations in the gallbladder include a phyrigian cap, septations, duplication, and ectopic location (intrahepatic, retrohepatic, or beneath the left lobe of the liver), all of which can be confidently recognized on MR imaging.

Gallbladder calculi are easily recognized as faceted signal voids on a background of T2 hyperintense bile. Pitfalls to the identification of gallstones include air bubbles, hemorrhage, and debris, but other clues can help differentiate these filling defects in the gallbladder. Air bubbles are located in the nondependent portion of the gallbladder and often create an air-bile level. T1-weighted images are helpful in differentiating clot or areas of hemorrhage and appear as T1 hyperintense foci. A decrease in signal intensity of the bile on out-of-phase T1-weighted images compared with in-phase images confirms the presence of T1 hyperintense material in the gallbladder, and can help diagnose this as concentrated bile rather than hemorrhage.[17]

Cholecystitis is routinely diagnosed with US; however, in certain equivocal situations, MR imaging can play a role in identifying cystic duct and gallbladder neck calculi not visible on US.[18] In most patients with cholecystitis, a hyperintense, thick, edematous wall with pericholecystic fluid and a distended gallbladder is seen on T2-weighted images. Gallstones are also commonly seen, in approximately 85% of cases (**Figs. 5 and 6**). Intense enhancement of the thickened gallbladder is a hallmark of acute cholecystitis on MR imaging. Transient pericholecystic hepatic enhancement is seen in 70% of cases of acute cholecystitis, and is caused by increased hepatic local inflammation and resultant hyperemia.[14] Conversely, chronic cholecystitis shows mild gallbladder wall enhancement, more commonly on delayed phase image. In chronic cholecystitis, the gallbladder is usually not so distended, but is contracted and shows wall thickening.[17]

A variant of chronic cholecystitis, xanthogranulomatous cholecystitis, is a rare disease caused by occlusion of Rokitansky-Aschoff sinuses with subsequent intramural rupture of bile and mucin

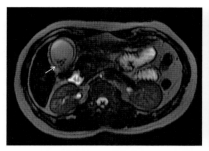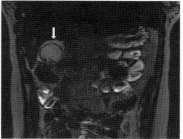

Fig. 5. Acute cholecystitis. Axial and coronal T2-weighted images show classic findings of acute cholecystitis: thickening of the gallbladder wall (*thick arrow*), pericholecystic fluid, and gallstones (*thin arrow*).

to form multiple intramural xanthogranulomatous nodules. This entity mimics gallbladder carcinoma on US and computed tomography (CT). MR imaging findings include focal or diffuse gallbladder wall thickening, enhancement, and intramural abscesses.[11] Loss of the normal fat plane between the liver and gallbladder is often seen, further confusing this diagnosis with gallbladder carcinoma. Xanthogranulomatous cholecystitis is therefore treated with surgery because of the resemblance to gallbladder carcinoma.[17]

Acalculous cholecystitis occurs in the absence of gallstones and is usually diagnosed with US or a hepatobiliary iminodiacetic acid scan. In certain patients, MR imaging may plan a role but these patients are often acutely ill, and MR imaging has limited usefulness. MR imaging findings of this entity are similar to the sonographic findings, and include gallbladder wall thickening, pericholecystic abscess, and marked gallbladder distension. A variant of this form of cholecystitis, hemorrhagic cholecystitis, presents with hemorrhage in the gallbladder, which has a characteristic appearance on

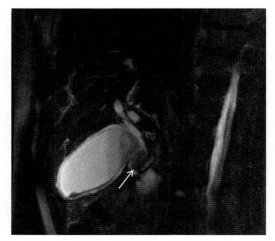

Fig. 6. Acute cholecystitis. Coronal MIP shows a gallstone impacted in the gallbladder neck (*arrow*) with distension of the gallbladder and thickening of the gallbladder wall.

MR imaging. Subacute hemorrhage is T1 hyperintense as a result of the T1 shortening effect of methemoglobin. Chronic hemorrhage is T2 hypointense as a result of the deposition of hemosiderin. Ischemia is also commonly associated with hemorrhagic cholecystitis.[17]

Functional imaging of the gallbladder analogous to nuclear hepatobiliary scintigraphy can also be concurrently performed with availability of hepatobiliary MR contrast agents such as Gd-benzyloxy propionic tetraacetic acid (Gd-BOPTA) (Multihance, Bracco, Milan, Italy) and Gd-ethoxybenzyl (EOB)-DTPA (Eovist, Bayer, Wayne, NJ, USA). These agents have initial extracellular distribution but are selectively taken up by hepatocytes and partially excreted into the bile. Although there is a paucity of literature on functional imaging of the gallbladder, a few studies have shown that filling of the intra- and extrahepatic biliary ducts but nonfilling of the gallbladder with Gd-BOPTA can be seen in cholecystitis.[19] Combining standard T2-weighted MRCP with hepatobiliary-specific contrast imaging can be used together to functionally diagnosis cholecystitis and provide anatomic information such as the location and cause of the gallbladder obstruction.[19]

Gallbladder wall thickening is associated with another benign entity of the gallbladder, adenomyomatosis, which can manifest as focal, segmental, or diffuse involvement of the gallbladder. This disease process is characterized by thickening of the muscularis layer of the gallbladder wall, proliferation of the surface epithelium, and formation of epithelial lined cytic spaces and Rokitansky-Aschoff sinuses. On MR imaging, these sinuses appear as T1 hypointense and T2 hyperintense intramural foci in a linear configuration. Early linear mucosal enhancement of the gallbladder wall in the involved segments is noted. Focal involvement is often present in the gallbladder fundus.[20] This diagnosis can also be confused with chronic cholecystitis or gallbladder carcinoma. Dynamic postcontrast MR imaging can help distinguish this disease from gallbladder carcinoma, which shows inconsistent nonlinear early enhancement (**Fig. 7**).[17]

Gallbladder polyps are usually incidental and asymptomatic, and are detected in 4% to 5% of the population. Most polyps are benign; however, 10% are adenomatous, and can become premalignant. Polyps are usually homogenously low-signal intensity on both T1- and T2-weighted images and show delayed contrast enhancement. Features that favor benign polyp include a diameter of less than 10 mm and a stalk. Sessile polyps, polyps greater than 10 mm, and adjacent wall thickening raise concern for malignancy, for which cholecystectomy should be considered.[17,21]

Mirizzi Syndrome

Mirizzi syndrome was first described in 1948 and is a rare condition in which there is extrinsic compression of the common hepatic duct from an impacted gallstone in the gallbladder neck, infundibulum, or Hartmann pouch (**Fig. 8**).[22] There can be associated inflammation, which contributes to the biliary obstruction. The frequency of Mirizzi syndrome ranges from 0.1% to 1.0% in patients with cholelithiasis. Patients with Mirizzi syndrome present with painless jaundice or symptoms of cholangitis.[23] Although the exact cause that predisposes a patient to developing Mirizzi syndrome is unknown, anatomic factors such as long parallel cystic duct or a low medial insertion of the cystic duct into the CBD are often associated.[22,23]

Mirrizi syndrome is classified into 4 types, based on the size and the presence of a cholecyst-choledochal fistula. Type I lesions have no fistula, with IA consisting of multiple small stones within a long cystic duct and IB consisting of a larger stone impacted within the Hartmann pouch. Types II to IV have a fistula, and are graded based on the size of the fistula. Patients with type I lesions are usually treated with cholecystectomy, whereas patients with types II to IV usually have a biliary-enteric anastamosis and cholecystectomy.[23]

Preoperative imaging is essential for diagnosis as well as determining the presence of a fistula. Traditionally, ERCP has been used, but it is invasive and associated with complications. ERCP also has limited usefulness in evaluating the degree of gallbladder inflammation, and ERCP interventions are generally not useful in Mirizzi syndrome.[22] MRCP can characterize the obstruction associated with Mirizzi syndrome as well as document the presence of other biliary conditions.[22] The MRCP appearance of Mirizzi syndrome may resemble tumors of the cystic duct, gallbladder, or hilar cancer. Recently, it has been suggested that patients with suspected Mirizzi syndrome may benefit from CT evaluation to improve diagnostic accuracy.[24]

Biliary Obstruction

Diseases associated with biliary obstruction are a major cause of morbidity and mortality in North America. Conditions that have a malignant cause are more likely to cause biliary obstruction.

Choledocholithiasis

Primary choledocholelithiasis results from stasis and infection within the CBD, and secondary choledocholelithiasis occurs when gallbladder stones pass into the CBD. The prevalence of acute cholecystitis associated with CBD stones is less than 5%.[25]

The overall prevalence of CBD stones in patients with cholelithiasis is between 8% and 15%.[26] The management of CBD stones has also evolved with the refinement of endoscopic approaches.

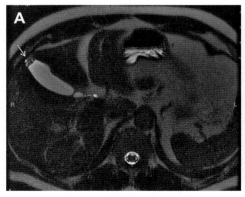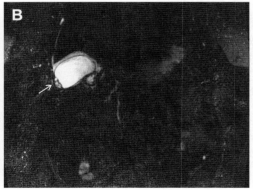

Fig. 7. Adenomyomatosis. (*A*) Axial MR cholangiography shows wall thickening and tiny hyperintense foci at the gallbladder fundus (*arrow*), a common location for focal adenomyomatosis. (*B*) Coronal thick-slab MRCP MIP image shows small hyperintense rounded structures at the fundus of the gallbladder, representing adenomyomatosis (*arrow*).

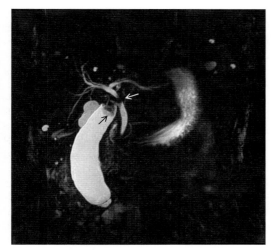

Fig. 8. Mirrizi syndrome. A gallstone in the gallbladder neck (*black arrow*) causes both dilation of the gallbladder and obstruction of the proximal CBD (*white arrow*), and is well depicted on this coronal thick-slab MIP image.

Endoscopic stone extraction followed by papillotomy remains a preferred approach in the acute setting. However, in stable patients, an open or laparoscopic surgical approach to remove the gallbladder with CBD exploration is generally performed.

US has lower sensitivity of only 21% to 63% for biliary ductal stones because of the limited acoustic window, anatomic variants, and ductal dilatation.[27] CT with multiplanar reconstructions has been shown to be sensitive for CBD stones.[28,29] However, noncalcified stones, tumefactive sludge, or clot can be missed.

Therefore, preoperative MRCP is increasingly being used to noninvasively image patients with suspected choledocholithiasis before subjecting them to ERCP. Because many complications can arise from choledocholithiasis, including cholangitis, abscess, pancreatitis, or biliary cirrhosis, MRCP can be useful for preoperative planning. Although it is noninvasive, the disadvantages of MRCP include the limitation of patient claustrophobia and patient motion.[30]

On MRCP images, stones are easily recognized as signal void T2 dark areas, contrasted with the background of high-signal bile (**Figs. 9–11**). The reported performance of MRCP in the diagnosis of choledocholelithiasis in one recent study is 91% sensitivity, 84% specificity, and diagnostic accuracy was 90%.[30] Causes of false-positive results include pneumobilia, hemobilia, crossing hepatic artery, and occasional intraductal tumors.[31] False-negative results can be considered in small stones (3–5 mm) or impacted calculi into the wall of the biliary tree that do not have bile surrounding the stones.[31] Reviewing the source images obtained in the other planes is helpful to minimize the false-positive and false-negative results. For example, air bubbles if present are seen nondependently in the bile ducts.

Biliary Strictures

A focal narrowing in the bile duct is defined as a stricture. Bile duct strictures can have a benign or malignant cause, with benign strictures more prevalent. The most common cause of biliary stricture is iatrogenic from surgical procedures. Additional causes of bile duct strictures include inflammatory conditions such as pancreatitis, infectious cholangitis, or primary sclerosing cholangitis (PSC). Bile duct strictures can be associated with complications

A   **B**

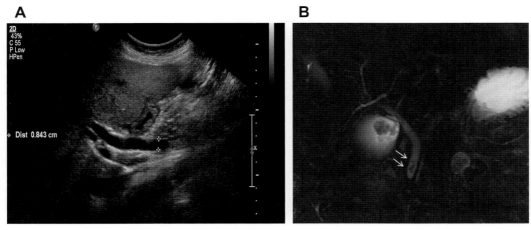

Fig. 9. Choledocholithiasis not detected by US. (*A*) Dilation of the CBD was initially seen on US of unknown cause. (*B*) A coronal MRCP image of the same patient shows at least 2 filling defects (*arrows*) in the distal CBD as the cause of the biliary obstruction.

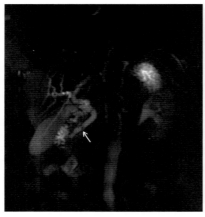
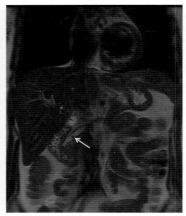

Fig. 10. Choledocholithiasis. Coronal MIP and SS fast spin echo images reveal filling defects (*arrows*) in the mid- to distal CBD consistent with choledocholithiasis.

such as ascending cholangitis, hepatic abscess, and biliary cirrhosis.[32]

Iatrogenic causes cause 95% of biliary structures.[33] Iatrogenic procedures that cause bile duct strictures fall into 2 groups: procedures involving the bile ducts themselves, or those that involve the epigastric region (most commonly Billroth II partial gastric resection). The most common surgical procedure associated with biliary stricture is cholecystectomy.[33] The incidence of a major bile duct injury, including stricture after open cholecystectomy, is 0.2% to 0.3%; after laparoscopic cholecystectomy it is 0.4% to 0.6%.[32]

Noniatrogenic causes for biliary strictures include a myriad of causes. Generally, any inflammatory process of the bile ducts creates a risk for stricture. Chronic pancreatitis is the cause of 10% of benign biliary strictures. Other causes include cholangitis associated with the human immunodeficiency virus (HIV), radiation, tuberculosis, chemotherapeutic drugs, and autoimmune causes

such as lupus and polyarteritis nodosa[32] (**Table 3**). Bile duct strictures can also affect patients who undergo orthotopic liver transplant. Strictures usually occur several months after the transplant and are related to hepatic artery ischemia.[34]

The most common clinical symptoms associated with bile duct stricture include symptoms of biliary obstruction, such as jaundice, fever, chills, and epigastric pain. Laboratory studies are usually suggestive of cholestasis (increased alkaline phosphatase levels), without an increase of hepatic enzymes.[33]

The imaging evaluation of patients with suspected biliary strictures usually begins with abdominal US, which can be used to assess the intra- and extrahepatic ducts for signs of dilation. US can also be used to look for complications of bile duct strictures. Traditionally, ERCP and percutaneous transhepatic cholangiography have been used to assess for bile duct strictures given the improved anatomic visualization of the bile ducts when compared with US. However, both techniques are invasive and operator dependent.

MRCP is a noninvasive method to assess for biliary duct stricture. In addition, MRCP studies include axial images through the upper abdomen, so assessment for complications from bile duct strictures can be performed.

A bile duct stricture causes a luminal narrowing and if complete, causes proximal biliary obstruction. Generally, a smooth, concentric, short-segment strictures favors a benign cause, whereas an abrupt, eccentric, long-segment stricture favors a malignant cause (**Fig. 12**).[35] However, these imaging characteristics are not specific. For example, malignant imaging features were associated with benign causes in 35% of cases.[36] MRCP has been shown to be accurate in the diagnosis of bile duct injuries, including strictures.[37]

Fig. 11. Choledocholithiasis. A calculus (*arrow*) is clearly seen in the mid-CBD on this coronal thick-slab MRCP.

Table 3
Types of biliary strictures

Type	Cause/Frequency
Iatrogenic	Postsurgical injury accounts for 90% of all strictures: laparoscopic cholecystectomy, biliary ductal or biliary-enteric anastomosis
Infectious	Infectious cholangitis, HIV cholangitis, tuberculosis
Inflammatory	Pancreatitis accounts for 10% of all strictures; PSC, autoimmune disease, stone perforation
Drugs/therapy related	Chemotherapy, radiation

The location of biliary strictures can also be described. Bismuth created a classification system to describe the location of strictures. Bismuth type I strictures are located more than 2 cm distal to the confluence of the left and right hepatic ducts (hepatic bifurcation). Type II strictures are located less than 2 cm from the hepatic bifurcation. Bismuth type III lesions are present at the bifurcation. Type IV lesions involve the right or left hepatic ducts, and type V lesions extend into the right or left hepatic branch ducts.[38]

Treatment of biliary strictures can be surgical, endoscopic, or percutaneous. Endoscopic management with sphincterotomy, balloon dilation, and stenting is preferred and has been show to be highly effective. Endoscopic complications include cholangitis, pancreatitis, perforation, and stent occlusion/migration. A recent study that followed patients after endoscopic therapy showed a 22% stricture recurrence rate, with more than half of these patients responding to repeat balloon dilation. Only 9% of

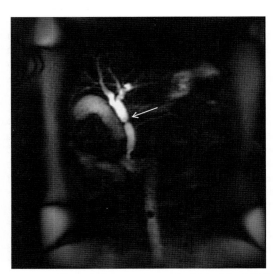

Fig. 12. Biliary stricture. Coronal thick-slab MRCP reveals a tight focal narrowing in the mid-CBD (*arrow*) associated with biliary ductal dilation caused by a benign stricture.

patients proceeded to surgical therapy.[39] Percutaneous dilation is effective 40% to 85% of the time, and potential complications include hemorrhage, bile leakage, and cholangitis, but it can be useful in treatment of high strictures or strictures of small diameter ducts.[33] Surgical therapy most commonly involves a hepaticojejunostomy and is usually considered in select patients who fail endoscopic or percutaneous radiological therapy.[33]

Cholangitis

Cholangitis, or inflammation of the bile ducts, can be caused by a variety of factors, both infectious and noninfectious.[40] Although many of these patients are initially diagnosed through a combination of laboratory values and clinical assessment, MRCP has been useful in diagnosing and monitoring the response to therapy in many of these patients.

Infectious Cholangitis

Bacterial cholangitis is usually the result of ascending infection from the intestine, and classically results in biliary obstruction.[40] The most commonly associated organisms associated with bacterial cholangitis are gram negative and include *Escherichia coli*, *Klebsiella*, *Enterococcus*, *Enterobacter*, *Pseudomonas*, and anaerobes.[40] Clinical symptoms include the Charcot triad of fever, jaundice, and right upper quadrant pain, but are seen in only 70% of patients.[40] Obstructive conditions, such as biliary stones, sludge, strictures, as well as instrumentation predispose patients to bacterial cholangitis. Treatment is usually with antibiotics and biliary decompression, if necessary.

Imaging in patients suspected to have infectious cholangitis generally begins with CT or US, usually to look for a cause of biliary obstruction. There is increased utilization of MRCP in diagnosing patients with suspected cholangitis. In a study of 13 patients who had clinically confirmed cholangitis, 100% of patients had evidence of biliary obstruction on MR imaging, with 54% showing central obstruction. Smooth, symmetric bile duct wall thickening was also observed.[41] Enhancement of the intrahepatic biliary walls is a common finding, especially on delayed images.[41] The advantage of using MRCP to assess these patients is the ability to assess the liver parenchyma, as geographic T2 signal changes were also observed in these patients.

HIV is well known to affect the liver and biliary tree.[42] AIDS cholangiopathy involves multiple biliary strictures, liked related to opportunistic infections such as cryptosporidium, cytomegalovirus, and microsporidium.[43] With the advent of highly active antiretroviral therapy, it is now a rare entity.[44] Most causes of AIDS cholangiopathy occur in patients with a CD4 count less than 200 mm³.[43] ERCP findings include papillary stenosis and long-segment biliary strictures.[42] ERCP treatment includes sphincterotomy, and is helpful in reducing symptoms, but not does not improve survival.[43] Given that ERCP is an invasive procedure, MRCP is a good modality to assess these patients and can be used to evaluate for liver parenchymal disease.[42] Typical MRCP findings include peripheral long-segment extrahepatic biliary stricture, similar to those found in patients with PSC.[43]

Recurrent Pyogenic Cholangitis

Recurrent pyogenic cholangitis (RPC) is characterized as multiple intrahepatic pigmented stones with associated cholangitis.[45] The cause is not definitely known, but it has been associated with recurrent parasitic infections, such as *Ascaris lumbricoides* and *Clonorchis sinensis*. Chronic infection is felt to cause inflammation of the bile ducts, leading to strictures and bile stasis, resulting in intrahepatic biliary stones. This condition was previously noted only in Asian countries, but there has been an increase in prevalence in Western countries as a result of population changes. Clinical presentation is nonspecific and includes fever, jaundice, and right upper quadrant pain.

Because RPC is less common than other causes of right upper quadrant pain, imaging generally begins with abdominal US. Usually, there is biliary dilation of the central intrahepatic ducts, with relative sparing of the peripheral ducts.[46] For unknown reasons, left-sided ducts are more affected than right-sided ducts. Pneumobilia is common in these patients, so intrahepatic biliary stones can be obscured on US imaging.[47] CT and ERCP findings resemble those seen on US.

MRCP findings show central ductal dilation in segmented or lobar distribution and decreased arborization. There are also multiple filling defects

in the dilated ducts, with a thickened, enhancing wall. In long-standing cases, atrophy of the affected liver segments is present.

MRCP has been shown to be more sensitive than ERCP in detecting the intrahepatic calculi associated with RPC.[48] In addition, MR is more useful in detecting the complications of RPC. For example, 20% of patients with RPC are found to have hepatic abscess.[47] Because of the bile stasis and increased infections, patients with RPC are also at an increased risk of malignancy, because cholangiocarcinoma is found in up to 5% of patients.[46]

Management of RPC is geared to controlling cholangitis and obstruction, and often requires a team of interventional radiologists, endoscopists, and surgeons.[45] Endoscopy can be used to remove intrahepatic stones and dilate strictures. Percutaneous techniques can also be used to extract stones and manage strictures that are inaccessible by endoscopy. Surgical therapy involves surgical removal of obstructed liver segments and biliary bypass. In rare cases, orthotopic liver transplantation can be used with chronic RPC that has led to hepatic failure.[45]

PSC

Diffuse fibrosing inflammation of the small, medium, and large intra- and extrahepatic biliary ducts is found in patients with PSC.[49] PSC is associated with inflammatory bowel disease in 75% of patients.[50] Laboratory findings that suggest PSC are nonspecific, but 80% of patients with PSC have perinuclear antineutrophil cytoplasmic antibodies.[49] On ERCP, the gold standard for evaluating PSC, multifocal strictures of the intra- and extrahepatic ducts with a beaded appearance are classically seen.[51] However, diagnosis and monitoring of PSC with ERCP is invasive and is associated with complications that are often seen at a higher rate in patients with PSC, including sepsis, hemorrhage, pancreatitis, bowel perforation, and cholangitis,[52,53] and can lead to progression of cholestasis in advanced PSC.[54] MRCP has also been shown to be equivalent to ERCP in the diagnosis of PSC.[55] Therefore ERCP is best reserved for essential therapeutic interventions in PSC.

The classic MRCP findings include multifocal dilations of biliary segments alternating with segments of stricture, peripheral wedge-shaped areas of increased T2 signal, and the presence of ductal calculi related to cholestasis or infection (**Figs. 13** and **14**).[56] MRCP has been shown to improve visibility of the bile ducts and associated strictures.

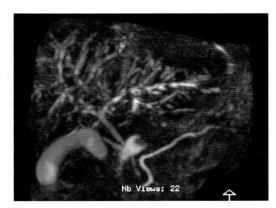

Fig. 13. PSC. Coronal MIP image from 3D fast spin echo T2-weighted MRCP shows dilated ducts with multiple strictures and areas of dilation.

MRCP is not only useful for diagnosis of PSC but in conjunction with contrast-enhanced MR imaging can also serve to evaluate disease progression and the effects of therapy.[56] In advanced PSC, in which there is worsened fibrosis, pruning of the biliary tree is seen in the periphery of the liver and segments of ductal obliteration. Morphologic changes of the liver are seen in cirrhosis that suggest a diagnosis of including hypertrophy of the caudate lobe and atrophy of the right posterior and left lateral segments of the liver.[57] Varying degrees of enhancement can be seen around the abnormal biliary ducts, but this finding is not associated with differences in survival.[58]

Twenty percent of patients with PSC die of cholangiocarcinoma, and MRCP and MR imaging with contrast offers the added benefit over ERCP of assessing the parenchymal organs for development of tumor. The classic MR findings of intraductal cholangiocarcinoma include polypoid lesions showing delayed contrast enhancement. Cholangiocarcinoma should also be suspected if there is rapid progression of biliary strictures or high-grade ductal narrowing associated with proximal ductal dilation. MRCP findings can be used to guide interventional procedures in these patients,

including the decision as to whether to perform an endoscopic or percutaneous biliary drainage procedure.

MRCP Imaging in Postoperative Patients

MRCP imaging of the postsurgical patient can be challenging, and careful attention should be paid to the type of surgery performed, altered anatomic relationships, as well as the most common immediate and delayed complications for major hepaticobiliary and pancreaticobiliary surgeries. Most injury to the extrahepatic biliary duct system is iatrogenic, and most commonly secondary to cholecystectomy (open and laparoscopic).[59] For the purposes of this article, we discuss complications related to 3 common surgeries affecting the biliary system: cholecystectomy, biliary-enteric anastomoses such as choledochojejunostomy and hepaticojejunostomy, and liver resection and transplantation.

CHOLECYSTECTOMY

After cholecystectomy, patients can present with various symptoms of bloating, nausea, and vague upper abdominal pain, often called postcholecystectomy syndrome. This syndrome is often more likely in the patient who initially presented with atypical right upper quadrant pain, suggesting that their pain may not have been caused by the presence of cholelithiasis or true biliary colic. Alternatively, operative complications should be considered. If these symptoms present in the immediate postoperative period, differential considerations include retained common bile duct stone, clipped or transected hepatic or CBD, bile leak, or possibly hepatic injury related to surgery (anatomic variant or intraoperative complication). If the patient presents weeks or months after surgery, differential considerations include CBD stricture, or dysfunction of the sphincter of Oddi.[59,60] MRCP can be an important diagnostic tool in evaluating and diagnosing these conditions.

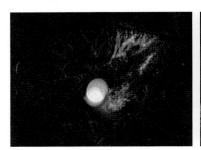
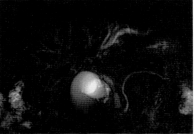

Fig. 14. PSC with history of Crohn disease. Two coronal 3D MIP images show focal irregular dilation and narrowing of bile ducts in the left hepatic lobe in a patient with Crohn disease who developed sclerosing cholangitis.

A common feature of both the initial and late postoperative complications of cholecystectomy is biliary dilatation. The postoperative CBD should measure maximally 13 mm, and taper slowly.[60] The imaging features of retained CBD stones are the same as for choledocholithiasis, which were discussed earlier. More specific to the postcholecystectomy patient, a clipped or transected hepatic or CBD is present with intrahepatic biliary ductal dilatation to the level of the occlusion with an abrupt cutoff (**Fig. 15**).[37] Susceptibility artifact can be seen on gradient echo sequences from metallic clips at the site of stricture. In addition, failure to recognize anatomic variants, such as the insertion of the right hepatic duct into the cystic duct, may cause focal or segmental right hepatic biliary dilatation from postoperative duct ligation.[61]

Biliary leaks are more likely to occur in patients with anatomic variants, chronic cholecystitis, or intrahepatic portion of the gallbladder.[62] If the right hepatic duct is mistaken for the cystic duct and transected without occlusion, the patient can present with a leak that requires the creation of a biliary-enteric anastomosis, such as hepaticojejunostomy. Patients with significant biliary leaks often present with fever and abdominal pain.

MRCP imaging features of postoperative biliary leak include increased T2 hyperintense fluid, commonly pooling preferentially at the site of the leak, and extending to the subhepatic space (**Figs. 16** and **17**).[37] If there is associated hemorrhagic component to the bile leak, variable T1 hyperintensity can be identified, typically of the peripheral rim of a hematoma. If imaging is performed with mangafodipir trisodium, which is excreted in the bile, the location of the leak may be more easily defined.[63]

Biliary strictures after cholecystectomy show similar imaging characteristics as those of other benign causes. These characteristics are more commonly seen after laparoscopic resection, and can be secondary to misplaced clips, the sequela of prior choledocholithiasis, or fibrosis or thermal injury. Typically, patients with stricture of the CBD present with diffuse intrahepatic biliary ductal dilatation, although single-lobe dilatation may be seen (more typically left lobe).[63] The stricture is typically abrupt with short-segment narrowing of the duct. MRCP can be useful in pretreatment planning of postoperative strictures, and to determine whether balloon dilatation/stenting or operative management would be better indicated.[37]

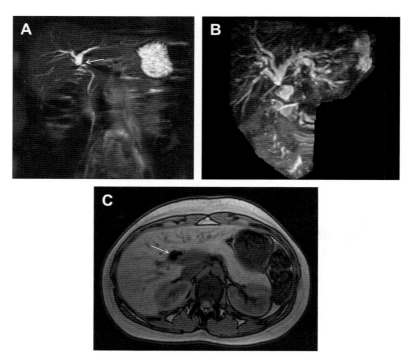

Fig. 15. Clipped CBD, status after cholecystectomy. (*A*) Coronal MIP MRCP images show intrahepatic biliary ductal dilatation, with abrupt change in caliber (*arrow*). Differential considerations based on this imaging appearance include retained stone, clipped CBD, and high-grade stricture. (*B*) 3D MRCP images show the extent of intrahepatic biliary dilatation. (*C*) Opposed phase axial T1 imaging shows metallic blooming artifact at the site of the narrowed CBD (*arrow*), consistent with a metallic clip.

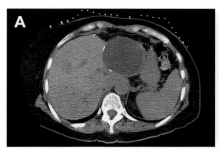
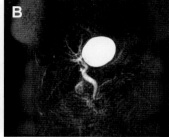

Fig. 16. Biloma. (*A*) A cystic structure abutting the liver seen on CT represented a biloma when seen on MRCP. (*B*) Coronal MIP image shows that the cystic structure communicates with an intrahepatic duct. The patient had a remote history of trauma and previous cholecystectomy.

BILIARY-ENTERIC ANASTOMOSIS

Surgery to create biliary-enteric anastomoses can be performed to treat both benign and malignant causes. Most commonly, a loop of jejunum is brought anteriorly and anastomosed to the common duct, usually with either a Roux-en-Y choledocho-jejunostomy or hepaticojejunostomy.[59] Common complications postbiliary-enteric anastomoses include obstruction, cholangitis, intrahepatic strictures, biliary leaks, and intrahepatic stones. MRCP plays an important role in the diagnosis of these patients, because the surgical anatomy precludes ERCP.[64]

In patients presenting with jaundice, conventional MRCP can detect the site and often the cause of the patient's stricture. However, because these postoperative patients can have both obstructive and nonobstructive biliary dilatation, conventional MRCP is limited by lack of functional information. MRCP performed with biliary-excreted contrast agents is advantageous because imaging provides both structural and functional information. In a study performed by Hottat and colleagues, patients with suspected stricture who showed delayed excretion of manganese dipyridoxyl diphosphate (>2 hours) were found to have significant stricture at percutaneous transhepatic cholangiography. Similar results can be seen with the use of Gd-EOB-DTPA-enhanced MR cholangiography.[65] In addition, in some patients with dilated bile ducts, Gd-EOB-DTPA MRCP was able to show patency of the anastomosis when contrast opacification was seen of the jejunum. In these cases, ductal dilatation was secondary to cholangitis or intrahepatic bile duct strictures rather than anastomotic strictures.[66]

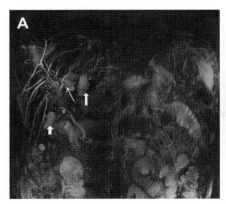
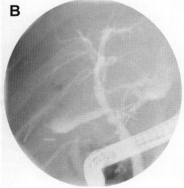

Fig. 17. Persistent bile leak with biloma and intrahepatic bile lakes, status 1 month after hepatic transplant. (*A*) Coronal MIP MRCP image shows intrahepatic biliary ductal dilatation with focal T2 hyperintense collections within the hepatic parenchyma, consistent with bile lakes (*thin white arrow*). Two focal collections are identified in the subhepatic space, consistent with biloma (*thick white arrows*). Nonvisualization of the midportion of the CBD is secondary to the presence of a stent, which was placed to treat the site of the identified leak. (*B*) ERCP image shows the origin of the leak at the site of the CBD anastomosis (choledochocholedochotomy).

LIVER TRANSPLANTATION AND PARTIAL HEPATECTOMY

Biliary complications after orthotopic liver transplant (OLT) are a major cause of transplant-related morbidity and mortality related. Two main biliary reconstruction patterns are commonly used in OLT: end-to-end anastomosis of donor and recipient CBDs (choledochocholedochostomy) and either choledochojejunostomy or hepaticojejunostomy. Duct-to-duct technique is more commonly used because it is technically easier and physiologic. Because this technique preserves the sphincter of Oddi, there is less incidence of cholangitis then would be seen with biliary-enteric anastomosis.[67]

The most common early complication status after OLT is bile leak at the anastomotic site, with subsequent development of biloma. The incidence of post-OLT bile leak has been described to be as high as 19%, and it generally occurs within 1 month of surgery. The bile leak may also occur from widespread biliary necrosis caused by ischemia from hepatic artery thrombosis, resulting in a nonanastomotic leak. In patients with partial liver transplant (split liver or living donor liver transplantation), the incidence of bile leak is higher because of cut surface leaks.[67] Regardless of the cause, MRCP shows the presence of T2 hyperintense subhepatic collection consistent with a biloma. This collection can sometimes be identified as extending from the anastomotic site.[68]

Stricture is the most common late biliary complication of OLT. It is more commonly seen in patients with Roux-en-Y choledochojejunostomy and the incidence is higher within the first year. These strictures are most often believed to be related to fibrosis/local ischemia at the anastomotic site. Imaging features of biliary stricture are described above notably short-segment narrowing with proximal intrahepatic biliary dilitiation.[67,68]

Biliary strictures occur rarely in patients after partial hepatectomy, but are more common in patients who have undergone extended right hepatectomies, and are believed to be secondary to displacement and rotation of hilar structures with hepatic regeneration. An important feature of biliary obstruction in the regenerative liver is smooth tapering of the bile duct attributed to the limited degree of possible intrahepatic biliary dilatation because of increased hepatic turgidity (**Fig. 18**).[69]

Ampullary Disorders

The anatomy of the ampulla of Vater consists of the ampullary bile duct, the ampullary pancreatic duct, a 1- to 8-mm-long common channel of the biliary and pancreatic duct and the major papilla surrounded by the sphincter of Oddi. It is common not to visualize the sphincteric portion of the common channel on SS MRCP in healthy patients, which can be related to the small caliber of the channel or normal physiologic contraction at the sphincter of Oddi. Similarly, the normal major papilla is also not well seen or is small in size. A normal papilla can be seen as an oval protruding structure less than 10 mm in diameter. An enlarged papilla greater than 10 mm with ampullary mucosal thickening of greater than 2 mm, or enhancement of the papilla more than the adjacent duodenal mucosa suggests abnormality at the ampulla.[5]

Papillitis is a benign acute inflammation of the mucosa overlying the papilla. Choledocholithiasis is the most common cause for acute papillitis. Other causes include cholangitis, acute pancreatitis, and rarely periampullary duodenal diverticulum. On MR imaging, one may see mild to moderate dilatation of the biliary duct to the level of the papilla, possibly along with an impacted calculus, an enlarged papilla, mild ampullary wall thickening less than 3 mm, and increased enhancement of the papilla. Smooth, symmetric wall thickening suggests a benign cause (**Fig. 19**).[5]

Dilatation of the biliary and pancreatic duct to the level of the ampulla should raise concern about an ampullary or periampullary lesion or mass. Benign causes that can also result in this ominous appearance include papillary stricture and sphincter of Oddi dysfunction (SOD). Benign strictures in the region of the papilla have a similar inflammatory cause to those found elsewhere in the biliary ducts, and cause structural partial or complete obstruction at the papilla and sphincter. Functional abnormalities

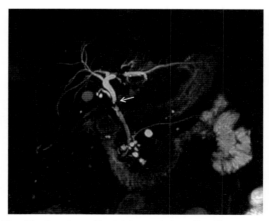

Fig. 18. Anastomotic stricture, status after liver transplant. Coronal MIP MRCP image shows a short-segment narrowing of the CBD at the level of the anastomosis (*arrow*), with mild intrahepatic biliary ductal dilatation.

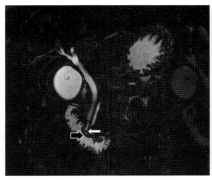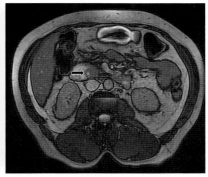

Fig. 19. Papillitis secondary to an impacted calculus in the ampulla. Coronal thick-slab MRCP reveals a calculus impacted in the ampulla. There is swelling of the ampulla (*thin and thick black arrows*) associated with the presence of the impacted stone (*white arrow*), which can be appreciated on the coronal MRCP images and axial opposed phase T1-weighted image.

of the sphincter of Oddi resulting in clinical symptoms of biliary or pancreatic obstruction, such as biliary pain or pancreatitis, constitute sphincter of Oddi dyskinesia. ERCP and sphincter of Oddi manometry are the gold standards for evaluation of this disorder. SOD can also be diagnosed with nuclear hepatobiliary imaging. Although MRCP is not the typical method of evaluating SOD, findings on standard MRCP imaging can suggest the diagnosis. If there is dilatation of the CBD, pancreatic duct or both to the level of the ampulla without a mass or stricture, SOD should be considered. Although function of the sphincter is assessed with manometry or nuclear imaging, the use of biliary-excreted MR contrast agents, specifically gadobenate dimeglumine (Gd-BOPTA) and gadxetic acid (Gd-EOD-DTPA), has been used to evaluate the sphincter.[5] Delayed drainage of bile can be seen with delayed passage of these agents through the ampulla of Vater on MR images obtained more than 0.5 to 1 hour after intravenous contrast administration, which can suggest the diagnosis of SOD.[66,70]

Table 4
MRCP standard protocol

Sequence	Usefulness of Sequence
2D axial T2 (TE 102, TR 2920, ETL 1)	Evaluation of biliary ducts and adjacent organs
Coronal SS FSE (TE 180, TR minimum, BW 62.50)	Evaluation of biliary ducts and adjacent organs
Gradient echo in and out of phase (TR 130, Flip angle 80, BW 31.25)	Evaluation of organs and useful to evaluate for hemorrhage/clot
Thick-slab 2D SS FSE (TE max, ETL 1, Flip angle 1, BW 32)	Overview of biliary ductal anatomy
Thin-slab 2D SS FSE (TE max, TR 150, Flip angle 0.25, BW 62.50)	Detailed evaluation of biliary ducts
Diffusion-weighted imaging (TE minimum, TR 2500)	Abdominal organs; malignant/pathologic processes
3D isotropic MRCP-fast recovery 3D FSE (RARE) (TR 1500, BW 62.50)	Detailed evaluation of biliary ducts
Dynamic axial T1 with fat saturation images after contrast (TE minimum, Flip angle 15, BW 31.25)	Biliary and abdominal organ disease
Axial T1 after contrast with fat saturation thin-section images (TE minimum, TR 150, Flip angle 80, BW 31.25)	Biliary and abdominal organ disease

Abbreviations: BW, bandwidth; FSE, fast spin echo.

Papillary and Ampullary Adenomas

Papillary adenomas are benign tumors of the biliary tree that have malignant potential. Multiple papillomas can be scattered in throughout the biliary tree in a condition called biliary papillomatosis., which shows an irregular pattern of biliary dilatation because of the random distribution of the papillomas. The most common benign tumor of the ampulla is an ampullary adenoma. Both papillary and ampullary adenomas are seen as small filling defects in the biliary ductal system and show homogenous enhancement.[11]

PROTOCOLS

MRCP relies on the high T2 signal intensity of bile in the biliary system. Therefore, heavily T2-weighted sequences are obtained to best visualize the ducts. Fat saturation is used for these images to suppress the background signal from the surrounding organs and tissues. 2D and thin-section 3D images are obtained using fast spin echo or turbo spin echo or SS fast spin echo techniques. A thick-slab section of 4 to 5 cm is obtained for an overview of the biliary tract, usually in the coronal and coronal oblique planes. Thin-slab multisection sequences of 3 to 4 mm are also acquired in the axial and coronal planes to allow for detailed evaluation of intraductal conditions.[11,35] 3D reconstructions can be created from the thin section source images using MIPs that generate images similar to conventional cholangiography.[71] Standard T1, in- and out-of-phase, T2, post-Gd T1 with fat saturation and diffusion-weighted images are also obtained to allow for evaluation of the biliary duct wall and surrounding organs. The use of biliary-excreted Gd contrast agents such as gadobenate dimeglumine (Gd-BOPTA) and gadoxetic acid dosodium (Gd-EOB-DTPA) can also provide functional information about the excretion of bile, anatomic detail for surgical planning, and transplant evaluation, and help determine if fluid signal lesions are connected to the biliary system.[66,72] High-signal magnets of 1.5 T or greater and parallel imaging allow for superb images and shorter scan times. Various breath holding, respiratory triggered, and navigator nonbreath-hold techniques can be used to minimize motion artifact.[35] The protocol for MRCP is summarized in **Table 4**.

REFERENCES

1. Palmucci S, Mauro LA, Coppolino M, et al. Evaluation of the biliary and pancreatic system with 2D SSFSE, breathhold 3D FRFSE and respiratory-triggered 3D FRFSE sequences. Radiol Med 2010; 115(3):467–82.
2. Sodickson A, Mortele KJ, Barish MA, et al. Three-dimensional fast-recovery fast spin-echo MRCP: comparison with two-dimensional single-shot fast spin-echo techniques. Radiology 2006;238(2):549–59.
3. Healet JE Jr, Schroy PC. Anatomy of the biliary ducts within the human liver; analysis of the prevailing pattern of branchings and the major variations of the biliary ducts. AMA Arch Surg 1953;66(5):599–616.
4. Yu J, Turner MA, Fulcher AS, et al. Congenital anomalies and normal variants of the pancreaticobiliary tract and the pancreas in adults: part 1, biliary tract. AJR Am J Roentgenol 2006;187(6):1536–43.
5. Kim TU, Kim S, Lee JW, et al. Ampulla of Vater: comprehensive anatomy, MR imaging of pathologic conditions, and correlation with endoscopy. Eur J Radiol 2008;66(1):48–64.
6. Mortelé KJ, Rocha TC, Streeter JL, et al. Multimodality imaging of pancreatic and biliary congenital anomalies. Radiographics 2006;26(3):715–31.
7. De Filippo M, Calabrese M, Quinto S, et al. Congenital anomalies and variations of the bile and pancreatic ducts: magnetic resonance cholangiopancreatography findings, epidemiology and clinical significance. Radiol Med 2008;113(6):841–59.
8. Suhocki PV, Meyers WC. Injury to aberrant bile ducts during cholecystectomy: a common cause of diagnostic error and treatment delay. AJR Am J Roentgenol 1999;172(4):955–9.
9. Turner MA, Fulcher AS. The cystic duct: normal anatomy and disease processes. Radiographics 2001;21(1):3–22.
10. Krausé D, Cercueil JP, Dranssart M, et al. MRI for evaluating congenital bile duct abnormalities. J Comput Assist Tomogr 2002;26(4):541–52.
11. Bilgin M, Shaikh F, Semelka RC, et al. Magnetic resonance imaging of gallbladder and biliary system. Top Magn Reson Imaging 2009;20(1):31–42.
12. Guy F, Cognet F, Dranssart M, et al. Caroli's disease: magnetic resonance imaging features. Eur Radiol 2002;12(11):2730–6.
13. Hosoki T, Hasuike Y, Takeda Y, et al. Visualization of pancreaticobiliary reflux in anomalous pancreaticobiliary junction by secretin-stimulated dynamic magnetic resonance cholangiopancreatography. Acta Radiol 2004;45(4):375–82.
14. Kamisawa T, Tu Y, Egawa N, et al. MRCP of congenital pancreaticobiliary malformation. Abdom Imaging 2007;32(1):129–33.
15. Norton KI, Glass RB, Kogan D, et al. MR cholangiography in the evaluation of neonatal cholestasis: initial results. Radiology 2002;222(3):687–91.
16. Chavhan GB, Babyn PS, Manson D, et al. Pediatric MR cholangiopancreatography: principles, technique, and clinical applications. Radiographics 2008;28(7): 1951–62.

17. Adusumilli S, Siegelman ES. MR imaging of the gallbladder. Magn Reson Imaging Clin N Am 2002; 10(1):165–84.

18. Park MS, Yu JS, Kim YH, et al. Acute cholecystitis: comparison of MR cholangiography and US. Radiology 1998;209(3):781–5.

19. Akpinar E, Turkbey B, Karcaaltincaba M, et al. Initial experience on utility of gadobenate dimeglumine (Gd-BOPTA) enhanced T1-weighted MR cholangiography in diagnosis of acute cholecystitis. J Magn Reson Imaging 2009;30(3):578–85.

20. Elsayes KM, Oliveira EP, Narra VR, et al. Magnetic resonance imaging of the gallbladder: spectrum of abnormalities. Acta Radiol 2007;48(5):476–82.

21. Levy AD, Murakata LA, Abbott RM, et al. From the archives of the AFIP. Benign tumors and tumorlike lesions of the gallbladder and extrahepatic bile ducts: radiologic-pathologic correlation. Armed Forces Institute of Pathology. Radiographics 2002; 22(2):387–413.

22. Kim PN, Outwater EK, Mitchell DG. Mirizzi syndrome: evaluation by MR imaging. Am J Gastroenterol 1999;94:2546–50.

23. Pemberton M, Wells AD. The Mirizzi syndrome. Postgrad Med 1997;73:487–90.

24. Yun EJ, Choi CS, Yoon DY, et al. Combination of magnetic resonance cholangiopancreatography and computed tomography for preoperative diagnosis of the Mirizzi syndrome. J Comput Assist Tomogr 2009;33:636–40.

25. Csendes A. Common bile duct stones: introduction. World J Surg 1998;22:1113.

26. Rosenthal RJ, Rossi RL, Martin RF. Options and strategies for the management of choledocholithiasis. World J Surg 1998;22:1125–32.

27. Stott MA, Farrands PA, Guyer PB, et al. Ultrasound of the common bile duct in patients undergoing cholecystectomy. J Clin Ultrasound 1991;19:73–6.

28. Anderson SW, Lucey BC, Varghese JC, et al. Accuracy of MDCT in the diagnosis of choledocholithiasis. AJR Am J Roentgenol 2006;187:174–80.

29. Jeffrey RB, Federle MP, Laing FC, et al. Computed tomography of choledocholithiasis. AJR Am J Roentgenol 1983;140:1179–83.

30. Calvo MM, Bujanda L, Calderon A, et al. Role of magnetic resonance cholangiopancreatography in patients with suspected choledocholithiasis. Mayo Clin Proc 2002;77:422–8.

31. Irie H, Honda H, Kuroiwa T, et al. Pitfalls in MR cholangiopancreatographic interpretation. Radiographics 2001;21:23–37.

32. Brugge W. Bile duct strictures. Emedicine. Available at: http://emedicine.medscape.com/article/186850-overview. Accessed March 16, 2010.

33. Jablonska B, Lampe P. Iatrogenic bile duct injuries: etiology, diagnosis and management. World J Gastroenterol 2009;15(33):4097–104.

34. Ward J, Sherdian MB, Guthrie JA, et al. Bile duct strictures after hepatobiliary surgery: assessment with MR cholangiography. Radiology 2004;231:101–8.

35. Yeh BM, Liu PS, Soto JA, et al. MR imaging and CT of the biliary tract. Radiographics 2009;29:1669–88.

36. Park M, Kim TK, Kim KW, et al. Differentiation of extrahepatic bile duct cholangiocarcinoma from benign stricture: findings at MRCP versus ERCP. Radiology 2004;233:234–40.

37. Khalid TR, Casillas VJ, Motalvo BM, et al. Using MR cholangiopancreatography to evaluate iatrogenic bile duct injury. AJR Am J Roentgenol 2001;177: 1347–52.

38. Bismuth H. Postoperative strictures of the bile ducts. In: Blumgart LH, editor. The Biliary Tract V. New York: Churchill Livingstone; 1982. p. 209–18.

39. Vitale GC, Tran TC, Davis BR, et al. Endoscopic management of postcholecystectomy bile duct strictures. J Am Coll Surg 2008;206:918–25.

40. Carpenter HA. Bacterial and parasitic cholangitis. Mayo Clin Proc 1998;73(5):473–8.

41. Bader TR, Braga L, Beavers KL, et al. MR imaging findings of infectious cholangitis. Magn Reson Imaging 2001;19:781–8.

42. Bilgin M, Balci NC, Erdogan A, et al. Hepatobiliary and pancreatic MRI and MRCP findings in patients with HIV infection. AJR Am J Roentgenol 2008;191: 228–32.

43. Ko W-F, Cello JP, Rogers SJ, et al. Prognostic factors for the survival of patients with AIDS cholangiopathy. Am J Gastroenterol 2003;98:2176–81.

44. Enns R. AIDS cholangiopathy: "an endangered disease." Am J Gastroenterol 2003;98(10):2111–2.

45. Hefferan EJ, Geoghegan T, Munk PL. Recurrent pyogenic cholangitis: from imaging to intervention. AJR Am J Roentgenol 2009;192:W28–35.

46. Okuno WT, Whitman GJ, Chew FS. Recurrent pyogenic cholangitis. AJR Am J Roentgenol 1996;167:484.

47. Kim MJ, Cha SW, Mitchell DG, et al. MR imaging findings in recurrent pyogenic cholangitis. AJR Am J Roentgenol 1999;173:1545–9.

48. Kim TK, Kim BS, Kim JH, et al. Diagnosis of intrahepatic stones: superiority of MR cholangiopancreatography over endoscopic retrograde cholangiopancreatography. AJR Am J Roentgenol 2002;179:429–34.

49. Gordon FD. Primary sclerosing cholangitis. Surg Clin North Am 2008;88:1385–407.

50. Lee YM, Kaplan MM. Primary sclerosing cholangitis. N Engl J Med 1995;332:924–32.

51. Vitellas KM, El-Dieb A, Vaswani KK. MR cholangiopancreatography in patients with primary sclerosing cholangitis: interobserver variability and comparison with endoscopic retrograde cholangiopancreatography. AJR Am J Roentgenol 2002;179:399–407.

52. Cohen SA, Siegel JH, Kasmin FE. Complications of diagnostic and therapeutic ERCP. Abdom Imaging 1996;21:385–94.

53. Silverman WB, Kaw M, Rabinovitz M, et al. Complication rate of endoscopic retrograde cholangiopancreatography (ERCP) in patients with primary sclerosing cholangitis: is it safe? Gastroenterology 1994;106:A359.

54. Beuers U, Spengler I, Sackmann M, et al. Deterioration of cholestasis after endoscopic retrograde cholangiography in advanced primary sclerosing cholangitis. J Hepatol 1992;15:140.

55. Berstad AE, Aabakken L, Smith HJ, et al. Diagnostic accuracy of magnetic resonance and endoscopic retrograde cholangiography in primary sclerosing cholangitis. Clin Gastroenterol Hepatol 2006;4(4):514–20.

56. Revelon G, Rashid A, Kawamoto S, et al. Primary sclerosing cholangitis: MR imaging findings with pathological correlation. AJR Am J Roentgenol 1999;173:1037–42.

57. Dodd GD III, Baron RL, Oliver JH III, et al. End-stage primary sclerosing cholangitis: CT findings of hepatic morphology in 36 patients. Radiology 1999;211: 357–62.

58. Petrovic BD, Nikolaidis P, Hammond NA, et al. Correlation between findings on MRCP and gadolinium-enhanced MR of the liver and a survival model for primary sclerosing cholangitis. Dig Dis Sci 2007;52(12):3499–506.

59. Oddsdottir M, Pham Thai H, Hunter JG. Gallbladder and the extrahepatic biliary system. In: Brunicardi FC, Andersen DK, Billiar TR, et al, editors. Schwartz's principles of surgery. 9th edition. Chapter 32. Available at: http://www.accessmedicine.com/content.aspx?aID=5026661. Accessed February 10, 2010.

60. Piccinni G, Angrisano A, Testini M, et al. Diagnosing and treating Sphincter of Oddi dysfunction: a critical literature review and reevaluation. J Clin Gastroenterol 2004;38(4):350–9.

61. Vitellas K, Keogan MT, Spritzer CE, et al. MR cholangiopancreatography of bile and pancreatic duct abnormalities with emphasis on single shot fast spin echo technique. Radiographics 2000;20: 939–57.

62. Hoeffel C, Azizi L, Lewin M, et al. Normal and pathologic features of the postoperative biliary tract at 3D MR cholangiopancreatography and MR imaging. Radiographics 2006;26:1603–20.

63. Thurley P, Dhingsa R. Laparoscopic cholecystectomy: postoperative imaging. AJR Am J Roentgenol 2008;191:794–801.

64. Pavone P, Laghi A, Catalano C, et al. MR cholangiography in the examination of patients with biliary-enteric anastomoses. AJR Am J Roentgenol 1997; 169:807–11.

65. Hottat N, Winant C, Metens T, et al. MR cholangiography with manganese dipyridoxyl diphosphate in the evaluation of biliary-enteric anastomoses: preliminary experience. AJR Am J Roentgenol 2005;184:1556–62.

66. Lee NK, Kim S, Lee JW, et al. Biliary MR imaging with Gd-EOB-DTPA and its clinical applications. Radiographics 2009;29(6):1707–24.

67. Girometti R, Cereser L, et al. Biliary complications after orthotopic liver transplantation: MRCP findings. Abdom Imaging 2008;33(5):542–54.

68. Novellas S, Caramella T, et al. MR cholangiopancreatography features of the biliary tree after liver transplantation. AJR Am J Roentgenol 2008;191(1):221–7.

69. Garcea G, Polimnovi N, et al. Diagnostic value of MRCP in the management of hilar strictures after extended liver resection. Clin Radiol 2004;59(9): 846–8.

70. Fayad LM, Holland GA, Bergin D, et al. Functional magnetic resonance cholangiography (FMRC) of the gallbladder and biliary tree with contrast-enhanced magnetic resonance cholangiography. J Magn Reson Imaging 2003;18(4):449–60.

71. Nandalur KR, Hussain HK, Weadock WJ, et al. Possible biliary disease: diagnostic performance of high-spatial-resolution isotropic 3D T2-weighted MRCP. Radiology 2008;249(3):883–90.

72. Seale MK, Catalano OA, Saini S, et al. Hepatobiliary-specific MR contrast agents: role in imaging the liver and biliary tree. Radiographics 2009;29(6):1725–48.

MR Imaging Evaluation of the Hepatic Vasculature

Rizwan Aslam, MB ChB[a,b], Benjamin M. Yeh, MD[a,b,]*,
Judy Yee, MD[b]

KEYWORDS

- Hepatic vasculature • Liver injury • MR imaging
- Portal veins • Hepatic veins

Routine hepatic magnetic resonance (MR) imaging provides an excellent assessment of the hepatic vasculature. Automated contrast detection methods in combination with fast breath-hold sequences allow reproducible capture of the arterial, portal venous, and delayed phases of enhancement. This reproducible capture enables improved vascular lesion detection and characterization. Sequences can also be dedicated to focus on specific aspects of the hepatic blood vessels, including the demonstration of flow physiology. High-resolution, 3-dimensional, gadolinium-enhanced imaging, including fat suppression and multiphasic reconstructions, can be used routinely without exposing patients to ionizing radiation. MR imaging is able to provide an accurate assessment of the hepatic vascular anatomy. This accurate assessment is essential for patients who are being considered for surgery, such as liver resection or transplantation. In addition, MR imaging can also provide a road map to guide radiological intervention, which can reduce procedural times and improve safety (**Fig. 1**). For diagnostic evaluation, relatively noninvasive techniques such as MR angiography and computed tomography (CT) angiography have largely replaced digital subtraction angiography (DSA).

Multidetector row CT (MDCT) angiography provides excellent detail of the hepatic arteries and their branches and is a robust, quick method for vascular assessment before surgery. MDCT also has the advantage of being readily accessible in most institutions. However, a significant advantage of contrast-enhanced MR angiography is the ability to assess the liver without irradiation. Both CT and MR imaging contrast agents have some associated risk of contrast-induced nephropathy as well as other adverse effects, including rare but potentially lethal reactions such as anaphylactic shock. More recently, there has been increased awareness of nephrogenic systemic fibrosis as a potential complication in patients with severe chronic renal insufficiency or acute renal failure who undergo gadolinium-enhanced MR imaging.[1,2] A further advantage of MR imaging compared with MDCT is the ability to selectively visualize the hepatic vasculature using noncontrast-enhanced MR angiography. Doppler ultrasonography also allows for such noninvasive imaging of vessels without ionizing radiation or contrast agents, but visualization may be limited for various reasons such as overlying bowel gas or large body habitus.

Historically, an important limitation of MR angiography compared with DSA and CT angiography has been lower spatial resolution. However, there have been recent significant improvements in the achievable spatial resolution owing to the introduction of newer image reconstruction algorithms and dedicated contrast agents. These developments have enabled MR angiography to achieve higher spatial resolution and better image quality.

[a] Department of Radiology and Biomedical Imaging, University of California, San Francisco, School of Medicine, 505 Parnassus Avenue, M372, Box 0628, San Francisco, CA 94143-0628, USA
[b] Department of Radiology, San Francisco Veterans Affairs Medical Center, 4150 Clement Street, San Francisco, CA 94121, USA
* Corresponding author.
E-mail address: ben.yeh@radiology.ucsf.edu

Magn Reson Imaging Clin N Am 18 (2010) 515–523
doi:10.1016/j.mric.2010.08.005
1064-9689/10/$ — see front matter © 2010 Elsevier Inc. All rights reserved.

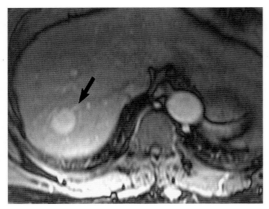

Fig. 1. Axial T1 contrast-enhanced image shows a feeding branch vessel from the right hepatic artery supplying a hypervascular lesion, later confirmed as hepatocellular carcinoma (*black arrow*).

The combination of multichannel, high field-strength MR systems, and the development of multielement angiography receiver coils has also helped to substantially improve the clinical utility of MR angiography.

HEPATIC ARTERIES
Contrast-Enhanced MR Angiography

Contrast-enhanced MR angiography is the preferred technique for MR imaging of the arterial vasculature. Contrast-enhanced MR angiography relies on timing scan acquisitions after contrast administration such that T1 shortening is maximal during the period when the center of k-space is acquired. Injection of conventional gadolinium contrast agents results in only a transient T1 shortening of the intra-arterial blood during which time data must be acquired, necessitating accurate timing of the scan with the injection of contrast material. Most routine MR imaging contrast agents rapidly diffuse from the vessels into the extracellular space. The intravascular half-life of such extracellular gadolinium-based contrast agents is approximately 90 seconds. Consequently, to optimize results, a sufficient volume of contrast needs to be injected in a short period to decrease the T1 of blood to values substantially less than those of adjacent tissues.

Until recent developments, breath-hold scan times exceeding 30 seconds were often required for standard 3-dimensional gradient-recalled echo (GRE) sequences. Such prolonged breath-hold times limit the quality of images obtainable in debilitated patients who have compromised respiratory function and are not capable of the multiple breath-holds required for dynamic GRE

MR imaging. Several approaches have been developed to reduce the breath-hold times in dynamic GRE MR imaging, such as decreasing the matrix size and the number of partitions. However, the introduction of such parameter changes to reduce acquisition time results in trade-offs including reduced spatial resolution or limited z-axis coverage.[3]

Parallel Imaging Techniques

Another approach that is presently applied to reduce breath-hold times is to use parallel imaging techniques. These methods use multiple radiofrequency receiver coils to acquire multiple data points simultaneously within a single phase-encoding gradient. In this approach, k-space is systematically undersampled by each coil, which conventionally would lead to aliasing or wrap-around artifacts. However, parallel imaging uses the redundant spatial information available from the multicoil configuration to restore the spatial resolution and avoid the aliasing artifact. Techniques that have been developed to correct for aliasing vary, depending on whether they work on image domain data, such as the sensitivity encoding method, or on the raw (k-space) data, such as the GeneRalized Autocalibrating Partially Parallel Acquisitions method.[3,4]

With parallel imaging, the maximum increase in speed is proportional to the number of coils. However, the signal-to-noise ratio (SNR) is reduced by shorter acquisition times and is further decreased by the amplification of noise that occurs in regions in which the geometry of coil sensitivities is suboptimal. This reduction in SNR can be partially overcome by faster rates of injection of the contrast bolus to achieve higher contrast concentrations during sampling.[4]

Shortened Scan Times

Advances in gradient hardware, pulse sequences, and computational power have allowed for greatly shortened scan times. By shortening the scan time to several seconds, it is possible to image arterial, portal, and venous contrast phases during individual breath-holds. The resultant images provide dynamic information on contrast arrival and rates of enhancement of vascular structures and organs. Regardless of the technique used, there is always a trade-off between spatial resolution and temporal resolution. Investigators have compared the diagnostic accuracy of dynamic parallel GRE MR imaging with contrast-enhanced 64-detector MDCT, which served as the noninvasive reference standard. Comprehensive hepatic vascular mapping of the hepatic arteries and the portal and hepatic veins was included. Image quality for depiction of most of the hepatic vessels was rated as high with the use of parallel GRE MR techniques. Furthermore, image quality was rated as good or excellent for 91.1% to 100% of vessels. The readers for this study were able to confidently diagnose variant hepatic vessels and arterial stenosis with 94% to 100% accuracy (**Fig. 2**). All portal and hepatic veins were visible for diagnostic purposes, and image quality was considered to be nondiagnostic in only 2.1% of the hepatic arteries evaluated.[4]

Noncontrast MR Angiography Techniques

It is technically feasible to image the hepatic arteries using specific sequences without the administration of MR contrast agents. The noncontrast technique, which is likely to be most effective in evaluating the hepatic arteries, is the respiratory-triggered, 3-dimensional, steady-state free-precession (SSFP) sequence, which is a fast MR technique that has been widely used in coronary MR angiography. SSFP can be used to rapidly produce images of acceptable resolution, and when time spatial labeling inversion pulse (T-SLIP) is combined with SSFP there is further improvement in the visualization of the hepatic arteries.[5,6] The T-SLIP sequence is a form of spin labeling that can provide quantitative and selective inflow information by placing the inversion pulse before data acquisition and suppressing the background tissue. The time-of-flight (TOF) technique, which can also be used to visualize vessel, is likely to be less effective because of in-plane saturation effects.[6] The SSFP sequence is a type of gradient-echo sequence applied with very short echo times, which allows imaging of blood vessels without the use of a contrast agent. SSFP depends on the ratio of T2 to T1. This ratio is relatively high for blood compared with the surrounding tissues and the short echo time renders the sequence flow insensitive.[7] T-SLIP is a type of arterial spin labeling technique, which can be used to further enhance the signal from the selected vessel in combination with SSFP by signal suppression of the background tissue and other vessels.[8]

These techniques are presently limited for routine clinical use because of the long acquisition times of up to 10 minutes. New methods to shorten acquisition times include the combination of this technique with parallel imaging and using techniques to counteract the reduction in signal that would occur. The combination of SSFP with short-tau inversion recovery (STIR) and T-SLIP enables greater background signal suppression to compensate for the signal reduction in the blood vessel induced by 2-dimensional parallel imaging.[7] The combination of 2-dimensional-PI, T-SLIP, and STIR has been shown to successfully shorten the acquisition time from 10 minutes to 6 minutes while allowing for selective hepatic artery visualization and maintaining diagnostic image quality.[5,7]

PORTAL VEIN
Contrast-Enhanced MR Portography

Several modalities are available to image the portal veins, and each modality has its strengths and limitations. Doppler ultrasonography (DUS) is particularly useful, as it is noninvasive, inexpensive, and provides information regarding portal flow. However, DUS is highly operator and subject dependent and, therefore, may be adversely affected by factors such as patient obesity, intestinal gas, and excessive abdominal ascites.

Any technique used to image the portal vein must be able to provide an accurate assessment of portal venous anatomy, which is essential for patients being evaluated for liver resection or transplantation. Studies have demonstrated the superiority of 3-dimensional MR portography over DUS.[9,10] The normal portal vein bifurcates into right and left branches in 89% of individuals.[11] The right portal vein divides into anterior and posterior branches, whereas the left divides into superior and inferior branches. Common anatomic variants are trifurcation of the main portal vein, in which the left portal vein arises at the bifurcation of the right portal vein. Other common variants are a left portal vein origin from the right anterior portal vein branch or an early origin of the right posterior portal vein branch seen in 4% and 6% of individuals, respectively.[11] Unfavorable congenital portal venous anomalies may preclude

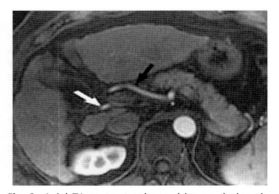

Fig. 2. Axial T1 contrast-enhanced image during the arterial phase shows an anomalous right hepatic artery (*white arrow*) that originates directly from the superior mesenteric artery (SMA). The left hepatic artery has a conventional origin from the celiac axis (*black arrow*).

individuals from liver donation.[12] It is also essential to evaluate the size and patency of the recipient portal vein prior to liver transplantation because the donor portal vein should optimally be no more than 3 to 4 mm different in size relative to that of the recipient's portal vein.[13]

Portal Vein Thrombosis

Portal vein thrombosis is another important clinical indication for portal venous evaluation. The diagnostic sensitivity of DUS for detecting portal vein thrombosis is reported to range from 66% to 100%.[9,10] Portal vein thrombosis may be associated with a variety of different disease processes such as severe intra-abdominal infections, hypercoagulable states, and various malignancies. Portal vein thrombosis may also be a complication of pregnancy, oral contraceptive use, or trauma. In such cases, portal vein thrombi appear as well-defined, nonenhancing, intraluminal filling defects on contrast-enhanced MR imaging, and may be associated with transient hepatic intensity differences caused by compensatory increased arterial flow to the thrombosed hepatic segments. Distinction between acute and chronic portal vein thrombosis is often of clinical value. In the acute setting, portal vein thrombus may resolve with anticoagulation therapy. However, once the occlusion is long-standing, the likelihood of therapeutic recanalization is greatly reduced. Acute thrombi may show increased signal on T2-weighted sequences relative to chronic thrombi. Chronic portal venous occlusion leads to cavernous transformation of the portal vein, which may preclude future transplantation or liver resections.

Although bland thrombus is the most common filling defect to be seen within the portal vein, it is prudent to consider alternative diagnoses. In particular thrombophlebitis, which is caused by infected venous clot, should be excluded because treatment requires antibiotics in addition to anticoagulation. At MR imaging, thrombophlebitis may be suggested when periportal edema, venous mural thickening, and venous mural enhancement is seen in a febrile patient or patient with sepsis. Another critical diagnosis to consider is tumor thrombus, which typically presents as portal vein expansion with enhancing tissue. The most common malignancy to present with portal venous tumor thrombus is hepatocellular carcinoma, which frequently exhibits direct tumor extension into the portal vein (**Fig. 3**).[13,14] The enhancement of tumor thrombus may be subtle, and for such cases subtraction images may be of benefit.[13] A notable pitfall is that tumor thrombus may show increased T2 signal, much like an acute thrombus,

and so evaluation for enhancement, which is seen only with tumor thrombus, is important.

Portal Vein Angiography Advantages

MR portography (portal vein angiography) compares favorably to other imaging modalities using contrast agents for the diagnosis of portal vein thrombus. Kreft and colleagues[15,16] described an overall sensitivity, specificity, and accuracy for the detection of thrombosis of 100%, 98%, and 99%, respectively, for 3-dimensional gadolinium-enhanced MR angiography and 91%, 100%, and 96%, respectively, for standard intra-arterial DSA. A 3-dimensional gadolinium-enhanced MR angiography also shows an efficacy similar to a 64-slice MDCT for portal vein thrombus detection, and is able to identify portal vein anatomic variants with sensitivities and specificities of 100%.[3,17] In this regard, MR imaging has a clear advantage when compared with MDCT or catheter-based angiography regarding concerns of irradiation and, in patients without renal insufficiency, the safety profile of the contrast agent.

Noncontrast MR Imaging of the Portal Vein

Gadolinium-based contrast agents are clinically contraindicated in some patients. In such patients, noncontrast-enhanced MR imaging techniques may help to provide useful diagnostic information. There are other drawbacks to the use of contrast agents, which can be overcome by noncontrast MR angiography techniques. For example, it is occasionally difficult to differentiate the portal vein and the surrounding liver parenchyma during the portal venous phase of enhancement because of insufficient difference in signal.[18,19] Furthermore, mistiming of image acquisition may result in suboptimal venous opacification relative to surrounding structures.[18]

TOF MR angiography is a well-established, noncontrast technique that can be used to assess patency as well as the direction of flow in the portal vein. TOF MR angiography produces saturation of stationary tissue by multiple repetitive radiofrequency pulses. Nonsaturated blood entering the imaging section is of higher signal than the surrounding saturated tissue. Imaging data can then be acquired as multiple overlapping sections that can be reconstructed to create angiographic images. Presaturation bands can be used to eliminate arterial signal and also provide information on whether flow is hepatopedal or hepatofugal.[6]

Patent blood vessels show high signal intensity on SSFP imaging, whereas thrombus is usually seen as a lower signal-filling defect within vessel.[16] Although slow-moving blood may occasionally

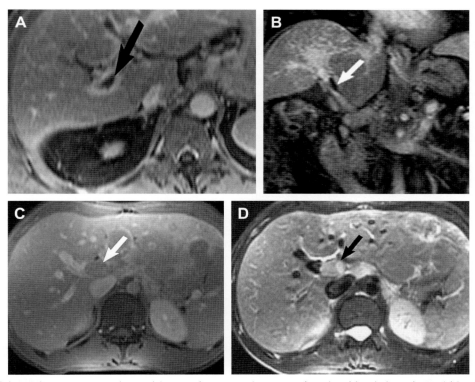

Fig. 3. (A) Axial T1 contrast-enhanced image demonstrating nonenhancing bland thrombus within the right portal vein (*black arrow*). (B) Coronal T1 postcontrast image of the same patient showing an enhancing mass (hepatocellular carcinoma) superior to the nonenhancing bland thrombus in the right portal vein (*white arrow*). (C) T1-weighted, contrast-enhanced, axial image showing enhancing tumor thrombus extending into the main portal vein (*arrow*). The tumor thrombus extends directly from the hepatocellular carcinoma located in the left lobe. The enhancement characteristics of the tumor thrombus are similar to the liver parenchyma. (D) T2-weighted axial image with fat saturation in the same patient. Note hyperintense tumor thrombus in the main portal vein (*arrow*).

result in ambiguous findings, SSFP may be repeated several times until a satisfactory image is obtained.[16] Therefore, SSFP imaging may provide helpful assessment of the portal vein in debilitated patients or those with poor venous access. In a study by Smith and colleagues,[16] SSFP imaging allowed correct diagnosis in 17 out of 17 patients as negative for portal vein thrombosis, achieving a specificity of 100%. In this study 4 of 6 patients were also found to be positive for portal vein thrombosis using SSFP imaging, and the diagnosis was inconclusive in 3 patients, of whom 2 were eventually found to be positive for portal vein thrombosis while 1 had portal vein stenosis. Thus, the sensitivity of SSFP for portal vein thrombus detection was only 67% when compared with contrast-enhanced MR imaging of the portal vein.[16] An important factor to remember is that overlapping hepatic arteries and veins may obscure the portal vein; therefore,

the combination of T-SLIP with SSFP is recommended for selective suppression of signal from blood vessels that are of no clinical interest. Furthermore, more than one T-SLIP can be placed in the imaging region, to enable selective visualization of the vessel of interest.[5] Another potential disadvantage of SSFP for evaluation of the portal vein is the insensitivity of SSFP to the direction of blood flow. If the direction of flow is of clinical relevance, TOF or phase contrast (PC) techniques can be used to image the portal veins.[16]

Half-Fourier fast spin echo (FSE) is a newer, T2-weighted, unenhanced MR angiography technique that has potential clinical applications.[18,20] Half-Fourier FSE allows for a coronal acquisition to enable shorter 3-dimensional acquisition times.[18] The T2-weighting results in relatively low background liver parenchymal signal intensity, resulting in greater portal vein conspicuity. Selective visualization of the portal vein with half-Fourier FSE may also require the addition of T-SLIP to improve results.[18]

Portal Blood Flow Evaluation

The 2 main noninvasive methods for the quantitative assessment of hepatic blood flow are duplex DUS and MR imaging.[21] Regarding MR imaging techniques, PC imaging is ideally suited for flow quantification. PC sequences use the intrinsic ability of MR imaging to detect tissue displacement. Whereas conventional MR imaging sequences represent only the combined magnetization vector amplitude, PC also computes the phase shift of this vector induced by flow direction and velocity.[6,21] Examples of clinical scenarios in which PC techniques may be helpful include the quantification of increases in portal flow after transhepatic shunting[22] or the noninvasive calculation of total hepatic blood flow rates.[21] Hepatic artery flow rate measurements can also be deduced by subtraction of the portal blood flow rate from that of the hepatic venous flow rate.[21] An alternative method to measure portal venous and hepatic arterial fraction flow is by the use of dynamic contrast-enhanced MR imaging with intravenous gadolinium boluses. Such methods have shown promise for the assessment of diffuse liver disease, in which the relative portal venous flow is reduced compared with control patients.[23]

Hepatic Veins

It is important to assess for anatomic variants of the donor hepatic veins before liver transplantation, as well as for patients who are to undergo partial hepatectomy. The hepatic veins in most individuals are usually composed of a right, middle, and left main hepatic veins. Common anatomic variants are accessory hepatic veins draining segments V and VIII in 43% and 49%, respectively.[13] Another common anatomic variant is a hepatic vein-draining segment VI directly into the inferior vena cava (IVC). The identification of these and other anatomic variants is critical prior to hepatic surgery. MR imaging is able to provide excellent evaluation of the hepatic anatomy for this purpose (**Fig. 4**).

Budd-Chiari Syndrome

The hepatic venous outflow tract may also become obstructed, resulting in Budd-Chiari

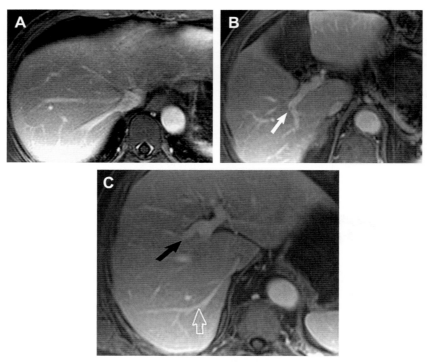

Fig. 4. (*A*) Axial T1 contrast-enhanced image showing an accessory hepatic vein-draining segment 7 of the liver directly in to the ICV. (*B*) Axial T1 postcontrast image showing an anomalous right portal vein branch from the main portal vein directly supplying only segments 5 and 6 (*arrow*). (*C*) Axial T1 contrast-enhanced image shows a portal vein branch supplying the right anterior segment of the liver arising from the left portal vein (*black arrow*). Note: an accessory hepatic vein-draining segment 6 of the liver (*white open arrow*).

syndrome. Although most commonly idiopathic, there are many causes of Budd-Chiari syndrome, including congenital hepatic venous webs, hypercoagulable states, tumor, and inflammatory and autoimmune diseases. Features seen on MR imaging in Budd-Chiari syndrome include: hepatic vein occlusion or narrowing, and IVC and/or hepatic vein thrombosis. The level of obstruction is described to be central if close to the IVC, and peripheral if at the level of the medium- or smaller-sized veins. The accurate identification of the level of obstruction may help to establish the cause. Intrahepatic collaterals may appear as comma-shaped enhancing vessels, and may develop spontaneously and bypass occlusions.[24] The caudate lobe often undergoes compensatory hypertrophy, as it has separate venous drainage directly into the IVC.

Early parenchymal imaging findings of the Budd-Chiari syndrome on MR imaging are usually seen in the liver periphery as areas of heterogeneous high signal on T2 and low signal on T1, related to hepatic congestion. These changes may spare the caudate lobe (**Fig. 5**A), or may result in caudate lobe hyperenhancement during arterial and venous phases of enhancement.[25] Congestive heart failure (CHF) may show liver parenchymal imaging features similar to those seen in Budd-Chiari syndrome, but the IVC and hepatic veins are markedly dilated in CHF (**Fig. 5**B) rather than diminutive or absent as in Budd-Chiari syndrome.[13]

Venoocclusive Disease

Venoocclusive disease is another type of venous outflow obstruction that typically affects patients who have undergone bone marrow transplantation. Venoocclusive disease results in nonthrombotic occlusion of the terminal hepatic venules and small sublobular hepatic veins and possible

fibrous obliteration of the veins in about 5% of patients who have undergone bone marrow transplantation.[13,26]

MR Blood Pool Contrast Agents

When performing MR imaging of the liver several types of contrast media are available, and their pharmacokinetics are worthwhile considering. Differences in contrast dynamics between the liver-specific agents may make them suitable for imaging different pathologic conditions. Conventional gadolinium chelates give excellent depiction of the hepatic vessels, but imaging depends on accurate timing of data acquisition after contrast injection to maximize visualization of the hepatic arteries, portal veins, and hepatic veins. The use of the hepatobiliary contrast agent gadoxetic acid may result in a relatively poorer depiction of the hepatic vasculature owing to the relatively smaller dose of gadoxetic acid (0.025 mmol/kg) compared with other agents (generally 0.1 mmol/kg), which results in much less flexibility in image acquisition timing than with other agents that are generally given at higher doses and volumes. Furthermore, the high extraction rate of gadoxetic acid into the hepatocytes and biliary tract compared with other agents may result in a higher background signal, which may interfere with vascular conspicuity and may also result in decreased concentrations of contrast material in the hepatic and portal veins relative to background liver parenchyma.

The agent gadobenate meglumine is also a hepatobiliary agent but has a lower excretion rate than gadoxetic acid, and exhibits some serum protein binding. This trait may result in better vascular images because of its greater T1-relaxivity and slightly higher intravascular retention time compared with conventional gadolinium chelates. Further along this spectrum, the newly approved

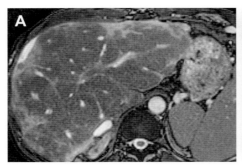
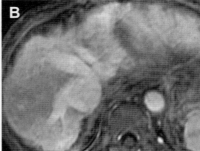

Fig. 5. (*A*) Budd-Chiari Syndrome. Axial T2 fat-saturated image of the liver demonstrates patchy areas of hyperintensity in the periphery of the liver and diminutive hepatic veins and IVC. Note is made of the hypertrophied caudate lobe. (*B*) Axial T1 contrast-enhanced image showing markedly dilated hepatic veins and IVC in a patient with CHF, which contrasts with the diminutive vessels seen in Budd-Chiari syndrome.

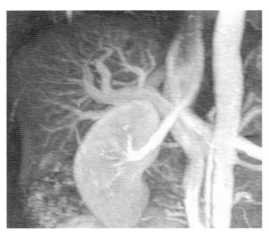

Fig. 6. A coronal, maximum-intensity projection image after the administration of gadofosveset trisodium (blood pool gadolinium contrast agent). Note the enhancement of the arteries, portal veins, and renal veins with minimal enhancement of the hepatic parenchyma.

blood pool agent, gadofosveset trisodium (Ablavar, Lantheus, Billerica, MA, USA), is even more strongly, though reversibly, bound to serum albumin, and is therefore retained in the vascular space for a much longer time[27] and exhibits an even higher T1 relaxation compared with other contrast agents.[28,29] Because gadofosveset trisodium has a long intravascular half-life, it enables greater flexibility in scan times and scan delays for vascular imaging (**Fig. 6**). However, because the contrast material has a variable and prolonged time to equilibration with the liver parenchyma, the clinical utility of gadofosveset trisodium needs to be further studied.

SUMMARY

MR imaging is a valuable tool for the evaluation of liver vasculature; it is particularly useful because it does not expose the patient to ionizing radiation. Compared with ultrasonography, MR imaging is a fairly robust technique and is less affected by patient- and operator-related factors. In addition, MR imaging is able to provide qualitative and quantitative data regarding the hepatic vasculature. When contrast agents are contraindicated, noncontrast MR angiography techniques can frequently provide useful vascular information.

REFERENCES

1. Thomsen HS, Marcos SK. Contrast-medium-induced nephropathy: is there a new consensus? A review of published guidelines. Eur Radiol 2006; 16(8):1835–40.

2. Dawson P. Nephrogenic systemic fibrosis: possible mechanisms and imaging management strategies. J Magn Reson Imaging 2008;28(4):797–804.

3. Heilmaier C, Sutter R, Lutz AM, et al. Mapping of hepatic vascular anatomy: dynamic contrast-enhanced parallel MR imaging compared with 64 detector row CT. Radiology 2007;245(3):872–80.

4. Chen Q, Quijano CV, Mai VM, et al. On improving temporal and spatial resolution of 3D contrast-enhanced body MR angiography with parallel imaging. Radiology 2004;231(3):893–9.

5. Shimada K, Isoda H, Okada T. Non-contrast-enhanced hepatic MR angiography with true steady-state free-precession and time spatial labeling inversion pulse: optimization of the technique and preliminary results. Eur J Radiol 2009;70(1):111–7.

6. Miyazaki M, Lee VS. Nonenhanced MR angiography. Radiology 2008;248(1):20–43.

7. Shimada K, Isoda H, Okada T, et al. Non-contrast-enhanced hepatic MR angiography: do two-dimensional parallel imaging and short tau inversion recovery methods shorten acquisition time without image quality deterioration? Eur J Radiol 2009. [Epub ahead of print].

8. Nishimura DG, Macovski A, Jackson JI, et al. Magnetic resonance angiography by selective inversion recovery using a compact gradient echo sequence. Magn Reson Med 1988;8(1):96–103.

9. Cakmak O, Elmas N, Tamsel S, et al. Role of contrast-enhanced 3D magnetic resonance portography in evaluating portal venous system compared with color Doppler ultrasonography. Abdom Imaging 2008;33(1):65–71.

10. Tessler FN, Gehring BJ, Gomes AS, et al. Diagnosis of portal vein thrombosis: value of color Doppler imaging. AJR Am J Roentgenol 1991;157(2):293–6.

11. Lee VS, Morgan GR, Lin JC, et al. Liver transplant donor candidates: associations between vascular and biliary anatomic variants. Liver Transpl 2004; 10(8):1049–54.

12. Atri M, Bret PM, Fraser-Hill MA. Intrahepatic portal venous variations: prevalence with US. Radiology 1992;184(1):157–8.

13. Rubin GD, Rofsky NM. CT and MR angiography comprehensive vascular assessment. Philadelphia (PA): Lippincott Williams & Wilkins; 2009. p. 830–40.

14. Sobhonslidsuk A, Reddy KR. Portal vein thrombosis: a concise review. Am J Gastroenterol 2002;97(3):535–41.

15. Kreft B, Strunk H, Flacke S. Detection of thrombosis in the portal venous system: comparison of contrast-enhanced MR angiography with intraarterial digital subtraction angiography. Radiology 2000;216(1):86–92.

16. Smith CS, Sheehy N, McEniff N, et al. Magnetic resonance portal venography: use of fast-acquisition

true FISP imaging in the detection of portal vein thrombosis. Clin Radiol 2007;62(12):1180–8.

17. Lee VS, Morgan GR, Teperman LW, et al. MR imaging as the sole preoperative imaging modality for right hepatectomy: a prospective study of living adult-to-adult liver donor candidates. AJR Am J Roentgenol 2001;176(6):1475–82.

18. Shimada K, Isoda H, Okada T, et al. Unenhanced MR portography with a half-Fourier fast spin-echo sequence and time-space labeling inversion pulses: preliminary results. AJR Am J Roentgenol 2009; 193(1):106–12.

19. Lee MW, Lee JM, Lee JY, et al. Preoperative evaluation of hepatic arterial and portal venous anatomy using the time resolved echo-shared MR angiographic technique in living liver donors. Eur Radiol 2007;17(4):1074–80.

20. Ito K, Koike S, Jo C, et al. Intraportal venous flow distribution: evaluation with single breath-hold ECG-triggered three-dimensional half-Fourier fast spin-echo MR imaging and a selective inversion-recovery tagging pulse. AJR Am J Roentgenol 2002;178(2):343–8.

21. Yzet T, Bouzerar R, Baledent O, et al. Dynamic measurements of total hepatic blood flow with phase contrast MRI. Eur J Radiol 2010;73(1): 119–24.

22. Debatin JF, Zahner B, Meyenberger C, et al. Azygos blood flow: phase contrast quantitation in volunteers and patients with portal hypertension pre- and postintrahepatic shunt placement. Hepatology 1996; 24(5):1109–15.

23. Baxter S, Wang ZJ, Joe BN, et al. Timing bolus dynamic contrast-enhanced (DCE) MRI assessment of hepatic perfusion: Initial experience. J Magn Reson Imaging 2009;29(6):1317–22.

24. Stark DD, Hahn PF, Trey C, et al. MRI of the Budd-Chiari syndrome. AJR Am J Roentgenol 1986; 146(6):1141–8.

25. Noone TC, Semelka RC, Siegelman ES, et al. Budd-Chiari syndrome: spectrum of appearances of acute, subacute, and chronic disease with magnetic resonance imaging. J Magn Reson Imaging 2000; 11(1):44–50.

26. Morrin MM, Pedrosa I, Rofsky NM. Magnetic resonance imaging for disorders of liver vasculature. Top Magn Reson Imaging 2002;13(3):177–90.

27. Parmelee DJ, Walovitch RC, Ouellet HS, et al. Preclinical evaluation of the pharmacokinetics, biodistribution, and elimination of MS-325, a blood pool agent for magnetic resonance imaging. Invest Radiol 1997;32(12):741–7.

28. Fink C, Goyen M, Lotz J. Magnetic resonance angiography with blood-pool contrast agents: future applications. Eur Radiol 2007;17(Suppl 2): B38–44.

29. Brismar TB, Dahlstrom N, Edsborg N, et al. Liver vessel enhancement by Gd-BOPTA and Gd-EOB-DTPA: a comparison in healthy volunteers. Acta Radiol 2009;50(7):709–15.

Magnetic Resonance Imaging of the Liver: Sequence Optimization and Artifacts

Geoffrey E. Wile, MD[a],*, John R. Leyendecker, MD[b]

KEYWORDS

- Liver • Imaging artifacts • Sequence optimization
- 1.5-T imaging protocol

INTRODUCTION AND CHALLENGES OF LIVER MR IMAGING

The liver is one of the most challenging organs of the body to image with magnetic resonance (MR). Much of the liver's posterior, lateral, and superior margins are subject to lung-related susceptibility effects, while bowel skirts its inferior and anterior edges. The left hemiliver lies just under the constantly moving heart, a liability for such motion-sensitive techniques as diffusion-weighted imaging (DWI). Pulsatile flow within the aorta and respiratory motion of the gallbladder can create phase errors that simulate disease. The dual hepatic blood supply and variability in tumor vascularity demand precise timing of multiphase contrast-enhanced acquisitions. These challenges are further compounded by the fact that the liver is one of the largest and most mobile organs of the abdomen. As a result, liver MR imaging requires many compromises, such as between signal-to-noise ratio (SNR), spatial and temporal resolution, artifact suppression, and lesion conspicuity.

In recent years, clever hardware and pulse sequence innovations and the introduction of new liver-specific contrast agents together have helped mitigate these many obstacles to push MR imaging to the forefront of liver imaging. Nonetheless, liver MR imaging is far from standardized. The plethora of available vendors, systems, coils, sequences, and imaging parameters that have made liver MR imaging so successful have also made it dauntingly complex. In fact, the title of this article is a misnomer. There is in essence no optimal union of imaging parameters, only a marriage of convenience subject to the laws of physics and the constraints of one's equipment, practice environment, and economics. In this article, the authors provide guidance regarding the development of a liver MR imaging protocol. For each protocol component (eg, T2-weighted sequence), the many available variations, with their strengths and weaknesses, are discussed. Along the way, the recognition and elimination of imaging pitfalls and artifacts frequently encountered during liver imaging with MR are also discussed. For simplicity, this discourse will primarily focus on imaging at a field strength of 1.5 Tesla (T), as a dedicated discussion of imaging the liver at 3.0 T can be found elsewhere in this issue.

BASIC PRINCIPLES OF SEQUENCE OPTIMIZATION

Obtaining images with MR requires both homogeneous static magnetic fields and transmitted radiofrequency (RF) fields, rapid and accurate spatial encoding, and clear signal reception. Static field (B_0) homogeneity is a function of both magnet design and patient anatomy, and is shimmed through active and passive means. The uniformity

[a] Body Imaging Section, Department of Radiology, Vanderbilt University Medical Center, 1161 21st Avenue South, Nashville, TN 37232, USA
[b] Abdominal Imaging Section, Department of Radiology, Wake Forest University School of Medicine, Medical Center Boulevard, Winston-Salem, NC 27157, USA
* Corresponding author.
E-mail address: geoffrey.wile@vanderbilt.edu

Magn Reson Imaging Clin N Am 18 (2010) 525–547
doi:10.1016/j.mric.2010.07.010

of the transmitted RF field (B_1) is a function of field strength, coil design, the transmitted RF pulse, and patient body habitus.[1] B_1 inhomogeneities become more problematic at higher field strengths, in larger patients, and in the presence of ascites.[2] Such B_1 inhomogeneities contribute to spatial variations in SNR and flip angle that can have an adverse effect on image contrast and uniformity of fat suppression. A variety of strategies have been developed to reduce the effects of B_1 nonuniformity, including the use of dielectric pads, RF shimming, and adiabatic pulses.[1–3] Because these issues are more relevant to a discussion of 3.0-T imaging, they are not discussed further here.

Clear signal reception requires use of an appropriate receiver coil. The development of dedicated receiver coils directly applied to the surface of the patient is considered a major advance in body MR imaging. Coils applied directly over the patient, conforming to the curvature of the body wall, dramatically improve SNR by bringing the receiver elements closer to the signal source (**Fig. 1**). The use of multicoil, multichannel arrays and quadrature coil geometry can further the potential gain in SNR, while improving efficiency by permitting applications such as parallel imaging.[4,5] Such is the improvement in image quality that the use of a surface coil is considered mandatory, when possible, for the performance of high-quality liver MR imaging.

Once a suitable environment for exciting protons and receiving signal has been established, imaging parameters are manipulated and compromises made between 5 main factors:

1. Signal-to-noise ratio (SNR)
2. Contrast-to-noise ratio (CNR)
3. Spatial resolution
4. Temporal resolution
5. Artifacts.

Signal-to-Noise Ratio

SNR is the strength of the signal relative to the noise inherent in the system. Signal is a function of the net transverse magnetization in the body as each echo is collected. Increases in B_0 field strength and voxel volume improve SNR, although the latter compromises spatial resolution. Voxel size can be increased in the through-plane (slice or partition thickness) or in-plane (matrix) axes, with the benefit of reducing acquisition time if all other parameters are kept constant. A reduction in receiver bandwidth improves SNR at the expense of temporal resolution (achievable echo and repetition times) and increased chemical shift artifact. For example, a typical 3-dimensional (3D) fat-suppressed T1-weighted gradient echo sequence used for liver imaging might use the following parameters:

> Marix = 320 × 160, Partition thickness 5 mm overlapping 50%, Flip angle 12°, Bandwidth + 62.5 kHz, Acceleration factor = 2

Total acquisition time to cover the liver with this sequence would be approximately 23 seconds. The acquisition time could be reduced to 13 seconds by reducing the matrix to 256 × 128, increasing the partition thickness from 5 mm to 6 mm, and increasing the receiver bandwidth to +100 kHz without affecting SNR (the loss of SNR caused by the increased bandwidth is compensated for by the gain in SNR caused by the decreased matrix and increased partition thickness).

The number of signal averages also affects SNR, and can be thought of as the amount of data stored in each line of k-space. Doubling the number of signal averages increases the signal by the square root of 2, but with the expense of doubling the imaging time. Imaging parameters

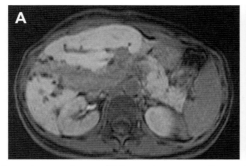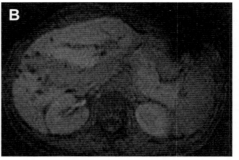

Fig. 1. Importance of a multichannel array receiver coil. (*A*) Three-dimensional gradient echo fat-suppressed sequence through the liver acquired with a multichannel surface coil using parallel imaging. (*B*) Image obtained in the same individual with nearly identical imaging parameters using the scanner's main body coil. The imaged volume was smaller and SNR lower for the same acquisition time without the surface coil.

repetition time (TR), echo time (TE), and flip angle also influence signal but are generally considered more important determinants of image contrast. While high SNR is desirable, it is not the ultimate goal of liver imaging. Rather, an abundance of signals facilitates additional strategies to improve spatial and temporal resolution.

Contrast-to-Noise Ratio

CNR is a far more critical measure than SNR of the clinical utility of an image. CNR is the difference in signal intensity between 2 different regions of interest in the same image, scaled to noise. CNR is a measure of lesion conspicuity and is affected, to an extent, by the same factors that influence SNR; however, because CNR determines how visible an abnormality will appear on an image, parameters affecting image contrast can have a profound influence on CNR. For example, increases in flip angle for a constant TR can reduce image SNR by preventing full recovery of tissue magnetization between excitation pulses. However, such a strategy can improve the CNR between enhancing vessels and background liver (to a point) after administration of gadolinium-based contrast material. Increasing the TE will improve liver lesion contrast for cysts, hemangiomas, bile, and other tissues and substances with long T2 relaxation times at the expense of SNR.

Spatial Resolution

Spatial resolution, the factor that controls detail discrimination, is primarily controlled by voxel size. In general, high-resolution images of the liver are desirable to resolve small focal lesions and anatomic structures; however, improvements in spatial resolution typically come with compromises in temporal resolution or SNR. When optimizing spatial resolution, one must determine the minimum acceptable SNR and maximum tolerable breath-hold duration for a sequence. As a general rule, lower spatial resolution is preferable to severe respiratory motion artifact, as the high contrast sensitivity inherent to MR imaging can compensate for larger voxel size. The use of respiratory triggering permits high-resolution imaging without compromising SNR but is not practical for imaging discrete vascular phases after intravenous contrast administration. An apparent increase in spatial resolution without significant time penalty can be achieved with zero fill interpolation, a technique that fills portions of k-space with zeros to interpolate the acquired matrix to one of higher apparent resolution.[6] In-plane or through-plane zero filling can be applied, and this technique is often employed in the fat-suppressed 3D sequences used for dynamic contrast-enhanced imaging.[7]

Temporal Resolution

Optimizing temporal resolution is critical to achieving motion-free breath-hold imaging of the liver, particularly during the dynamic phases of contrast enhancement. Dynamic contrast-enhanced liver imaging is typically performed with a 3D fat-suppressed T1-weighted gradient echo sequence. In most cases, the TR is kept as short as possible, with T1 contrast for this short TR maintained by use of a reduced flip angle. With the exception of newer dual-echo techniques, many manufacturers use an opposed-phase echo time for their dynamic liver sequence, leaving little room for further reduction of the TE at 1.5 T. Despite being reasonably optimized for breath-hold imaging, further improvements in temporal resolution can be gained over the "out-of-the-box" configuration, albeit at a price.

The simplest strategy to reduce scan time is to lower spatial resolution. Aside from potentially obscuring small structures and abnormalities, decreasing resolution can exacerbate truncation artifact (edge ringing that propagates through the images in the phase-encoding direction). The use of zero filling can help mitigate some of the effects of lower imaging matrices but can also exacerbate truncation artifact.[8] Fortunately, truncation artifacts are rarely of clinical significance when imaging the liver using currently available pulse sequences and typical matrices (256 × 128 or higher). The SNR gained by lower spatial resolution can offset SNR lost by increasing the receiver bandwidth to further reduce acquisition time. Additional time savings can be achieved through the use of a reduced-phase field of view and partial Fourier methods.

Parallel Imaging

Parallel imaging has become a mainstay of hepatic MR imaging, allowing dramatic improvements in temporal resolution with a few trade-offs. These techniques save time by decreasing the number of individual phase-encoding steps necessary to create a complete image, which is accomplished by using the spatial information from individual coil elements in tandem with conventional gradient-based spatial encoding.[9–11] These sequences are known as sensitivity encoding (SENSE), modified SENSE (mSENSE), or generalized autocalibrating partially parallel acquisition (GRAPPA), depending on the vendor and the method of data manipulation, either within k-space (GRAPPA) or within image space.[9] In addition, these techniques vary with respect to calibration techniques. GRAPPA and mSENSE are autocalibrating, acquiring calibration data during image acquisition, whereas other techniques require dedicated calibration scans.[12]

The use of parallel imaging can significantly reduce acquisition times, and is now considered routine for liver imaging. The reduction in scan time is related to the number of lines of k-space that are acquired in parallel during the phase encoding process (often referred to as the acceleration factor). This factor is higher for single-shot T2-weighted sequences (sometimes as high as 4). Signal, in this case, is maintained by the shorter echo train length. An acceleration factor of 2 or less is common for most abdominal applications, although higher factors are becoming more achievable on newer platforms. Some newer 3D sequences and coils allow for parallel imaging to be applied in the in-plane and through-plane direction simultaneously.

One downside of parallel imaging can be a reduction in SNR that worsens as the parallel imaging acceleration factor increases. This trend can be offset in many cases by adjustments in other parameters, although the signal gain through the use of gadolinium-based contrast media minimizes the impact of signal loss at typical acceleration factors of 2 or less. Another potential hazard associated with the use of parallel imaging is related to artifacts generated during image reconstruction. SENSE-based techniques reduce the number of phase encoding steps by acquiring data with a reduced phase field of view. The resulting aliased image is "unwrapped" using coil sensitivity profiles obtained during the calibration process.[11] However, if the prescribed field of view is too small in the phase encoding direction, the unwrapping is incomplete and residual signal contaminates the central portion of the image.[13] In addition, when there are too few phase-encoding steps acquired to maintain signal, or if the patient is large, noise amplification can be severe in the central portion of the image. When the field of view is increased in the phase direction in both cases, these artifacts can be reduced (**Fig. 2**). Misregistration between the calibration scan and the image acquisition can also lead to artifacts (**Fig. 3**), a common occurrence with breath-hold techniques when respiration is suspended inconsistently between the calibration scan and the image acquisition. Calibration artifacts can be corrected by recalibrating or by using one of the autocalibrating methods of parallel imaging.[14] **Table 1** provides an overview of the effects of changes in the some of the key parameters of sequence optimization.

Additional Artifacts

Parallel imaging is just one potential source of artifacts encountered during image acquisition and

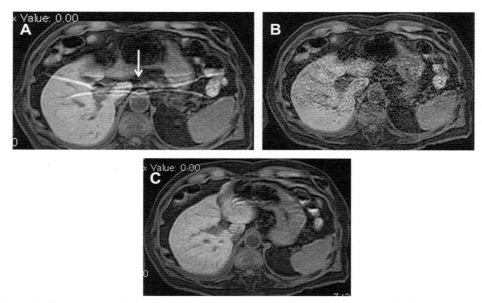

Fig. 2. Example of parallel imaging artifact. (*A*) Image acquired using SENSE-based parallel imaging and too small a field of view. Note the presence of phase wrap artifact (*arrow*) in the center of the image. (*B*) Image acquired with a slightly larger field of view in the same patient shows less artifact but noise amplification in the central portion of the image. (*C*) After increasing the field of view further, both artifacts are eliminated.

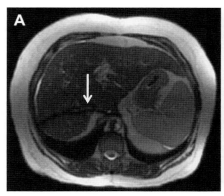
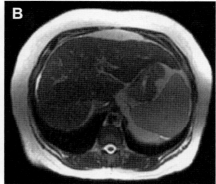

Fig. 3. Parallel imaging calibration artifact. (*A*) This single-shot fast spin echo (ssFSE) image shows an artifact (*arrow*) overlying the liver due to mismatch between calibration scan and image acquisition using SENSE-based parallel imaging. (*B*) Artifact becomes much less conspicuous after recalibration.

interpretation. One of the most common sources of artifacts encountered in liver imaging is motion-induced phase errors. Motion is problematic because it can introduce phase shifts that are not induced by the spatial encoding gradients, resulting in misplaced signal on the image. Motion occurring between phase-encoding steps or during application of the imaging gradients can result in "ghost" artifacts along the phase encoding axis.[12] The two most common sources of ghost artifacts are respiratory motion (**Fig. 4**) and vascular flow. The former source can be addressed with careful respiratory triggering, breath-hold imaging, fat suppression, or placement of saturation bands over high signal fat in the anterior abdominal wall.[12,15] Vascular flow-related artifacts can be mitigated through the use of gradient moment nulling (also known as flow compensation) or saturation bands placed above and below the imaging volume.[14] However, gradient moment nulling, as typically used, only corrects for phase errors induced by flow at constant velocity (ie, first order flow). Phase ghosts are problematic because they can mimic hepatic lesions, particularly within the left lateral section of the liver (**Fig. 5**). The anatomic structures most likely to produce motion-related ghost artifacts in the liver include the anterior abdominal wall, gallbladder, inferior vena cava, and aorta.

Wraparound artifact occurs when objects or body parts outside the field of view are spatially mismapped to within the image. Wraparound artifact occurs because the image is only encoded for a maximum of 360° of phase shift. Any phase shift outside of this range (due to the object's location outside the field of view) is misrepresented on the image. Protons experiencing higher degrees of phase shift, for example 365°, will appear to

have experienced only 5° of shift, resulting in their being spatially mapped to the low-shift side of the image (**Fig. 6**). Because 3D acquisitions use phase encoding to distinguish partitions in the slice direction, wraparound can occur in this axis as well as in the in-plane phase-encoding direction (typically anterior to posterior for a liver acquisition). Wraparound artifact can be eliminated or reduced by increasing the field of view, to move the offending structure out of the imaging region where wraparound occurs. or through the use of saturation bands to reduce signal in the source of the artifact. Alternatively, one can use an option known as phase oversampling or "no-phase-wrap" to sample outside the field of view in the phase encoding direction. However, this method is not preferred for breath-hold imaging, as it can increase acquisition time significantly. By swapping the phase and frequency directions, wraparound artifact can be shifted off of structures of interest, but this eliminates the time-saving benefit of using a rectangular field of view. The use of SENSE-based parallel imaging techniques can cause a distinctive wraparound artifact near the center of the image, as the image cannot be completely unwrapped if the field of view is too small (see **Fig. 2**).

Differing magnetic susceptibilities of tissues and substances within the abdomen is a common source of artifacts during liver imaging. Substances, such as air or metal, cause magnetic field inhomogeneities that result in local signal loss, geometric distortion, and failure of spectrally selective forms of fat suppression. In this manner, cholecystectomy clips can obscure the porta hepatis region, and gas within the colon can create the appearance of tumors within the adjacent liver (**Fig. 7**). Gradient echo—based

Table 1
Overview of effects of changes in some of the key parameters of sequence optimization

Parameter	Scan Time	Spatial Resolution	SNR	Artifact
Receiver bandwidth	An increase in bandwidth increases sampling rate and allows shorter TE, decreasing scan time	No direct effect on spatial resolution	SNR is decreased with increasing bandwidth	Water/fat misregistration is exacerbated at lower bandwidths
Acceleration factor (parallel imaging)	Increasing acceleration factor decreases scan time	No direct effect but may allow for improved spatial resolution for a given scan time	Increasing the parallel imaging factor decreases SNR	Artifacts related to aliasing and callibration are propagated in the phase-encoding direction
Field of view	Increasing field of view increases scan time if spatial resolution is kept constant	If the matrix is kept constant, voxel size will increase, resulting in decreased spatial resolution	If the matrix is kept constant, SNR increases due to larger voxel size	Most commonly associated with aliasing when the field of view is decreased and excludes anatomy. Artifact appears in the center of an image with parallel imaging if anatomy is excluded in phase-encoding direction
Matrix	Scan time is increased with a finer matrix in the phase-encoding axis	Spatial resolution is increased with an increase in matrix for constant field of view	SNR is decreased with smaller voxel size	Truncation artifact may be seen with marked reduction in matrix
Slice thickness	Increasing slice thickness decreases scan time for constant anatomic coverage	Through-plane resolution is decreased when slice thickness is increased	SNR increases with increasing slice thickness	Degradation of multiplanar reconstructions and worsened volume averaging effects with increased slice thickness
Number of signal averages (NEX, NSA)	Increasing NSA increases scan time	No effect on spatial resolution	SNR increases with increasing NSA	May introduce image blurring with higher NSA

Abbreviations: NEX, number of excitations; NSA, number of acquisitions; SNR, signal-to-noise ratio; TE, echo time.

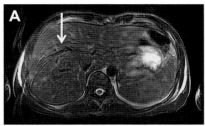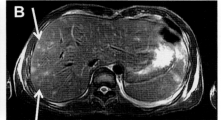

Fig. 4. Respiratory motion. (*A*) Respiratory-triggered fast spin echo (FSE) T2-weighted image shows respiratory motion-induced phase ghosting (*arrow*) obscuring foci of hepatic lymphoma. (*B*) The sequence was repeated with better patient coaching. Note how better motion suppression improves lesion visibility (*arrows*).

sequences are most sensitive to susceptibility differences, as the lack of RF refocusing pulses prevents correction for T2* decay. Susceptibility artifact can be reduced by minimizing TE as gas and ferromagnetic particles such as clips, wires, and ballistic fragments create local field inhomogeneities that become more pronounced over time. Shorter echo times may be achieved by using fractional echo sampling and higher receiver bandwidths.

The Difficult Patient

Some patients present unique challenges due to habitus, claustrophobia, or limited breath-holding capacity. The most important factor to be considered initially for all patients is comfort. A comfortable patient is more likely to remain still and comply with instructions. For patients with lung disease, supplemental oxygen can improve comfort and increase breath-holding compliance. Dramatic reductions in scan time can be achieved through simple sequence modifications such as increased slice or partition thickness, reduced matrix, and increased bandwidth. Because of the high contrast sensitivity of MR imaging,

a low-resolution, motion-free image is often more clinically useful than a high-resolution image degraded by motion.

For dynamic enhanced imaging of the liver, diagnostic data sets covering the entire liver can be obtained in less than 10 seconds when necessary. For patients who cannot suspend respirations for more than a few seconds, acquiring data during shallow continuous breathing or with respiratory triggering might be an option. When respiratory triggering is not an option, motion-resistant sequences such as single-shot echo train spin echo, steady-state free precession (SSFP), and magnetization-prepared gradient echo can be considered. Protocols should be as efficient as possible to prevent patient fatigue, and critical breath-hold sequences should be accomplished as soon as possible in the imaging protocol.

Coil positioning and clearance within the magnet can be challenging in large patients. Normal landmarks for coil positioning may not be apparent to the technologist; therefore, scout imaging with special attention to coil placement relative to the area of interest is important. The technologist should not hesitate to reposition the surface coil when necessary. Failure to do so

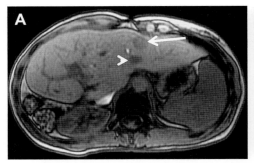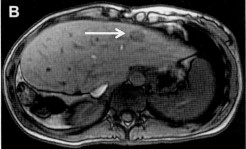

Fig. 5. Pseudolesion caused by vascular flow artifact propagated in the phase direction into the left hemiliver. (*A*) Pseudolesion (*arrow*) adjacent to a true lesion (epithelioid hemangioendothelioma, *arrowhead*) on this 2D gradient echo T1-weighted image. (*B*) An image at a different level shows persistence of the ghost artifact (*arrow*) but not the true lesion.

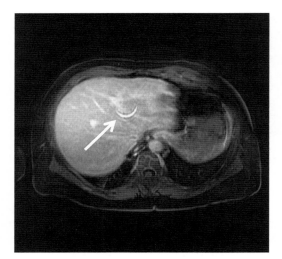

Fig. 6. Intravenous tubing "wrapped" into an image (*arrow*). The actual tubing was draped over the anterior abdomen outside the field of view but mimics a vessel within the liver.

results in signal-starved areas at the coil margins. A patient with a protuberant abdomen may require additional padding under the free ends of the surface coil to prevent movement that can contribute to calibration errors when using parallel imaging. In those patients for whom coil placement is not possible because of insufficient magnet clearance, the intrinsic body coil can be used with sequence modifications to compensate for relative loss of signal. In all cases, excellent communication between the patient and technologist is essential to ensuring patient compliance and satisfactory image quality. Coaching the patient and attention to respiratory waveforms can improve acquisition timing, and communication with the patient helps keep the patient calm and focused on the examination. Light sedation can be helpful, but heavy sedation can hinder patient compliance.

THE BASIC LIVER IMAGING PROTOCOL

The typical liver MR imaging protocol consists of the following basic components: localizer, T1-weighted gradient echo sequence with in-phase and opposed-phase echo times, fat-suppressed T2-weighted sequence, and multiphase dynamic gadolinium-enhanced series using a fat-suppressed gradient echo sequence. Optional sequences include diffusion-weighted echo-planar and hepatobiliary phase images (provided a hepatobiliary contrast agent is administered). Every MR system provides the user with an "out-of-the-box" 3-plane localizer that provides limited data for image planning, which confirms appropriate patient and coil positioning before further imaging. This initial localizer is typically performed during free breathing and provides only limited views of the liver. For this reason, many practitioners augment the 3-plane localizer with a coronal breath-hold localizer using either a T2-weighted single-shot echo train spin echo or SSFP sequence. Both of these latter sequences are resistant to motion and are acquired quickly in 1 or 2 breath-holds, providing motion-resistant imaging of all abdominal organs within the field of view. The use of fat suppression with these sequences is optional. Edge blurring can be problematic with long echo train sequences, but this can be minimized by optimizing the TE, minimizing the interecho spacing, and using parallel imaging (**Fig. 8**).[9]

SSFP techniques provide motion-free images with the highest possible SNR per unit time of any sequence[16]; these images are not truly T2-weighted, but rather T2/T1-weighted, and display unique properties. Blood, bile ducts, and pancreatic ducts are bright, allowing for noncontrast evaluation of vessels and ducts.[17] In the authors' experience, SSFP has only limited utility for hepatic lesion detection, although this type of

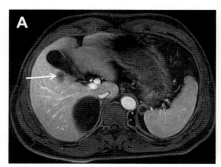
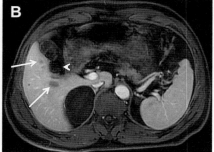

Fig. 7. (*A* and *B*) Pseudolesions (*arrows*) created by bowel gas (*arrowhead, B*) causing susceptibility artifact in liver on enhanced fat-suppressed T1-weighted image. All lesions with *arrows* were caused by bowel gas along inferior liver margin.

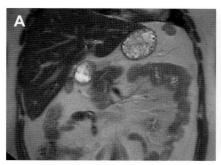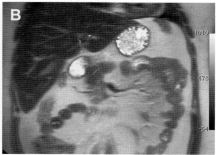

Fig. 8. Coronal single-shot echo train spin-echo images. (*A*) ssFSE image with parallel imaging factor optimized. (*B*) Edge blurring noted on an image from the same patient with an acceleration factor of 1 as opposed to 4; this resulted in an increased echo train length (93 to 314).

sequence has been shown to perform similarly to T2-weighted single-shot echo train spin echo (eg, single-shot turbo spin echo [TSE], single-shot fast spin echo [FSE], half-Fourier single-shot turbo spin echo [HASTE]) images when incorporated into a body imaging protocol.[18] SSFP methods are very sensitive to magnetic field inhomogeneities and suffer from off-resonance artifacts, which manifest as alternating bands of bright and dark signal (referred to as "banding"), (**Fig. 9**).[16]

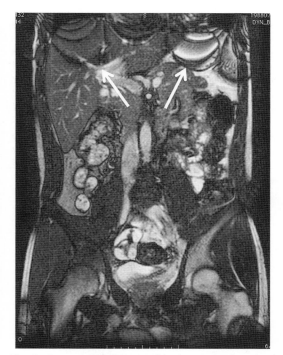

Fig. 9. Coronal SSFP image with alternating bands of bright and dark signal, "banding" or off-resonance artifact (*arrows*) caused by magnetic field inhomogeneity.

Unenhanced Gradient Echo T1-Weighted Imaging

In addition to serving as a precontrast baseline, T1-weighted sequences aid in tissue characterization based on T1 relaxation times and lipid content. This latter capability is made possible by the difference in precessional frequency between fat and water protons (approximately 3.5 ppm). Protons in water precess at a predictably higher frequency than those in fat, and this difference, which is field strength dependent, leads to two forms of chemical shift artifact.

The first type of chemical shift artifact occurs in all sequences at fat/water interfaces as a result of spatial misregistration of fat and water protons along the frequency-encoding direction. This misregistration results in bright and dark bands on opposite sides of an organ surrounded by fat or of fat surrounded by water-containing soft tissue (as in the case of a lipoma within a solid organ).[19] The prominence of this artifact is influenced by magnetic field strength, receiver bandwidth, and matrix.

The second type of chemical shift is of far more importance to hepatic imaging, and is caused by cancellation of the transverse magnetization vectors of fat and water protons when 180° out of phase. This phenomenon occurs with gradient echo sequences using specific echo times that are field strength dependent.[14] On an opposed-phase image, a dark border occurs at fat/water interfaces (where fat and water protons are present in similar amounts within the same voxels). Areas of hepatic steatosis and neoplasms containing intracellular lipid, such as some hepatic adenomas and hepatocellular carcinomas, lose signal on opposed-phase images relative to in-phase images (**Fig. 10**). When the presence of intracellular lipid is in doubt, subtraction imaging can be helpful.[20]

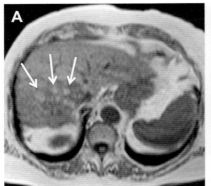
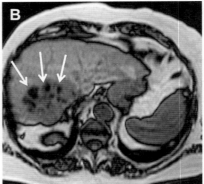

Fig. 10. Hepatocellular carcinoma (HCC) with foci of lipid. (*A*) T1-weighted in-phase gradient echo image shows mass (HCC) in right hemiliver that contains high signal intensity foci (*arrows*). (*B*) Foci of marked signal dropout are noted within the mass on the opposed-phase image, consistent with lipid-containing regions (*arrows*).

Hepatic steatosis revealed by chemical shift imaging can be diffuse, focal, multifocal, geographic, or perivascular in distribution. Occasionally, steatosis serves as a contrast agent of sorts, making focal neoplasms more conspicuous (**Fig. 11**). The presence of lipid within focal nodular hyperplasia or metastatic disease is extremely rare, making lipid a useful discriminator between hepatic neoplasms.[21]

The utility of chemical shift imaging is not restricted to detection of lipid.[22] In particular, susceptibility artifacts related to the presence of gas (as in the case of pneumobilia or hepatic abscess) or iron (as in the case of hemosiderosis and genetic hemochromatosis) will become more conspicuous with the longer echo time of a dual-echo gradient echo sequence. Most vendors offer opposed-phase and in-phase acquisitions as part of a dual-echo sequence using echo times of approximately 2.1 to 2.3 milliseconds and 4.2 to 4.6 milliseconds, respectively, at 1.5 T. More recently, 3D dual-echo sequences have become available.[22] At 3.0 T, the precessional frequency is twice as fast with theoretical opposed-phase echo times of 1.1, 3.4, and 5.6 milliseconds, and in-phase times of 2.2, 4.5, and 6.7 milliseconds. To capture the first opposed-phase and in-phase echoes as is typically done at 1.5 T, a high bandwidth is needed. Therefore, many 3.0-T dual-echo sequences are set to collect the first in-phase echo at 2.2 milliseconds and the opposed-phase at approximately 5.6 milliseconds. This situation potentially complicates the distinction between iron deposition and hepatic steatosis (**Fig. 12**). In addition, T2* effects become more pronounced at longer echo times, potentially confounding signal intensity measurement comparisons between in-phase and opposed-phase images.

Opposed-phase and in-phase echo times can be further exploited to create "water-only" and

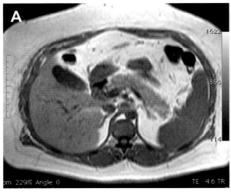
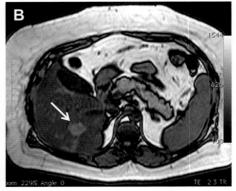

Fig. 11. Diffuse hepatic steatosis and hepatic adenoma. (*A*) In-phase T1-weighted gradient echo image through the right hemiliver of a patient with hepatic adenoma shows no focal abnormality. (*B*) Note that the adenoma (*arrow*) becomes conspicuous on this opposed-phase image because of signal loss in the surrounding steatotic liver.

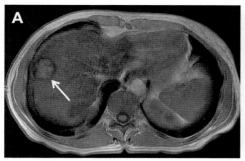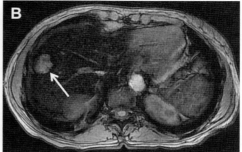

Fig. 12. Lung carcinoma metastasis in patient with hemochromatosis imaged at 3.0 T. (*A*) In-phase T1-weighted gradient echo image shows metastasis (*arrow*). (*B*) Opposed-phase image shows signal loss in the liver parenchyma causing liver lesion (*arrow*) to be more conspicuous. In this case the in-phase image was acquired with a TE of 2.2 milliseconds and the opposed-phase image was acquired at with a longer echo time of 5.6 milliseconds. The signal loss on the opposed-phase image in this case was caused by the presence of hepatic parenchymal iron, not steatosis.

"fat-only" images using modifications of the technique originally described by Dixon.[23] In the simplest sense, these additional images are created by adding or subtracting the in-phase and opposed-phase data sets. To correct for imperfections in B_0, the two-point Dixon technique was modified to include an additional in-phase image (3-point Dixon), relying on the supposition that any difference between the two in-phase images are the result of field inhomogeneity.[24–26] 2D and 3D modifications of these techniques can potentially improve imaging efficiency by simultaneously providing opposed-phase and in-phase images as well as a precontrast "fat-suppressed" (water-only) image. As a result, they are becoming increasingly popular for precontrast- and postcontrast-enhanced imaging of the liver.[27]

T2-Weighted Imaging

T2-weighted imaging of the liver serves for both lesion detection and characterization. Its utility for lesion detection stems from the relatively low signal intensity of normal liver parenchyma on T2-weighted sequences and the relatively high signal intensity of many liver abnormalities. Basic lesion characterization is possible because benign lesions such as cysts, hemangiomas, and biliary hamartomas have significantly longer T2 relaxation times than most solid hepatocellular and metastatic lesions. Although the utility of T2-weighted imaging for detection of hepatocellular carcinoma and cirrhotic nodule characterization has been questioned in this era of dynamic enhanced MR imaging, most liver MR protocols continue to include T2-weighted imaging routinely for both cirrhotic and noncirrhotic livers.[28,29] Of all the routine liver imaging sequences, the choice of

T2-weighted sequence varies the most from institution to institution. This variation is due to the large number of potential variations in respiratory motion and fat suppression techniques and echo train length. Some studies comparing different fat-suppressed T2-weighted imaging techniques for hepatic lesion detection are summarized in **Table 2**.

With improvements in multiphase dynamic imaging and DWI techniques, the choice of T2-weighted imaging technique has become less critical, and many institutions choose in favor of efficiency. Imaging times can be shortened by using longer echo trains, partial Fourier techniques, or some form of fast recovery technique. Fast recovery–type FSE sequences use a 180° refocusing pulse followed by a −90° flip-back pulse, forcing recovery of longitudinal magnetization.[30] One study performed by Augui et al[31] evaluated the performance of breath-hold fast-recovery FSE T2 compared with respiratory-triggered FSE T2 images and also with single-shot echo train spin echo techniques. The investigators found higher SNR and CNR in the breath-held T2 FSE with fast recovery, due to decreased motion-related image degradation. However, they also showed higher overall lesion signal in the standard respiratory-triggered FSE T2 sequences. Solid lesion detection was inferior with single-shot FSE images, likely related to image blurring and magnetization transfer effects. Another study[32] looked at this same question with a somewhat different outcome, and showed that TSE with respiratory triggering or navigator pulse was superior to HASTE or breath-held TSE with fast recovery. The investigators surmised that lesion conspicuity was decreased in part by magnetization transfer effects seen at higher echo train

Table 2
Studies comparing different fat-suppressed T2-weighted imaging techniques for hepatic lesion detection

Study	Techniques Compared	Conclusions
Tang et al[92] Radiology 1997;203:776	Fast HASTE Conventional HASTE BH TSE RT TSE	Diagnostic performance was significantly higher with the fast HASTE and RT TSE sequences than with the conventional HASTE and BH TSE sequences
Coates et al[93] JMRI 1998;8:642	HASTE TSE SE	HASTE demonstrated lower liver-spleen and liver lesion CNR than TSE and CSE
Kanematsu et al[33] Radiology 1999;211:363	EPI BH FSE RT FSE SE	RT FSE images had significantly better or comparative detectability of lesions compared with the other types of images. Image quality was best on the RT FSE images
Lee et al[94] Abdom Imaging 2000;25:93	HASTE IR HASTE BH TSE	BH TSE had the highest liver/lesion CNR but lesion detection was not statistically different for these techniques
Katayama et al[95] JMRI 2001;14:439	ssFSE BH FRFSE RT FSE	BH FRFSE provided the highest tumor detection, although the mean lesion-to-liver CNRs were inferior to RT FSE and ssFSE
Augui et al[31] Radiology 2002;223:853	ssFSE BH FRFSE RT FSE	CNRs for hepatic lesions were higher with BH FRFSE than with RT FSE, and BH FRFSE displayed better lesion clarity than ssFSE
Huang et al[91] AJR 2005;184:842	BH FRFSE RT FSE	Better image quality with BH FSE but no difference in lesion detection or characterization
Lee et al[32] JMRI 2007;26:323	NT TSE RT TSE BH restore TSE HASTE	NT TSE and RT TSE were superior to BH restore TSE and HASTE for the detection of focal hepatic lesions
Kim et al[96] AJR 2008;190:W19	NT TSE NT HASTE RT TSE	Sensitivity for lesion detection was highest for navigator-triggered TSE

Abbreviations: BH, breath-hold; CNR, contrast-to-noise ratio; EPI, echo-planar imaging; FRFSE, fast recovery fast spin echo; FSE, fast spin echo; HASTE, half-Fourier single-shot turbo spin echo; IR, inversion recovery; NT, navigator-triggered; RT, respiratory-triggered; SE, spin echo; ssFSE, single-shot fast spin echo; TSE, turbo spin echo.
Data from Refs.[31–33,91–96]

lengths. It is entirely possible that similar sequences from different vendors perform differently, accounting for some of the confusion regarding the best choice of T2-weighted sequence.

Regardless of the type of T2-weighted sequence chosen, the use of fat suppression and some form of respiratory motion suppression or compensation are recommended for routine T2-weighted imaging of the liver. Fat suppression helps to decrease motion-related phase ghosting, exacerbated by high signal intensity fat in the body wall.[12] Fat suppression also serves to improve the display dynamic range, improving the conspicuity of subtle findings.[33,34] As with the choice of T2-weighted pulse sequence, the choice of fat suppression technique varies between institutions. Chemically selective fat saturation is in common use, but is sensitive to magnetic field inhomogeneities. Short-tau inversion recovery (STIR) is less dependent on magnetic field homogeneity and provides more uniform fat suppression, but images tend to be signal starved.[35] Spectrally adiabatic inversion recovery (SPAIR) combines chemically selective inversion recovery with an adiabatic pulse that improves the uniformity of fat suppression.[36]

One additional tool used first in neurologic imaging to decrease motion artifact is the PROPELLER (Periodically Rotated Overlapping Parallel Lines with Enhanced Reconstruction) (BLADE, MULTIVANE) technique that employs echo trains in an FSE/TSE sequence ("blades") that rotate around k-space with partial overlap, filling the center of k-space with each dataset (**Fig. 13**). The SNR is increased by oversampling the central portion of k-space, and respiratory motion is reduced by translocating mobile structures to an estimated position based on data from the multiple overlapping "blades".[37] One study[38] showed that the use of BLADE with a navigator-triggered T2-weighted sequence improved image quality without affecting lesion detection or characterization over navigator-triggered T2-weighted imaging alone. Another study by Hirokawa et al.[39] observed improved image quality and lesion detection with a similar technique after administration of super paramagnetic iron oxides. Recently, Bayramoglu and colleagues[40] compared a navigator-triggered, fat-suppressed sequence using a form of fast recovery and BLADE with a variety of other fat-suppressed T2-weighted sequences, finding that the images acquired with the BLADE technique showed higher relative

SNR, CNR, decreased artifacts, and improved depiction of edge detail compared with similar sequences performed without BLADE.

Multiphase Dynamic Enhanced Imaging

Contrast-enhanced images are a critical component of a comprehensive liver MR protocol.[41] The effectiveness of contrast-enhanced imaging for hepatic lesion detection and characterization has diminished the relative role of T2-weighted imaging.[42,43] In addition to improving the detection and characterization of focal hepatic lesions, the appropriate use of intravenous contrast agents can reveal the presence of inflammation, fibrosis, and alterations in hepatic blood flow. However, extracting the maximal amount of clinically useful information from MR imaging requires careful attention to the details of contrast administration and acquisition timing.

Intravenous contrast agents used to image the liver can be categorized as extracellular,

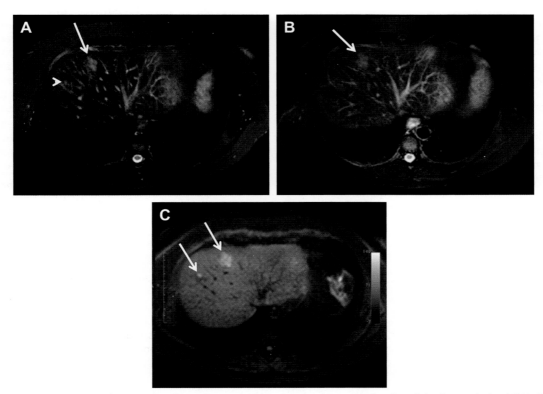

Fig. 13. Comparison of T2-weighted imaging techniques in a patient with focal nodular hyperplasia. (*A*) Turbo spin echo (TSE) T2-weighted image with fat suppression acquired with respiratory triggering shows a mildly hyperintense lesion in the right hepatic lobe (*arrow*). A smaller adjacent lesion (*arrowhead*) is faintly seen. (*B*) TSE T2-weighted image also acquired with fat suppression and triggering, using a PROPELLER-type technique, shows the larger lesion well (*arrow*) but the smaller lesion was not clearly seen on this sequence. (*C*) Spin-echo echo-planar image obtained with a b value of 50 shows both lesions clearly (*arrows*). Note the lack of signal in the hepatic veins on this "black blood" image.

hepatocyte specific (or hepatobiliary), and reticuloendothelial. The extracellular agents are in widespread use, and this article focuses most of its discussion on these agents. Currently approved hepatocyte specific agents are either gadolinium-based or manganese-based.[44] This latter class of agents includes mangafodipir trisodium (Mn-DPDP), an agent that cannot be administered as an intravenous bolus, precluding multiphase dynamic imaging. In part because of this limitation, this agent failed to gain significant market share and is no longer marketed in the United States. Gadolinium-based hepatobiliary contrast agents include gadobenate dimeglumine (Gd-BOPTA) and gadoxetate disodium (Gd-EOB-DTPA). These agents can be administered as an intravenous bolus, providing the opportunity to image the liver during the dynamic phases of enhancement as well as during the hepatobiliary phase. Reticuloendothelial contrast agents include the superparamagnetic iron oxide (SPIO) agents. Only one SPIO agent (ferumoxides) is approved for use in the United States, but as with mangafodipir, dynamic enhanced imaging is not an option with this agent, and this agent is no longer marketed in the United States for liver imaging.

Multiphase dynamic imaging with gadolinium-based contrast agents has become the standard for liver MR imaging, and should be routinely performed when possible. Dynamic contrast-enhanced imaging should include, at a minimum, a precontrast data set followed by arterial dominant, portal venous, and equilibrium or late dynamic phase acquisitions. Gadolinium-based contrast material is administered as an intravenous bolus, and a fat-suppressed T1-weighted gradient echo sequence is performed at the appropriate time intervals during breath-holding.

For this purpose, a 3D acquisition provides satisfactory in-plane and through-plane spatial resolution, adequate SNR, and a temporal resolution sufficient to permit breath-hold imaging and resolution of distinct enhancement phases.[45,46]

Precise and accurate arterial phase timing is critical to hepatic lesion detection and characterization (Fig. 14).[47–51] The window of opportunity for the arterial phase of enhancement is relatively narrow, as one attempts to acquire images at a time when hypervascular tumors, or other transiently enhancing phenomena (such as can be seen with hepatitis), are maximally enhanced relative to the background liver. The optimal time to capture arterially enhancing lesions of the liver is slightly later than the time at which the aorta and hepatic artery enhancement peaks (sometimes referred to as the angiographic phase).[48,49]

Subsequent phases of enhancement are also important for accurate lesion detection and characterization.[52–54] During the portal venous or equilibrium phase some hepatocellular carcinomas and hepatic adenomas will become hypointense to background liver, while lesions of focal nodular hyperplasia will generally remain isointense or slightly hyperintense to liver. Hemangiomas will demonstrate nodular enhancement that becomes progressively more confluent, while some cholangiocarcinomas and metastases will progress from rim-enhancing to peripherally hypointense with central enhancement. This appearance, commonly referred to as "peripheral washout," occurs several minutes after contrast administration. Additional features useful for lesion characterization, such as an enhancing pseudocapsule, central scar, or fibrosis, are also best demonstrated on latter phases of enhancement.

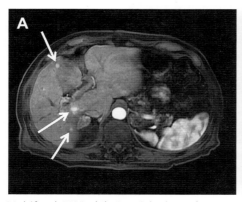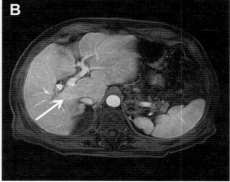

Fig. 14. Multifocal HCC. (*A*) Arterial phase fat-suppressed T1-weighted image shows several small, avidly enhancing HCCs (*arrows*). (*B*) Lesions are much less conspicuous on portal venous phase image. Note enhancing rim on larger lesion (*arrow*) on portal venous phase image.

Because of the critical importance of well-timed arterial phase images, various strategies have been developed for reliably capturing this phase. Using a fixed time delay between contrast administration and image acquisition is discouraged because of the variability in contrast arrival times between patients with differing venous access sites and hemodynamic status. Many centers currently employ a timing bolus strategy that involves repeated acquisitions of the region of interest after administration of a small test dose of the contrast agent.[50] The subsequent image acquisition timing is based on the arrival time of the test dose. Although this method is easily implemented and generally successful, it is less time efficient than bolus tracking techniques and could potentially alter subsequent image contrast, particularly with hepatobiliary agents such as Gd-EOB-DTPA. Using this method, Goshima and colleagues[47] determined the optimal acquisition delay for hypervascular hepatocellular carcinoma (HCC) to be 9 to 12 seconds between peak enhancement in the abdominal aorta (at the level of L1 vertebral body) and the filling of the center of k-space.

Bolus tracking methods initiate image acquisition when the full diagnostic dose of intravenous contrast arrives at the target organ.[51,55] To accomplish this, a large vessel, such as the abdominal aorta, is monitored and the scan triggered after a temporary pause to allow the patient to suspend respiration. The scan can be triggered either automatically, once a signal intensity threshold is reached in the monitored vessel, or manually by a technologist observing a low spatial, high temporal resolution gradient echo acquisition (real-time monitoring or fluoroscopic triggering). This latter method of triggering the acquisition requires that technologists be facile at multitasking, as they are responsible for monitoring the contrast bolus, providing breathing instructions, and triggering the scan. In general, the abdominal aorta at or below the level of the diaphragm is a convenient vessel to monitor, although the exact location can be adjusted based on the desired time delay between contrast arrival and scan initiation.

Hypervascular liver tumors have been shown to demonstrate peak CNR relative to background approximately 6 seconds after peak aortic enhancement (at the same level as the tumor) and, on average, 26 to 31 seconds after contrast infusion.[48] Other investigators have reported a time delay between peak enhancement of the abdominal aorta at the level of the celiac axis and peak enhancement of a hypervascular liver mass to be approximately 9 seconds. Ideally, the subsequent arterial phase acquisition should be timed such that the center of k-space is acquired around the time of maximal lesion CNR relative to liver.[49]

Successful timing of the arterial dominant phase acquisition can be easily recognized. A well-timed image reveals contrast enhancement of the hepatic artery and portal vein without evidence of hepatic vein enhancement.[49] Absence of portal vein enhancement implies that imaging commenced too early to capture peak lesion enhancement.[41,50,56,57] On a well-timed arterial phase image, the spleen often demonstrates heterogeneous enhancement.

With the advent of multiarterial phase imaging, some centers have reverted back to the use of a fixed scan delay.[56,58–60] This strategy employs a 3D T1-weighted gradient echo sequence with sufficient temporal resolution to permit 2, 3, or even 4 acquisitions during a single breath-hold (generally less than 30 seconds in total) (Fig. 15). Because multiple complete data sets are acquired in rapid succession, this method ensures that at least one image set will coincide with the period of maximal lesion enhancement relative to liver. Of course, some degree of SNR or spatial resolution must be sacrificed to accomplish this, although newer, more efficient sequences minimize the necessary trade-offs.

Regardless of which timing strategy is employed, most MR practitioners use a fat-suppressed, T1-weighted, 3D gradient echo sequence for postcontrast imaging.[45] This type of sequence permits breath-hold imaging while maintaining satisfactory SNR and spatial resolution. The use of fat suppression is considered extremely important for improving the conspicuity of gadolinium enhancement. Because respiratory motion is potentially so detrimental, it may be necessary to modify this sequence to accommodate a patient with limited breath-holding capacity. Most centers now routinely use parallel imaging to minimize scan duration. Further improvements in temporal resolution can be accomplished by sacrificing in-plane or through-plane resolution and the use of slice interpolation (also often done routinely).[45] The increase in SNR achieved by lowering spatial resolution permits implementation of additional strategies, such as partial Fourier techniques and increases in receiver bandwidth, that shorten scan time at the expense of SNR. The phase field of view can also be reduced, although this approach is limited by undesirable artifacts when the field of view is reduced too far with some forms of SENSE-based parallel imaging techniques.[13]

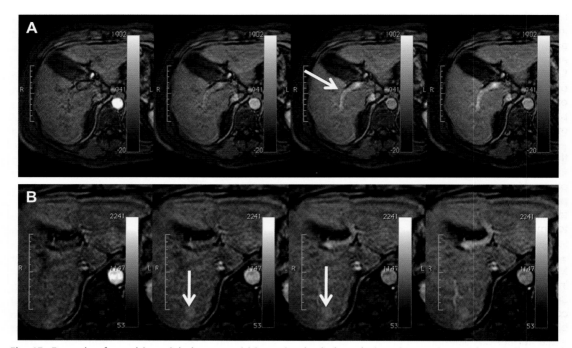

Fig. 15. Example of a multiarterial phase acquisition using keyhole technique in a patient with a small HCC. (*A*) On this single acquisition early to late arterial phases are acquired through the entire liver in a single breath-hold with a total of 4 phases. These images show early arterial phase on the left to late arterial phase on the right. The third and fourth images likely display the best example the "sweet spot" of the late arterial phase. Early portal venous enhancement (*arrow*) is usually a good indicator of proper timing for the arterial phase. (*B*) On the image set showing the HCC, lesion conspicuity (*arrows*) is best when there is portal venous enhancement.

Gadolinium-Based Hepatobiliary Agents

Gadobenate dimeglumine (Gd-BOPTA) and gadoxetate disodium (Gd-EOB-DTPA) are gadolinium-based contrast agents that have been used for liver imaging, although only gadoxetate was approved for this indication by the Food and Drug Administration at the time of preparation of this article. Both agents are transported to some extent across hepatocyte membranes and are eliminated by both renal and biliary pathways.[44] The hepatocyte uptake is significantly greater for gadoxetate than for gadobenate in normal livers (approximately 50% vs <5%, respectively).[44] Both agents can be administered via intravenous bolus, thereby permitting multiphase dynamic imaging in addition to hepatobiliary phase imaging. Furthermore, both agents have relatively high T1 relaxivity (r1).[61] Peak hepatic parenchymal enhancement occurs between 1 and 3 hours after administration of gadobenate, whereas peak enhancement after gadoxetate administration occurs between 20 and 120 minutes.[44,62–64] Both of these agents have been used to improve detection of metastases and to differentiate between hepatic adenoma and focal nodular hyperplasia.[65–67] Gadobenate administered at a dose of 0.1 mmol/kg body weight has been shown to provide a higher degree of hepatic vasculature enhancement than gadoxetate administered at a dose of 0.025 mmol/kg body weight, although the 2 agents have been shown to provide a similar degree of hepatic enhancement in normal volunteers.[68] When compared with a 0.1 mmol/kg body weight dose of gadobenate, gadoxetate administered at a dose of 0.025 mmol/kg body weight demonstrated lower liver parenchymal enhancement during early dynamic phases in normal volunteers.[69]

Because gadobenate is typically administered at a dose of 0.1 mmol/kg body weight, similar to extracellular gadolinium-based contrast media, no modifications are recommended for dynamic imaging with this agent. The currently approved dose of gadoxetate is 0.025 mmol/kg body weight. In its current formulation, the administered volume of this agent is one-half that of other gadolinium-based agents. At a comparable injection rate (eg, 2 mL/s), this results in a shorter bolus and a need for very accurate timing of the arterial phase acquisition. Various strategies that have been investigated to overcome this potential limitation include diluting the agent with saline to increase the administered volume, increasing the administered dose, multiarterial phase imaging, and reducing the injection rate (**Fig. 16**).[70–72] Despite its high relaxivity, the relatively low dose of gadoxetate resulted in reduced enhancement of abdominal organs during the early dynamic phases of imaging in one study comparing gadoxetate with gaobutrol.[73]

The sequences used to image the liver during the hepatobiliary phase are similar to those used for dynamic imaging. Because the hepatobiliary phase of parenchymal enhancement is typically prolonged, a wide window of opportunity exists for imaging this phase. Therefore, one can choose to image the liver in segments with a higher resolution breath-hold sequence or to employ a respiratory-triggered sequence if available. Modifications in flip angle (typically modest increases over the standard 10° to 15° used for 3D dynamic imaging) can improve the image contrast between enhancing parenchyma and bile ducts or focal lesions, although the optimal angle for lesion detection remains an area of investigation.

As the hepatobiliary phase after gadobenate administration begins at approximately 1 hour, many centers choose to remove the patient from the scanner between dynamic and hepatobiliary phase imaging. With gadoxetate, the imaging protocol can be reordered to complete T2-weighted and diffusion-weighted sequences after dynamic imaging, thereby making efficient use of the time interval between dynamic and hepatobiliary phase imaging.[74,75] In this manner, a complete liver imaging protocol can be completed in 25 to 35 minutes depending on the number and type of sequences run between the dynamic and hepatobiliary phases. Although gadoxetate can have a measurable effect on signal intensity of liver on T2-weighted and single-shot echo-planar images, Kim and colleagues[75] showed comparable diagnostic capability for detection of HCC and metastases with postgadoxetate-enhanced T2-weighted imaging compared with precontrast T2-weighted images.[69,76] There are data to suggest that many patients do not benefit from imaging beyond 10 minutes after gadoxetate administration, particularly those with normal liver function who achieve a high signal intensity contrast ratio between liver and spleen.[77]

Diffusion-Weighted Imaging

Recently, interest has grown in abdominal DWI. Potential applications such as liver lesion detection and characterization, grading of hepatic fibrosis, and assessment of treatment response to systemic and local therapies for malignant liver tumors have been investigated. Much of the recent interest has stemmed from widespread availability of breath-hold and respiratory-triggered DWI sequences and improvements in image quality as vendors have slowly overcome such problems as motion, susceptibility artifacts, and eddy currents. A new reluctance to administer gadolinium-based contrast agents to patients with advanced renal disease has further fueled interest as radiologists seek unenhanced alternatives to detecting and characterizing liver lesions with MR imaging.

DWI uses powerful gradients to probe the molecular motion of water molecules in tissue, allowing for qualitative and quantitative analysis. These symmetric dephasing and rephasing gradients are applied on either side of a 180° pulse (for

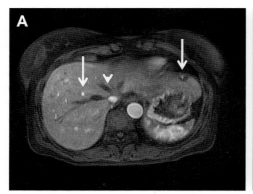
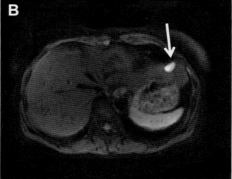

Fig. 16. (*A*) Gadoxetate-enhanced, arterial phase 3D gradient echo image of patient with hepatic hemangioma using injection rate of 1 mL/s. Note enhancement of the portal veins (*left arrow*) but not the hepatic veins (*arrowhead*). A hemangioma is beginning to enhance in the left hemi-liver (*right arrow*). (*B*) Diffusion-weighted image (b = 50) acquired after dynamic phase images shows hemangioma clearly (*arrow*).

a spin-echo echo-planar imaging–based DWI sequence). Abnormalities in tissue cellularity or structure, membrane permeability, or fluid composition can restrict the random diffusion of water molecules. Restricted water molecules experience less phase dispersion induced by the diffusion-sensitizing gradients than freely diffusing water molecules, and therefore maintain higher signal intensity on DW images. The strength of the diffusion-sensitizing gradients is controlled by b value. Images obtained at low b value resemble black-blood T2-weighted images. As the b value increases, SNR falls while the conspicuity of pathologic lesions such as metastases increases, as image contrast becomes based more on differences in diffusivity and less on other tissue characteristics such as T2 relaxation time (**Fig. 17**).[78]

Most currently available body diffusion applications are based on the spin-echo echo-planar technique. For this reason, DWI sequences are very sensitive to magnetic field inhomogeneities and susceptibility artifacts particularly at high b values[78] (**Fig. 18**). The basic sequence is also T2-weighted, allowing for "T2 shine-through" to contribute to signal intensity, especially at low b values.

The optimal choice of b value for liver imaging will depend in part on one's tolerance for image noise and susceptibility artifact. Many practitioners obtain images at multiple b values. A low b value image (<100 s/mm^2) serves as a black-blood T2-weighted-like image with minimal susceptibility artifact and high sensitivity for lesions of all types. A higher b-value image (≥500 s/mm^2) can better discriminate between cysts and hemangiomas versus solid neoplasms at the expense of SNR and increased sensitivity to susceptibility differences and motion. For liver imaging, at least one set of images is typically performed with a b value between 500 and 1000 s/mm^2, the higher b values minimizing the effects of tissue perfusion and showing greater specificity for diffusion-related signal changes. To extend beyond the realm of lesion detection to that of lesion characterization, it is necessary to acquire data at multiple b values. These data permit a qualitative assessment of lesion composition (cysts will be very bright at b50 but generally not at b800, as the effects of T2 shine-through become less apparent at higher b-values) and also allow for calculation of apparent diffusion coefficient (ADC) values. ADC maps aid in distinguishing T2 shine-through from areas of restricted diffusion. Lesions with true restricted diffusion show low signal on the ADC map and areas of T2 shine-through will remain bright (**Fig. 19**). Numerous studies have shown that ADC values can help distinguish between benign cysts and solid neoplasms of the liver.[79–84] On average, hemangiomas also tend to have higher ADC values than solid neoplasms, although some overlap exists. Slow-flowing blood has been hypothesized as one possible explanation for the low ADC value seen in some hemangiomas.[78] In addition, the utility of diffusion has been investigated in the setting of diffuse liver disease with some promise but with limitations due to acquisition time, background steatosis, inflammation, tissue perfusion, and hepatic iron deposition.[78,85,86]

DWI sequences can be combined with a variety of motion suppression techniques. Breath-hold techniques using parallel imaging are efficient, and sequences are available that can provide images through the liver at multiple b values during a single breath-hold. Improvements in SNR can be

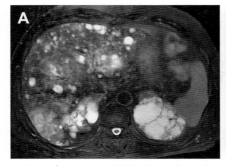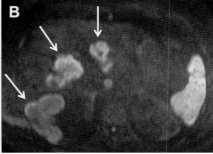

Fig. 17. Illustration of suppressed "T2 shine-through" on high b-value diffusion-weighted images in a patient with a polycystic kidney disease and metastatic colon cancer. (*A*) Fat-suppressed T2-weighted image shows innumerable areas of increased signal. (*B*) b1000 diffusion-weighted image shows suppression of the signal from the simple cysts, leaving only the metastatic lesions as bright (*arrows*).

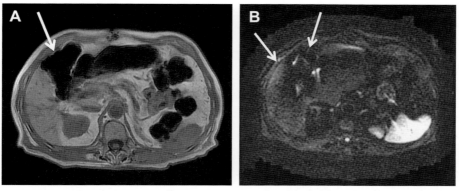

Fig. 18. Susceptibility artifact. (*A*) Gradient echo T1-weighted image shows air-filled colon (*arrow*) adjacent to caudal right hemiliver. (*B*) Note signal loss and geometric distortion (*arrows*) caused by susceptibility differences on this diffusion-weighted image in the same patient (b500).

gained through the use of respiratory triggering and multiple signal averages at the expense of time. Recent observational studies have shown improved lesion conspicuity on sequences using respiratory triggering or a navigator pulse, but with variable reproducibility of ADC values produced on navigator or triggered sequences as compared with breath-held sequences or those

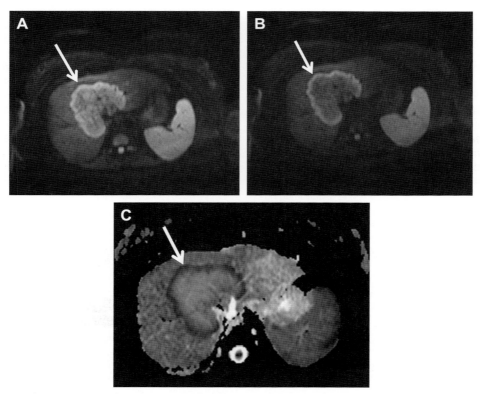

Fig. 19. Large liver metastasis demonstrated with diffusion-weighted imaging and ADC map. (*A*) Spin-echo echo-planar image obtained with a b value of 500 shows diffusely increased signal within the metastasis (*arrow*). (*B*) The b1000 image shows the central portion of the lesion to be of lower signal intensity than the periphery (*arrow*). (*C*) The ADC map from this acquisition generated with data from b0 and b500 shows restricted diffusion that is most pronounced at the periphery (*arrow*).

acquired during free breathing.[87–89] As with T2-weighted imaging, DWI has been combined with PROPELLER, with some success.[90]

SUMMARY

In the past several years, improvements in MR imaging technology have improved the quality and consistency of liver MR images that can be obtained, with careful attention to sequence optimization and protocol design and implementation (to include contrast selection and timing). Despite these technological advances, recognition and elimination of artifacts remains a critical part of liver MR imaging. No single sequence, protocol or list of imaging parameters can be considered optimal for all users, considering the wide variety of available hardware, sequences, and sequence modifications. Therefore, the reader is encouraged to use the information provided here to tailor his or her liver imaging protocol to achieve an appropriate balance between image quality, disease detection and characterization, and efficiency.

ACKNOWLEDGMENTS

The authors would like to thank Alastair J. Martin, PhD, for his editorial comments on the manuscript.

REFERENCES

1. Lattanzi R, Sodickson DK, Grant AK, et al. Electrodynamic constraints on homogeneity and radiofrequency power deposition in multiple coil excitations. Magn Reson Med 2009;61(2):315–34.
2. Merkle EM, Dale BM. Abdominal MRI at 3.0 T: the basics revisited. Am J Roentgenol 2006;186(6): 1524–32.
3. Kataoka M, Isoda H, Maetani Y, et al. MR imaging of the female pelvis at 3 Tesla: evaluation of image homogeneity using different dielectric pads. J Magn Reson Imaging 2007;26(6):1572–7.
4. Roemer PB, Edelstein WA, Hayes CE, et al. The NMR phased array. Magn Reson Med 1990;16(2): 192–225.
5. Hoult DI, Chen CN, Sank VJ. Quadrature detection in the laboratory frame. Magn Reson Med 1984; 1(3):339–53.
6. Du YP, Parker DL, Davis WL, et al. Reduction of partial-volume artifacts with zero-filled interpolation in 3-dimensional MR-angiography. JMRI 1994;4(5): 733–41.
7. Sodickson DK, Hardy CJ, Zhu YD, et al. Rapid volumetric MRI using parallel imaging with order-of-magnitude accelerations and a 32-element RF coil array: feasibility and implications. Acad Radiol 2005;12(5):626–35.
8. Elgavish RA, Twieg DB. Improved depiction of small anatomic structures in MR images using Gaussian-weighted spirals and zero-filled interpolation. Magn Reson Imaging 2003;21(2):103–12.
9. Bammer R, Schoenberg SO. Current concepts and advances in clinical parallel magnetic resonance imaging. Top Magn Reson Imaging 2004;15(3): 129–58.
10. Sodickson DK, Manning WJ. Simultaneous acquisition of spatial harmonics (SMASH): fast imaging with radiofrequency coil arrays. Magn Reson Med 1997;38(4):591–603.
11. Pruessmann KP, Weiger M, Scheidegger MB, et al. Sense: sensitivity encoding for fast MRI. Magn Reson Med 1999;42(5):952–62.
12. Yang RK, Roth CG, Ward RJ, et al. Optimizing abdominal MR imaging: approaches to common problems. Radiographics 2010;30(1):185–U210.
13. Glockner JF, Hu HH, Stanley DW, et al. Parallel MR imaging: a user's guide. Radiographics 2005;25(5): 1279–97.
14. Rescinito G, Sirlin C, Cittadini G Jr. Body MRI artefacts: from image degradation to diagnostic utility. Radiol Med 2009;114(1):18–31.
15. Wood ML, Runge VM, Henkelman RM. Overcoming motion in abdominal MR imaging. Am J Roentgenol 1988;150(3):513–22.
16. Chavhan GB, Babyn PS, Jankharia BG, et al. Steady-state MR imaging sequences: physics, classification, and clinical applications. Radiographics 2008;28(4):1147–60.
17. Keogan MT, Edelman RR. Technologic advances in abdominal MR imaging. Radiology 2001;220(2): 310–20.
18. Dutka MV, Bergin D, O'Kane PL, et al. Rapid multiplanar abdominal survey using MRI with the steady-state free-precession technique. J Magn Reson Imaging 2008;27(1):198–203.
19. Babcock EE, Brateman L, Weinreb JC, et al. Edge artifacts in MR images: chemical shift effect. J Comput Assist Tomogr 1985;9(2):252–7.
20. Ito K, Mitchell DG, Matsunaga N. MR imaging of the liver: techniques and clinical applications. Eur J Radiol 1999;32(1):2–14.
21. Mortele KJ, Praet M, Van Vlierberghe H, et al. CT and MR imaging findings in focal nodular hyperplasia of the liver: radiologic-pathologic correlation. AJR Am J Roentgenol 2000;175(3):687–92.
22. Merkle EM, Nelson RC. Dual gradient-echo in-phase and opposed-phase hepatic MR imaging: a useful tool for evaluating more than fatty infiltration or fatty sparing. Radiographics 2006;26(5):1409–18.
23. Dixon WT. Simple proton spectroscopic imaging. Radiology 1984;153(1):189–94.
24. Glover GH, Schneider E. Three-point Dixon technique for true water/fat decomposition with B0 inhomogeneity correction. Magn Reson Med 1991;18(2):371–83.

25. Ma J. Dixon techniques for water and fat imaging. J Magn Reson Imaging 2008;28(3):543–58.

26. Low RN, Ma JF, Panchal N. Fast spin-echo triple-echo Dixon: initial clinical experience with a novel pulse sequence for fat-suppressed T2-weighted abdominal MR imaging. J Magn Reson Imaging 2009;30(3):569–77.

27. Saranathan M, Rettmann D, Bayram E, et al. Multiecho time-resolved acquisition (META): a high spatio-temporal resolution Dixon imaging sequence for dynamic contrast-enhanced MRI. J Magn Reson Imaging 2009;29(6):1406–13.

28. Kondo H, Kanematsu M, Itoh K, et al. Does T2-weighted MR imaging improve preoperative detection of malignant hepatic tumors? Observer performance study in 49 surgically proven cases. Magn Reson Imaging 2005;23(1):89–95.

29. Hussain HK, Syed I, Nghiem HV, et al. T2-weighted MR imaging in the assessment of cirrhotic liver. Radiology 2004;230(3):637–44.

30. Masui T, Katayama M, Kobayashi S, et al. T2-weighted MRI of the female pelvis: comparison of breath-hold fast-recovery fast spin-echo and nonbreath-hold fast spin-echo sequences. J Magn Reson Imaging 2001;13(6):930–7.

31. Augui J, Vignaux O, Argaud C, et al. Liver: T2-weighted MR imaging with breath-hold fast-recovery optimized fast spin-echo compared with breath-hold half-Fourier and non-breath-hold respiratory-triggered fast spin-echo pulse sequences. Radiology 2002;223(3):853–9.

32. Lee SS, Byun JH, Hong HS, et al. Image quality and focal lesion detection on T2-weighted MR imaging of the liver: comparison of two high-resolution free-breathing imaging techniques with two breath-hold imaging techniques. J Magn Reson Imaging 2007;26(2):323–30.

33. Kanematsu M, Hoshi H, Itoh K, et al. Focal hepatic lesion detection: comparison of four fat-suppressed T2-weighted MR imaging pulse sequences. Radiology 1999;211(2):363–71.

34. Lu DS, Saini S, Hahn PF, et al. T2-weighted MR imaging of the upper part of the abdomen: should fat suppression be used routinely? AJR Am J Roentgenol 1994;162(5):1095–100.

35. Delfaut EM, Beltran J, Johnson G, et al. Fat suppression in MR imaging: techniques and pitfalls. Radiographics 1999;19(2):373–82.

36. Lauenstein TC, Sharma P, Hughes T, et al. Evaluation of optimized inversion-recovery fat-suppression techniques for T2-weighted abdominal MR imaging. J Magn Reson Imaging 2008;27(6):1448–54.

37. Hirokawa Y, Isoda H, Maetani YS, et al. MRI artifact reduction and quality improvement in the upper abdomen with PROPELLER and prospective acquisition correction (PACE) technique. AJR Am J Roentgenol 2008;191(4):1154–8.

38. Nanko S, Oshima H, Watanabe T, et al. Usefulness of the application of the BLADE technique to reduce motion artifacts on navigation-triggered prospective acquisition correction (PACE) T2-weighted MRI (T2WI) of the liver. J Magn Reson Imaging 2009;30(2):321–6.

39. Hirokawa Y, Isoda H, Maetani YS, et al. Hepatic lesions: improved image quality and detection with the periodically rotated overlapping parallel lines with enhanced reconstruction technique. Evaluation of SPIO-enhanced T2-weighted MR images. Radiology 2009;251(2):388–97.

40. Bayramoglu S, Kilickesmez O, Cimilli T, et al. T2-weighted MRI of the upper abdomen: comparison of four fat-suppressed T2-weighted sequences including PROPELLER (BLADE) technique. Acad Radiol 2010;17(3):368–74.

41. Martin DR, Semelka RC. Magnetic resonance imaging of the liver: review of techniques and approach to common diseases. Semin Ultrasound CT MR 2005;26(3):116–31.

42. Hecht EM, Holland AE, Israel GM, et al. Hepatocellular carcinoma in the cirrhotic liver: gadolinium-enhanced 3D T1-weighted MR imaging as a stand-alone sequence for diagnosis. Radiology 2006;239(2):438–47.

43. Coulam CH, Chan FP, Li KC. Can a multiphasic contrast-enhanced three-dimensional fast spoiled gradient-recalled echo sequence be sufficient for liver MR imaging? AJR Am J Roentgenol 2002;178(2):335–41.

44. Seale MK, Catalano OA, Saini S, et al. Hepatobiliary-specific MR contrast agents: role in imaging the liver and biliary tree. Radiographics 2009;29(6):1725–48.

45. Rofsky NM, Lee VS, Laub G, et al. Abdominal MR imaging with a volumetric interpolated breath-hold examination. Radiology 1999;212(3):876–84.

46. Lee VS, Lavelle MT, Rofsky NM, et al. Hepatic MR imaging with a dynamic contrast-enhanced isotropic volumetric interpolated breath-hold examination: feasibility, reproducibility, and technical quality. Radiology 2000;215(2):365–72.

47. Goshima S, Kanematsu M, Kondo H, et al. Optimal acquisition delay for dynamic contrast-enhanced MRI of hypervascular hepatocellular carcinoma. Am J Roentgenol 2009;192(3):686–92.

48. Van Beers BE, Materne R, Lacrosse M, et al. MR imaging of hypervascular liver tumors: timing optimization during the arterial phase. J Magn Reson Imaging 1999;9(4):562–7.

49. Sharma P, Kitajima HD, Kalb B, et al. Gadolinium-enhanced imaging of liver tumors and manifestations of hepatitis: pharmacodynamic and technical considerations. Top Magn Reson Imaging 2009;20(2):71–8.

50. Earls JP, Rofsky NM, DeCorato DR, et al. Hepatic arterial-phase dynamic gadolinium-enhanced MR

imaging: optimization with a test examination and a power injector. Radiology 1997;202(1):268–73.

51. Materne R, Horsmans Y, Jamart J, et al. Gadolinium-enhanced arterial-phase MR imaging of hypervascular liver tumors: comparison between tailored and fixed scanning delays in the same patients. J Magn Reson Imaging 2000;11(3):244–9.

52. Elsayes KM, Narra VR, Yin Y, et al. Focal hepatic lesions: diagnostic value of enhancement pattern approach with contrast-enhanced 3D gradient-echo MR imaging. Radiographics 2005;25(5): 1299–320.

53. Martin DR, Semelka RC. Imaging of benign and malignant focal liver lesions. Magn Reson Imaging Clin N Am 2001;9(4):785–802, vi–vii.

54. Quillin SP, Atilla S, Brown JJ, et al. Characterization of focal hepatic masses by dynamic contrast-enhanced MR imaging: findings in 311 lesions. Magn Reson Imaging 1997;15(3):275–85.

55. Shen XY, Chai CH, Xiao WB, et al. Diagnostic value of the fluoroscopic triggering 3D LAVA technique for primary liver cancer. Hepatobiliary Pancreat Dis Int 2010;9(2):159–63.

56. Kanematsu M, Semelka RC, Matsuo M, et al. Gadolinium-enhanced MR imaging of the liver: optimizing imaging delay for hepatic arterial and portal venous phases—a prospective randomized study in patients with chronic liver damage. Radiology 2002;225(2):407–15.

57. Martin DR, Seibert D, Yang M, et al. Reversible heterogeneous arterial phase liver perfusion associated with transient acute hepatitis: findings on gadolinium-enhanced MRI. J Magn Reson Imaging 2004;20(5):838–42.

58. Kanematsu M, Goshima S, Kondo H, et al. Double hepatic arterial phase MRI of the liver with switching of reversed centric and centric K-space reordering. AJR Am J Roentgenol 2006;187(2):464–72.

59. Mori K, Yoshioka H, Takahashi N, et al. Triple arterial phase dynamic MRI with sensitivity encoding for hypervascular hepatocellular carcinoma: comparison of the diagnostic accuracy among the early, middle, late, and whole triple arterial phase imaging. AJR Am J Roentgenol 2005;184(1):63–9.

60. Yoshioka H, Takahashi N, Yamaguchi M, et al. Double arterial phase dynamic MRI with sensitivity encoding (SENSE) for hypervascular hepatocellular carcinomas. J Magn Reson Imaging 2002;16(3): 259–66.

61. Rohrer M, Bauer H, Mintorovitch J, et al. Comparison of magnetic properties of MRI contrast media solutions at different magnetic field strengths. Invest Radiol 2005;40(11):715–24.

62. Vogl TJ, Kummel S, Hammerstingl R, et al. Liver tumors: comparison of MR imaging with Gd-EOB-DTPA and Gd-DTPA. Radiology 1996;200(1): 59–67.

63. Spinazzi A, Lorusso V, Pirovano G, et al. Safety, tolerance, biodistribution, and MR imaging enhancement of the liver with gadobenate dimeglumine: results of clinical pharmacologic and pilot imaging studies in nonpatient and patient volunteers. Acad Radiol 1999;6(5):282–91.

64. Spinazzi A, Lorusso V, Pirovano G, et al. Multihance clinical pharmacology: biodistribution and MR enhancement of the liver. Acad Radiol 1998;5(Suppl 1):S86–9 [discussion: S84–93].

65. Huppertz A, Haraida S, Kraus A, et al. Enhancement of focal liver lesions at gadoxetic acid-enhanced MR imaging: correlation with histopathologic findings and spiral CT—initial observations. Radiology 2005;234(2):468–78.

66. Zech CJ, Grazioli L, Breuer J, et al. Diagnostic performance and description of morphological features of focal nodular hyperplasia in Gd-EOB-DTPA-enhanced liver magnetic resonance imaging: results of a multicenter trial. Invest Radiol 2008;43(7): 504–11.

67. Zech CJ, Herrmann KA, Reiser MF, et al. MR imaging in patients with suspected liver metastases: value of liver-specific contrast agent Gd-EOB-DTPA. Magn Reson Med Sci 2007;6(1):43–52.

68. Brismar TB, Dahlstrom N, Edsborg N, et al. Liver vessel enhancement by Gd-BOPTA and Gd-EOB-DTPA: a comparison in healthy volunteers. Acta Radiol 2009;50(7):709–15.

69. Tamada T, Ito K, Sone T, et al. Dynamic contrast-enhanced magnetic resonance imaging of abdominal solid organ and major vessel: comparison of enhancement effect between Gd-EOB-DTPA and Gd-DTPA. J Magn Reson Imaging 2009;29(3): 636–40.

70. Akai H, Kiryu S, Takao H, et al. Efficacy of double-arterial phase gadolinium ethoxybenzyl diethylenetriamine pentaacetic acid-enhanced liver magnetic resonance imaging compared with double-arterial phase multi-detector row helical computed tomography. J Comput Assist Tomogr 2009;33(6): 887–92.

71. Motosugi U, Ichikawa T, Sou H, et al. Dilution method of gadolinium ethoxybenzyl diethylenetriaminepentaacetic acid (Gd-EOB-DTPA)-enhanced magnetic resonance imaging (MRI). J Magn Reson Imaging 2009;30(4):849–54.

72. Zech CJ, Vos B, Nordell A, et al. Vascular enhancement in early dynamic liver MR imaging in an animal model: comparison of two injection regimen and two different doses Gd-EOB-DTPA (gadoxetic acid) with standard Gd-DTPA. Invest Radiol 2009;44(6):305–10.

73. Kuhn JP, Hegenscheid K, Siegmund W, et al. Normal dynamic MRI enhancement patterns of the upper abdominal organs: gadoxetic acid compared with gadobutrol. AJR Am J Roentgenol 2009;193(5): 1318–23.

74. Choi JS, Kim MJ, Choi JY, et al. Diffusion-weighted MR imaging of liver on 3.0-Tesla system: effect of intravenous administration of gadoxetic acid disodium. Eur Radiol 2010;20(5):1052–60.

75. Kim YK, Kwak HS, Kim CS, et al. Detection and characterization of focal hepatic tumors: a comparison of T2-weighted MR images before and after the administration of gadoxetic acid. J Magn Reson Imaging 2009;30(2):437–43.

76. Gulani V, Willatt JM, Blaimer M, et al. Effect of contrast media on single-shot echo planar imaging: implications for abdominal diffusion imaging. J Magn Reson Imaging 2009;30(5):1203–8.

77. Motosugi U, Ichikawa T, Tominaga L, et al. Delay before the hepatocyte phase of Gd-EOB-DTPA-enhanced MR imaging: is it possible to shorten the examination time? Eur Radiol 2009;19(11):2623–9.

78. Qayyum A. Diffusion-weighted imaging in the abdomen and pelvis: concepts and applications. Radiographics 2009;29(6):1797–810.

79. Parikh T, Drew SJ, Lee VS, et al. Focal liver lesion detection and characterization with diffusion-weighted MR imaging: comparison with standard breath-hold T2-weighted imaging. Radiology 2008;246(3):812–22.

80. Bruegel M, Holzapfel K, Gaa J, et al. Characterization of focal liver lesions by ADC measurements using a respiratory triggered diffusion-weighted single-shot echo-planar MR imaging technique. Eur Radiol 2008;18(3):477–85.

81. Erturk SM, Ichikawa T, Sano K, et al. Diffusion-weighted magnetic resonance imaging for characterization of focal liver masses: impact of parallel imaging (SENSE) and b value. J Comput Assist Tomogr 2008;32(6):865–71.

82. Holzapfel K, Bruegel M, Eiber M, et al. Characterization of small (</=10mm) focal liver lesions: value of respiratory-triggered echo-planar diffusion-weighted MR imaging. Eur J Radiol June 8, 2009 [online].

83. Kilickesmez O, Bayramoglu S, Inci E, et al. Value of apparent diffusion coefficient measurement for discrimination of focal benign and malignant hepatic masses. J Med Imaging Radiat Oncol 2009;53(1):50–5.

84. Sandrasegaran K, Akisik FM, Lin C, et al. The value of diffusion-weighted imaging in characterizing focal liver masses. Acad Radiol 2009;16(10):1208–14.

85. Taouli B, Tolia AJ, Losada M, et al. Diffusion-weighted MRI for quantification of liver fibrosis: preliminary experience. Am J Roentgenol 2007;189(4):799–806.

86. Luciani A, Vignaud A, Cavet M, et al. Liver cirrhosis: intravoxel incoherent motion MR imaging—pilot study. Radiology 2008;249(3):891–9.

87. Nasu K, Kuroki Y, Sekiguchi R, et al. The effect of simultaneous use of respiratory triggering in diffusion-weighted imaging of the liver. Magn Reson Med Sci 2006;5(3):129–36.

88. Taouli B, Sandberg A, Stemmer A, et al. Diffusion-weighted imaging of the liver: comparison of navigator triggered and breathhold acquisitions. J Magn Reson Imaging 2009;30(3):561–8.

89. Kwee TC, Takahara T, Koh DM, et al. Comparison and reproducibility of ADC measurements in breath-hold, respiratory triggered, and free-breathing diffusion-weighted MR imaging of the liver. J Magn Reson Imaging 2008;28(5):1141–8.

90. Deng J, Miller FH, Salem R, et al. Multishot diffusion-weighted PROPELLER magnetic resonance imaging of the abdomen. Invest Radiol 2006;41(10):769–75.

91. Huang J, Raman SS, Vuong N, et al. Utility of breath-hold fast-recovery fast spin-echo T2 versus respiratory-triggered fast spin-echo T2 in clinical hepatic imaging. Am J Roentgenol 2005;184(3):842–6.

92. Tang Y, Yamashita Y, Namimoto T, et al. Liver T2-weighted MR imaging: comparison of fast and conventional half-Fourier single-shot turbo spin-echo, breath-hold turbo spin-echo, and respiratory-triggered turbo spin-echo sequences. Radiology 1997;203(3):766–72.

93. Coates GG, Borrello JA, McFarland EG, et al. Hepatic T2-weighted MRI: a prospective comparison of sequences, including breath-hold, half-Fourier turbo spin echo (HASTE). J Magn Reson Imaging 1998;8(3):642–9.

94. Lee MG, Jeong YK, Kim JC, et al. Fast T2-weighted liver MR imaging: comparison among breath-hold turbo-spin-echo, HASTE, and inversion recovery (IR) HASTE sequences. Abdom Imaging 2000;25(1):93–9.

95. Katayama M, Masui T, Kobayashi S, et al. Fat-suppressed T2-weighted MRI of the liver: comparison of respiratory-triggered fast spin-echo, breath-hold single-shot fast spin-echo, and breath-hold fast-recovery fast spin-echo sequences. J Magn Reson Imaging 2001;14(4):439–49.

96. Kim BS, Kim JH, Choi GM, et al. Comparison of three free-breathing T2-weighted MRI sequences in the evaluation of focal liver lesions. J Am J Roentgenol 2008;190(1):W19–27.

Imaging at Higher Magnetic Fields: 3 T Versus 1.5 T

Daniel T. Boll, MD*, Elmar M. Merkle, MD

KEYWORDS

- Higher magnetic fields • 3 T • 1.5 T
- Diffusion-weighted hepatobiliary imaging
- Contrast-enhanced imaging
- Non—contrast-enhanced imaging

Magnetic resonance (MR) imaging has proved to be a comprehensive modality for assessment of morphologic and functional characteristics of the hepatobiliary system in clinical scenarios of focal and diffuse liver disease. Concurrent technical improvements, such as amplification of the static magnetic field, development of powerful gradient systems, and multichannel phased-array body coils, as well as implementation of advanced imaging sequence designs using respiratory-triggered and three-dimensional data acquisition schemes, realize high-quality examinations of the hepatobiliary system with T1-, T2-, and also diffusion-weighted pulse sequences.[1]

This article highlights the basic concepts of MR imaging of the hepatobiliary system using high static magnetic fields and its imaging effects in noncontrast, as well as contrast-enhanced, imaging.

GAINS IN CONTRAST FROM AN INCREASE OF THE MAGNETIC FIELD

The strengthening of the static magnetic field of clinical imaging systems affects MR phenomena through various contrast mechanisms; however, doubling the magnetic field does not necessarily double the parenchymal contrast on MR imaging series on high-field MR imagers because of counteracting MR contrast phenomena.[2,3] General estimations of signal/noise ratios (SNR) for spin-echo—based (SNR$_{SE}$) and gradient-echo—based (SNR$_{GE}$) sequence designs are approximated according to

$$SNR_{SE} \, \alpha \, B_0 \, V \left(\sqrt{\frac{N_{PE} N_{PA} N_{AV}}{BW}} \right) \left(1 - e^{-\frac{TR}{T2}} \right) e^{-\frac{TE}{T2}}$$

and

$$SNR_{GE} \, \alpha \, B_0 \, V \left(\sqrt{\frac{N_{PE} N_{PA} N_{AV}}{BW}} \right) \frac{\sin(\theta)(1 - e^{-\frac{TR}{T_1}})}{\left(1 - e^{-\frac{TR}{T_1}} \cos(\theta)\right)} e^{-\frac{TE}{T_2^*}}$$

with B_0 representing the static magnetic field in T, V the voxel volume in mm^3, N_{PE} the number of phase-encoding steps, N_{PA} the number of partitions, N_{AV} the number of signal averages, BW the receiver bandwidth in Hz/pixel, θ the flip angle, TE the echo time in milliseconds, as well as T_1 the longitudinal, and T_2 the transverse, relaxation times in milliseconds. These multifactorial estimations outline the effect of cross-dependent imaging parameters that contribute to the overall SNR.

Initially, both approximations for SNR$_{SE}$ and SNR$_{GE}$ sequence designs emphasize that the attained SNR has proportional relationships with the static magnetic field B_0 and the voxel volume V, if the fine print in the square root and exponential functions is being ignored; doubling the magnetic field or voxel volume seems to proportionally increase SNR. Although the square root

Department of Radiology, Duke University Medical Center, DUMC 3808, Durham, NC 27710, USA
* Corresponding author.
E-mail address: daniel.boll@duke.edu

Magn Reson Imaging Clin N Am 18 (2010) 549–564
doi:10.1016/j.mric.2010.08.008

mri.theclinics.com

function establishes a square root proportionality between estimated SNR and acquisition time, it is the final exponential function, incorporating sequence- and tissue-specific parameters, that introduces signal components with an inverse proportionality to the static magnetic field B_0.

Sequence parameters like repetition time (TR) and TE, essential for defining pulse sequences, are based on tissue-specific relaxation times T1 and T2, which in turn are strongly dependent on the surrounding magnetic field B_0. At 0.5 T, liver parenchyma possesses a T1 relaxation time of approximately 327 to 518 milliseconds and a tissue-specific T2 relaxation time of 55 to 62 milliseconds as a result of protons' base precession frequency and spin-lattice and spin-spin interactions. At 1.5 T, hepatic tissue's relaxation time has substantially increased for T1 to 547 to 568 milliseconds and minimally decreased for T2 to 51 to 56 milliseconds. At 3.0 T, with a Larmor frequency of approximately 128 MHz, liver-specific T1 relaxation time has further increased to 809 milliseconds, whereas liver-specific T2 relaxation time has further decreased to approximately 45 to 50 milliseconds.[4]

The underlying principle of liver-specific T1-weighted imaging is to use the shortest possible TE in order to maximize hepatobiliary contrast as well as the number of slices attainable in a limited breath-hold period. The doubling in precession frequency at 3 T compared with 1.5 T also affects the precise timing of T1-weighted in- and opposed-imaging phases. The interecho spacing between the in- and opposed-phase echo pairs decreases substantially when the magnetic field B_0 is doubled, and thereby either requires shortening of TE when the first in and opposed pair is targeted, eventually forcing a wider bandwidth or, alternatively, prolonging TE if a later in and opposed pair is selected for imaging. These parameter adjustments may at least partially counteract prior contrast gains achieved by the stronger B_0 field (**Fig. 1**).[5,6]

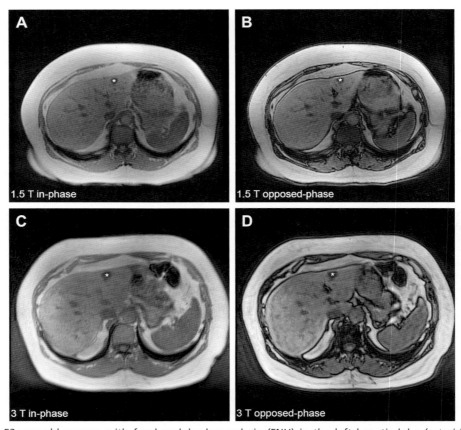

Fig. 1. A 53-year-old woman with focal nodular hyperplasia (FNH) in the left hepatic lobe (*asterisks*) on T1-weighted in-phase (A, C) and opposed-phase (B, D) imaging at 1.5 T (A, B) and 3 T (C, D). Interscan interval: 3 weeks. Note the increased conspicuity of the FNH and improved hepatic parenchymal contrast on the 3 T image series.

Although the changes in T2 relaxation times at low magnetic fields are insignificant, in high-field MR imaging, T2 relaxation times can decrease by up to 10%, and may potentially reduce the gain in estimated SNR. Hepatic T2-weighted spin-echo imaging requires a TR of at least 4 times the tissue's specific T1 relaxation time, and a TE that approximates the tissue's specific T2 relaxation time (**Fig. 2**).[4,7,8] Tissue susceptibility effects also increase substantially with higher B_0 fields, thereby accentuating field inhomogeneities and shimming difficulties, and result in a significant decrease in T2* that mainly affects gradient-echo sequences.[5,9]

After taking into account the linear increase of the Larmor frequency caused by the high B_0 field, and the subsequent necessity to alter the radiofrequency (RF) pulse profiles/strength accordingly, and after satisfying the general requirements for T1- and T2-weighted sequences, in particular the magnetic field–dependent timing parameters TE and TR, unacceptable specific absorption rates (SAR) may result if a linear translation of imaging parameters optimized for 1.5 T imaging was used. SAR is a measure to quantify and limit energy deposition within the body defined by

$$SAR = \frac{\sigma |E|^2}{2\rho}\left(\frac{\tau}{TR}\right)N_p N_s$$

with σ representing the conductivity in S/m, E the electric field in V/m, ρ the tissue density in kg/m³, τ the pulse duration in milliseconds, TR in milliseconds, and N_P and N_S representing the number of pulses and slices, respectively.[5,10] Because the electric field E and magnetic field B_0 grow

proportionally, a quadratic increase in energy deposition is to be expected if additional steps to reduce overall SAR are not initiated. Doubling of the RF frequency at 3 T is an exacerbating factor; even though ionizing energy is not deposited, tissue heating may be enhanced. Because of the decreased wavelength of the RF pulses used in high-field MR imaging, a more inhomogeneous distribution of power deposition may eventually lead to formation of hot spots at areas of increased conductivity such as medical implants and incorporated ferromagnetic particles.[5] Limiting the energy deposition at higher magnetic fields requires protocol adjustments such as prolongation of TR and flip angle θ reduction, both of which result in an overall decrease in expected SNR and alteration of tissue contrasts. Alternatively, reducing the number of image slices reduces SAR, but also reduces the anatomic coverage or increases the overall acquisition time. New approaches in RF pulse and gradient design propose the implementation of variable flip angles and allow a significant reduction of SAR.[11] Combining time-variant gradients with modified RF pulse waveforms achieves high flip angles while meeting SAR limits **Fig. 3**.[12]

CONTRAST AGENTS IN HEPATOBILIARY MR IMAGING

Although contrast-enhanced hepatobiliary MR imaging uses a wide range of gadolinium-based contrast agents, the essential mechanism of contrast enhancement dependency based on surrounding magnetic field B_0 remains a function of only the relaxivity of the paramagnetic

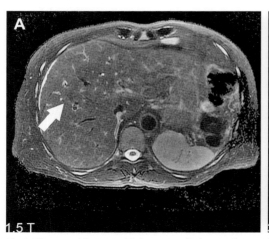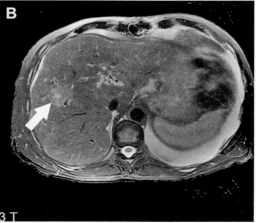

Fig. 2. A 52-year-old man with hepatocellular carcinoma (HCC) in the right hepatic lobe (*arrows*) on T2-weighted imaging at 1.5 T (*A*) and 3 T (*B*). Interscan interval: 6 days. Note the increased conspicuity of the HCC on the 3 T image series and no discernable lesion on the 1.5 T image series.

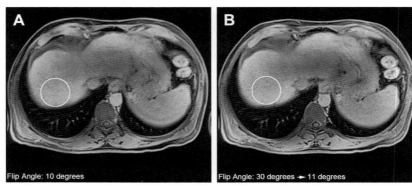

Fig. 3. A 59-year-old woman with hepatic cirrhosis on contrast-enhanced fat-saturated T1-weighted imaging following the administration of a hepatocyte-specific, gadolinium-based contrast agent on a delayed imaging phase using a flip angle of 10° (*A*). The flip angle was then manually increased to 30°; however, because of SAR limitations, the MR scanner adjusted the flip to the maximum 11°, and essentially no additional enhancement of image contrast (*circles*) was achieved as seen in (*B*). Interscan interval: 1 minute.

gadolinium ion complex and the tissue relaxation times.[13] The different relaxivities for various gadolinium chelates decrease only minimally as the magnetic field B_0 doubles from 1.5 T to 3 T, whereas the hepatic T1 relaxation times are prolonged substantially, resulting in an apparent contrast gain on high-field MR studies[5,14] (**Fig. 4**) estimated by

$$\frac{1}{T1_{Postcontrast}} = \frac{1}{T1_{Precontrast}} + r \times C$$

with $T1_{Precontrast}$ and $T1_{Postcontrast}$ representing hepatic longitudinal relaxation times before and after contrast administration in milliseconds, r the relaxivity of the gadolinium chelate in sec^{-1} $mmol^{-1}$, and C being the molar in vivo concentration of the contrast agent.

Different gadolinium chelates are responsible for different biodistributions of contrast material, ranging from nonspecific agents with a predominantly extracellular distribution to contrast materials that are taken up specifically by hepatocytes and are partially excreted through the biliary system; different biodistributions of contrast material also require specific hepatobiliary imaging protocols, as shown in the sequences in **Tables 1** to **3**. In general, the paramagnetic effect of gadolinium shortens tissue-specific relaxation times, leading to an increase in hepatic tissue signal intensities, particularly on T1-weighted sequences.

Gadolinium chelates without specific biodistribution are primarily confined to the extracellular space. Rapid redistribution of gadolinium chelates from intravascular to extracellular spaces requires that the contrast agent be infused intravenously as a small-volume bolus injection at up to 2 mL/s at a dose of 0.1 to 0.2 mmol/kg body weight. These

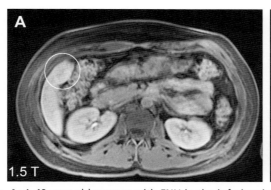
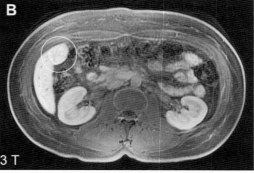

Fig. 4. A 49-year-old woman with FNH in the inferior right hepatic lobe (*circles*) on contrast-enhanced fat-saturated T1-weighted imaging using a hepatocyte-specific, gadolinium-based contrast agent on delayed phase imaging at 1.5 T (*A*) and 3 T (*B*). Interscan interval: 6 months. Note the increased conspicuity of the enhancing FNH on the 3 T image series compared with the 1.5 T image series.

Table 1
Hepatobiliary imaging protocol using nonspecific extracellular Gd-chelates

	T2w	T1w 2pt or 3pt Dixon	T2w Fat Saturated	Diffusion b 50 b 800	T1w Fat Saturated Triple Arterial Phase	T1w Fat Saturated Portal Venous Phase	T2w Fat Saturated MRCP	T1w Fat Saturated Equilibrium Phase
Sequence								
Acquisition Scheme	Single-shot fast spin echo	Spoiled gradient echo	Fast spin echo	Diffusion	Dynamic, multiphase spoiled gradient echo	Spoiled gradient echo	Single-shot fast spin echo	Spoiled gradient echo
Coverage	2D	3D	2D	2D	3D	3D	3D	3D
Triggering / Breath Hold	(Non) Breath hold	Breath hold	Respiratory triggered	Free breathing	Breath hold	Breath hold	Respiratory triggered	Breath hold
TR	1339 ms	5.026 ms	8571.4 ms	4900 ms	3.536 ms	4.364 ms	3529.4 ms	4.364 ms
TE	141.312 ms	1.336/2.622 ms	90.22 ms	77 ms	1.72 ms	2.1 ms	810.92 ms	2.1 ms
Pixel Bandwidth	325.5 Hz	651.1 Hz	244.1 Hz	1302 Hz	651 Hz	244.1 Hz	162.8 Hz	244.1 Hz
Slice Thickness	10 mm	5 mm	5 mm	5 mm	6 mm	4.4 mm	1.6 mm	4.4 mm
Imaging Plane	Transverse & coronal	Transverse	Transverse	Transverse	Transverse	Transverse & coronal	Coronal	Transverse
Matrix	384 × 128	320 × 192	384 × 224	192 × 75	256 × 128	288 × 192	288 × 288	288 × 192
Acquisition Time	2 × 20 s	24 s	3 – 5 min	2:14 min	3 × 8 s	25 s	2 – 5 min	25 s

Contrast administration

agents are available in various compositions, including gadopentetate dimeglumine (Gd-DTPA), gadoteridol (Gd-HP-DO3A), gadodiamide (Gd-DTPA-BMA), gadoversetamide (Gd-DTPA-BMEA), gadoterate meglumine (Gd-DOTA), and gadobutrol (Gd-BT-DO3A), with approval for various imaging applications from governmental health care authorities (**Fig. 5**; sequence **Table 1**). Gadofosveset trisodium represents a new class of blood-pool contrast agents specifically designed for visualization of abdominal or extremity vessels in patients with vascular diseases; contrast-enhanced hepatobiliary MR imaging occurs, at least partially, when the abdominal aorta is targeted for evaluation (**Fig. 6**).[15]

All hepatocyte-targeted contrast agents are characterized by active transport of the gadolinium chelates into hepatocytes; they are partly eliminated through the biliary system and subsequently allow parenchymal as well as biliary assessment by T1-weighted pulse sequences. Hepatocyte-selective contrast agents differ in the degree of biliary excretion, with gadobenate dimeglumine (Gd-BOPTA) showing a minor biliary excretion fraction (5), (sequence **Table 2**), compared with gadoxetate disodium (Gd-EOB-DTPA), which has a rapid and specific hepatocellular uptake and biliary excretion (~50%) (sequence **Table 3**). Gd-EOB-DTPA and Gd-BOPTA allow imaging during the arterial phase, the portal venous phase, and equilibrium phase, comparable with the other gadolinium chelates, and may allow for the addition of a hepatocyte phase to the contrast-enhanced liver imaging protocol. Because Gd-EOB-DTPA features a T1 relaxivity higher than conventional gadolinium-based agents, in addition to the marked hepatic uptake, an overall contrast dose of 0.025 mmol/kg body weight is sufficient for adequate parenchymal enhancement. Furthermore, increased transient protein interactions lead to higher T1 relaxivities with more effective T1 shortening compared with other gadolinium-based contrast materials (**Fig. 7**).[14,16]

Table 2
Hepatobiliary imaging protocol using hepatocyte-specific (limited biliary elimination), intracellular Gd-chelates

	T2w	T1w	T2w	Diffusion	T1w	T1w	T2w	T1w	T1w
Sequence		2pt or 3pt Dixon	Fat Saturated	b 50 / b 800	Fat Saturated Triple Arterial Phase	Fat Saturated Portal Venous Phase	Fat Saturated MRCP	Fat Saturated Equilibrium Phase	Fat Saturated 2 h Delay Phase
Acquisition Scheme	Single-shot fast spin echo	Spoiled gradient echo	Fast spin echo	Diffusion	Dynamic, multiphase spoiled gradient echo	Spoiled gradient echo	Single-shot fast spin echo	Spoiled gradient echo	Spoiled gradient echo
Coverage	2D	3D	2D	2D	3D	3D	3D	3D	3D
Triggering / Breath Hold	(Non) Breath hold	Breath hold	Respiratory triggered	Free breathing	Breath hold	Breath hold	Respiratory triggered	Breath hold	Breath Hold
TR	1339 ms	5.026 ms	8571.4 ms	4900 ms	3.536 ms	4.364 ms	3529.4 ms	4.364 ms	4.364 ms
TE	141.312 ms	1.336/2.622 ms	90.22 ms	77 ms	1.72 ms	2.1 ms	810.92 ms	2.1 ms	2.1 ms
Pixel Bandwidth	325.5 Hz	651.1 Hz	244.1 Hz	1302 Hz	651 Hz	244.1 Hz	162.8 Hz	244.1 Hz	244.1 Hz
Slice Thickness	10 mm	5 mm	5 mm	5 mm	6 mm	4.4 mm	1.6 mm	4.4 mm	4.4 mm
Imaging Plane	Transverse & coronal	Transverse	Transverse	Transverse	Transverse	Transverse & coronal	Coronal	Transverse	Transverse & coronal
Matrix	384 × 128	320 × 192	384 × 224	192 × 75	256 × 128	288 × 192	288 × 288	288 × 192	288 × 192
Acquisition Time	2 × 20 s	24 s	3 – 5 min	2:14 min	3 × 8 s	25 s	2 – 5 min	25 s	25 s

Contrast administration

ADVANCED IMAGING SEQUENCE DESIGNS

Doubling of the magnetic field to improve tissue contrast has led to extensive innovations in MR technology. Integration of hardware developments such as powerful gradient systems and multi-channel phased-array body coils, as well as modified sequence parameters that take into account the unique variations in hepatic T1 and T2 relaxation times occurring at magnetic fields of 3 T, must be achieved and harmonized by new imaging sequence designs. To maintain reasonable acquisition times within strict SAR limitations while maximizing parenchymal tissue contrast, the implementation of parallel imaging techniques and transition from two-dimensional to three-dimensional imaging schemes represent 2 of the most successful innovations in high-field hepatobiliary MR imaging.[5,17]

Parallel Imaging Techniques

Parallel imaging acceleration techniques use spatial information from individual elements of a phased-array coil set to perform a portion of the spatial encoding normally accomplished by time-consuming gradients, thereby significantly reducing acquisition times. Different approaches, either k-space or image-space based, such as simultaneous acquisition of spatial harmonics (SMASH) and sensitivity encoding (SENSE) have been introduced that realize spatial encoding with multiple distinct receiver coils for a sparse sampling of k-space. Linear combinations of component coil signals are used to emulate the effects of phase-encoding gradients. However, parallel imaging techniques must be calibrated using detailed and time-consuming coil mapping procedures and coil sensitivity profile acquisitions.

More recently, improvements for faster and more advanced calibration techniques have been developed, allowing for the acquisition of additional lines in the center of k-space. Data from multiple lines of all circumferentially distributed coils are used to fit the autocalibration signal for each individual coil. This fit gives the weights that can be used to generate the missing lines from that coil. Once all of the lines are reconstructed for a particular coil, a Fourier transformation is used to generate the

Table 3
Hepatobiliary imaging protocol using hepatocyte-specific (substantial biliary elimination), intracellular Gd-chelates

	T2w	T1w	T2w	Diffusion	T1w	T1w	T2w	T1w	T1w	T1w
Sequence		2pt or 3pt Dixon	Fat Saturated	b 50 / b 800	Fat Saturated Triple Arterial Phase	Fat Saturated Portal Venous Phase	Fat Saturated MRCP	Fat Saturated Equilibrium Phase I	Fat Saturated Equilibrium Phase II	Fat Saturated Equilibrium Phase III
Acquisition Scheme	Single-shot fast spin echo	Spoiled gradient echo	Fast spin echo	Diffusion	Dynamic, multiphase spoiled gradient echo	Spoiled gradient echo	Single-shot fast spin echo	Spoiled gradient echo 6 min p.i.	Spoiled gradient echo 12 min p.i.	Spoiled gradient echo 18 min p.i.
Coverage	2D	3D	2D	2D	3D	3D	3D	3D	3D	3D
Triggering / Breath Hold	(Non) Breath hold	Breath hold	Respiratory triggered	Free breathing	Breath hold	Breath hold	Respiratory triggered	Breath hold	Breath hold	Breath hold
TR	1339 ms	5.026 ms	8571.4 ms	4900 ms	3.536 ms	4.364 ms	3529.4 ms	4.364 ms	4.364 ms	4.364 ms
TE	141.312 ms	1.336/2.622 ms	90.22 ms	77 ms	1.72 ms	2.1 ms	810.92 ms	2.1 ms	2.1 ms	2.1 ms
Pixel Bandwidth	325.5 Hz	651.1 Hz	244.1 Hz	1302 Hz	651 Hz	244.1 Hz	162.8 Hz	244.1 Hz	244.1 Hz	244.1 Hz
Slice Thickness	10 mm	5 mm	5 mm	5 mm	6 mm	4.4 mm	1.6 mm	4.4 mm	4.4 mm	4.4 mm
Imaging Plane	Transverse & coronal	Transverse	Transverse	Transverse	Transverse	Transverse & coronal	Coronal	Transverse	Transverse	Transverse & coronal
Matrix	384 × 128	320 × 192	384 × 224	192 × 75	256 × 128	288 × 192	288 × 288	288 × 192	288 × 192	288 × 192
Acquisition Time	2 × 20 s	24 s	3 – 5 min	2:14 min	3 × 8 s	25 s	2 – 5 min	25 s	25 s	25 s

Contrast administration

uncombined image for that coil. This process is repeated for each coil of the array and the full set of images can be postprocessed using a sum-of-squares reconstruction; this approach is known as the generalized autocalibrating partially parallel acquisition (GRAPPA) technique.[18–21] Generally greater parenchymal contrast achieved with 3 T hepatobiliary MR imaging enables the implementation of higher parallel imaging acceleration factors without compromising image quality because of unacceptable noise levels possibly experienced at 1.5 T imaging.

Volumetric Acquisition Combined with Parallel Acceleration

The combination of volumetric acquisition schemes with parallel acceleration allows the implementation of three-dimensional T1-weighted gradient-echo breath-hold in- and opposed-phase MR sequences with 2-point Dixon postprocessing.[22,23] The echo spacing results in 2 imaging series, 1 with water and lipid signals in phase coherence, and another with water and lipid signals with an opposing phase configuration.[24] Subsequent summation and subtraction of in-phase and opposed-phase datasets enables generation of fat-only and water-only

image series (**Fig. 8**). Three-dimensional T1-weighted gradient-echo sequences such as volumetric interpolated breath-hold examination (VIBE) or liver acquisition with volume acceleration (LAVA) obtain a near-simultaneous acquisition of in- and opposed-phase MR series, using next-neighbor and vote-counting corrections to allow calculation of artifact-suppressed fat-only and water-only MR series. Acquisition of multiple in-phase echoes allows the derivation of T2* maps and fat-percentage calculations (**Fig. 9**). Raw-data interpolation of acquired in-phase and opposed-phase echoes without substantial signal loss is achieved by asymmetric echo sampling in the readout direction, thereby effectively reducing the number of phase-encoding steps, whereas sinc interpolation is used for completion of the k-space matrix.[25]

Contrast Gains

An increase of the flip angle (+20°) may prove particularly beneficial in contrast-enhanced imaging, because larger excitation angles on delayed phase series following the administrations of hepatocyte-specific contrast agents tends to enhance detectability of regional contrast distributions and increase the conspicuity of smaller

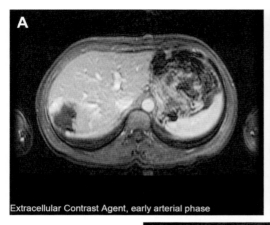

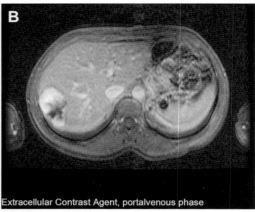

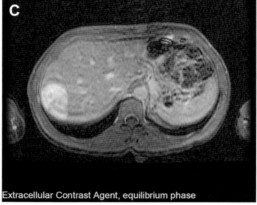

Fig. 5. A 45-year-old man with a large hemangioma in the right hepatic lobe on contrast-enhanced, fat-saturated, T1-weighted imaging using a extracellular gadolinium-based contrast agent on early arterial (*A*), portalvenous (*B*), and equilibrium (*C*) phases at 1.5 T (*B*). Note the hyperintense appearance of the hemangioma compared with the hepatic parenchyma on the equilibrium phase image series.

lesions (**Fig. 10**). However, SAR limitations, individually affected by the patients' body habitus, reduce the applicability of this approach, in particular on 3 T field MR imaging systems.

For many of the reasons described earlier, three-dimensional T1-weighted gradient-echo sequences can achieve a potential gain in contrast by a factor of up to 1.7, but the theoretic twofold

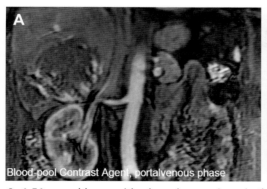

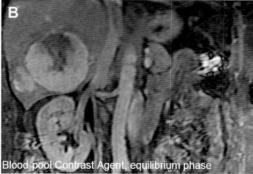

Fig. 6. A 54-year-old man with a large hemangioma in the right hepatic lobe on contrast-enhanced fat-saturated T1-weighted imaging using a blood-pool gadolinium-based contrast agent on portalvenous (*A*), and equilibrium (*B*) phases at 3 T (*B*). Note the hyperintense appearance of the hemangioma compared with the hepatic parenchyma on the equilibrium phase image series.

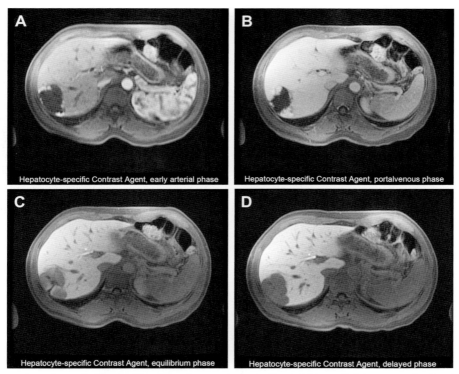

Fig. 7. The patient shown in **Fig. 5** with a large hemangioma in the right hepatic lobe on contrast-enhanced fat-saturated T1-weighted imaging using a hepatocyte-specific gadolinium-based contrast agent on early arterial (*A*), portalvenous (*B*), equilibrium (*C*), and delayed (*D*) phases at 3 T. Interscan interval: 4 months. Note the biliary excretion of the contrast agent and the hypointense appearance of the hemangioma compared with the hepatic parenchyma on the equilibrium and delayed phases.

contrast increase caused by amplification of the magnetic field from 1.5 T to 3 T is not generally obtained.[3,5]

A combination of three-dimensional sequence designs with respiratory triggering allows acquisition of heavily T2-weighted fast spin-echo sequences using variable flip angle excitations such as sampling perfection with application-optimized contrast using different flip angle evolution (SPACE), volumetric isotropic TSE acquisition

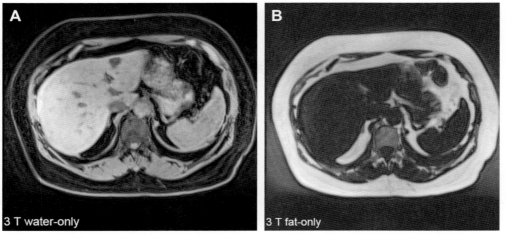

Fig. 8. The patient shown in **Fig. 1** with FNH in the left hepatic lobe on T1-weighted water-only (*A*) and fat-only (*B*) imaging at 3 T. Note the lack of fatty components within the lesion on the fat-only image series.

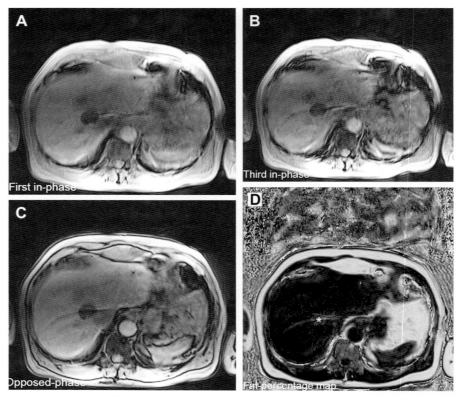

Fig. 9. A 49-year-old woman with a hepatic adenoma in the right hepatic lobe on 3-point T1-weighted Dixon imaging on first (*A*) and third (*B*) in-phase as well as initial opposed-phase (*C*) series. Fat components within the adenoma (*asterisk*) are confirmed on the fat-percentage series (*D*).

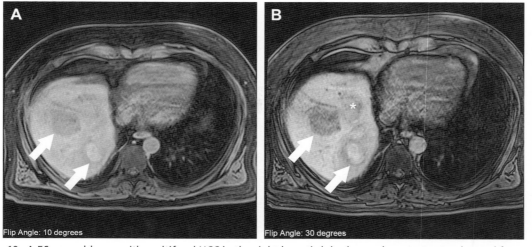

Fig. 10. A 56-year-old man with multifocal HCC in the right hepatic lobe (*arrows*) on contrast-enhanced fat-saturated T1-weighted imaging using a hepatocyte-specific gadolinium-based contrast agent on delayed phases at 3 T with flip angles of 10° (*A*) and 30° (*B*). Note the increased conspicuity of the HCCs on the 30° flip angle image series (*asterisk*). Interscan interval: 1 minute.

(VISTA) or Cube. These high-resolution MR chol-angiopancreatography (MRCP) image datasets can be further postprocessed with maximum intensity projection (MIP) techniques, **Fig. 11**. However, SAR limitations may potentially reduce the range of usable flip angle variations and lead to unacceptably poor T2 contrast on 3 T imaging systems executing fast spin-echo sequences with variable flip angle excitations.

Ultimately, T2-weighted sequences acquired at 3 T are expected to achieve signal gains of up to 1.8 times the signal attained by 1.5 T MR systems.[3,5]

Diffusion-weighted MR Imaging

Diffusion-weighted MR imaging (DWI) has become a routine component of abdominal MR sequence protocols. DWI offers molecular information that complements the morphologic information obtained by conventional pulse sequences.

In general, DWI is performed as an echo-planar imaging sequence with additional gradients implemented during the acquisition process. Following a typical RF excitation pulse, spins undergo dephasing mainly because of effects of the external MR field inhomogeneities. However, a small part of this dephasing is related to diffusion of water molecules. This effect is enhanced in DWI, which is usually based on a T2-weighted sequence with an additional symmetric pair of diffusion-sensitive gradients enveloping the refocusing pulses. Water molecules with restricted diffusion undergo an initial phase shift as a result of the first diffusion gradient, which will be completely reversed by the second diffusion gradient without residual phase shift at time of readout. In contrast, water molecules without substantial diffusion restriction acquire phase information from the first gradient but, because of their motion, their signal is not be completely rephased by the second gradient, leading to a signal loss. Hence, the diffusion of water molecules is apparent as attenuation of the measured signal intensity at DWI. The degree of water motion has been found to be inversely related to the degree of signal attenuation.

The sensitivity of the DWI sequence to water motion can be varied by changing the amplitude of the diffusion-weighted gradient, the duration of the applied gradient, and the time interval between the paired gradients. These variations in gradient characteristics are expressed in a numerical parameter, referred to as the b-value. The sensitivity for detecting restrictions in diffusion is varied by changing the b-value, which is measured in s/mm^2. The b-value is typically varied by altering the gradient amplitude, rather than the duration or time interval between gradients. Larger b-values are required to perceive more slow-moving molecules. Because DWI sequences are based on T2-weighted sequence designs, hepatic hemangiomas or cysts appear bright on standard T2-weighted imaging sequences and may also appear bright on a DWI sequence. This phenomenon is known as the T2 shine-through effect, and should not be misconstrued as an area of restricted diffusion.

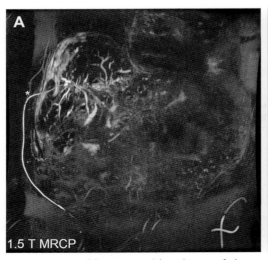
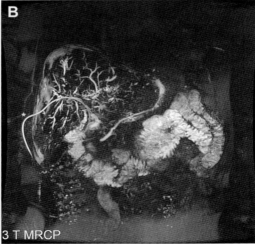

Fig. 11. A 42-year-old woman with stricture of the common bile duct following the placement of an inside-outside percutaneous biliary drain (*asterisk*) on an MIP based on an MRCP series at 1.5 T (*A*) and 3 T (*B*). Interscan interval: 1 week. Note the increased conspicuity of the intrahepatic biliary and pancreatic ducts on the later acquired 3 T image series (*B*) compared with the earlier acquired 1.5 T image series (*A*).

To resolve T2 shine-through effects, apparent diffusion coefficient (ADC) maps can be calculated to obtain pure diffusion information. In order to calculate ADC maps for each pixel in a DWI image series, at least two DWI datasets with differing b-values must be obtained. The ADC maps represent grayscale encoded ratios of logarithmic differences in signal intensities, as well as differences of b-values, of the two sequential DWI sequences. Areas of true restricted diffusion show high signal intensity on DWI with corresponding low signal intensity on the ADC map; areas of free diffusion also appear bright on DWI, corresponding to T2 shine-through effects, but are also bright on the ADC map (**Fig. 12**). DWI has proved to be useful in the detection of both benign and malignant hepatic lesions, with early clinical studies even suggesting DWI to be superior to breath-hold T2-weighted imaging for lesion detection.[26,27]

ARTIFACTS AT HIGHER FIELD STRENGTH

Only a few MR artifacts essentially interfere with the diagnostic quality of abdominal MR studies as the magnetic field B_0 doubles. These artifacts may become more apparent at 3 T compared with 1.5 T or, in some cases, may render individual sequences of a 3 T hepatobiliary MR study uninterpretable.

Susceptibility Artifacts

Magnetic susceptibility describes the phenomenon of magnetization of materials exposed to an external magnetic field B_0. Susceptibility artifacts occur at the interfaces of materials with different degrees of susceptibility as a result of induced microscopic gradients or variations in magnetic field strength. The extent of susceptibility artifacts depends on the differences in susceptibility between the materials and on the magnetic flux density of the external magnetic field B_0.[2,5,28] Susceptibility, in particular from ingested or implanted metallic objects, may lead to substantial variations in the magnetic field B_0, leading to image distortions with localized areas of signal loss caused by substantial T2* shortening effects.[5] The increased blooming of susceptibility artifacts on T1-weighted in- and opposed-phase

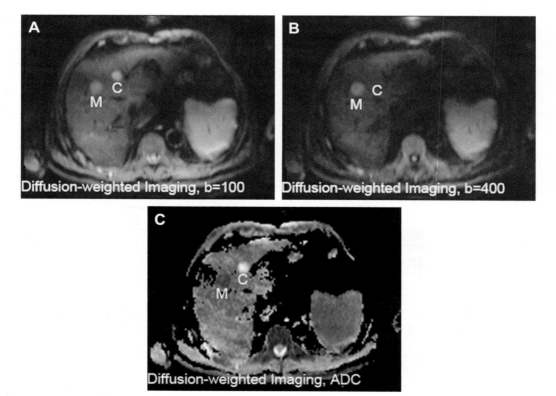

Fig. 12. A 49-year-old man with metastatic renal cell cancer (M) to the liver as well as hepatic cyst (C) on diffusion-weighted imaging at 3 T showing low b-value series (*A*), high b-value series (*B*), and ADC map (*C*). Note the T2 shine-through effect on (*A*), absent on (*B*) for the cyst (C) and the confirmation of restricted diffusion on (*C*) for the metastasis (M).

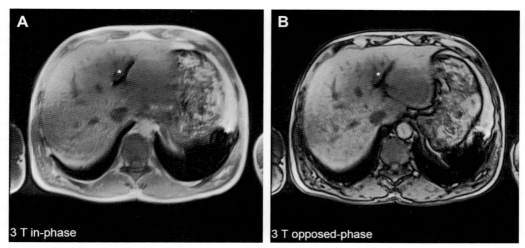

Fig. 13. A 52-year-old woman after endoscopic retrograde cholangiopancreatography with pneumobilia in the left biliary duct (*asterisks*) on T1-weighted in-phase (*A*) and opposed-phase (*B*) imaging at 3 T. Note the increased blooming of the intraductal air on the in-phase image series with the longer TE (2.2 milliseconds) compared with the opposed-phase image series with the sorter TE (1.2 milliseconds).

imaging sequences can be of benefit in the detection of pneumobilia and surgical clips along hepatic resection margins in post-interventional or post-surgical patients **Fig. 13.**[29–31] High-field gradient echo, as well as echo-planar imaging sequences, are most severely affected by the phenomenon of susceptibility, because neither perform 180° refocusing pulses and gather image data through long echo trains. Shortening TEs and combining parallel imaging acceleration to shorten the echo train length helps to reduce the effect of susceptibility artifacts.[5]

Chemical Shift Artifacts

Another artifact type whose severity increases with the doubling of the magnetic field and is readily apparent on high-field hepatobiliary MR imaging is based on the difference in resonance frequency between water and fat. The difference in precession frequency, also known as chemical shift, develops in proportion to the magnetic field strength, resulting in a frequency shift of 225 Hz at 1.5 T and 450 Hz at 3 T.[2,5]

The chemical shift artifact of the first kind is noted along the frequency-encoding axis and the slice selection dimension as a hypointense band extending toward the lower side and a hyperintense band extending toward the higher side of the readout gradient field (**Fig. 14**A).[5] Doubling the magnetic field increases the hypo/hyperintense bands to twice its thickness when comparing 1.5 T with 3 T imaging. Increasing the receiver bandwidth decreases the extent of this

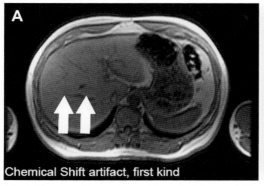

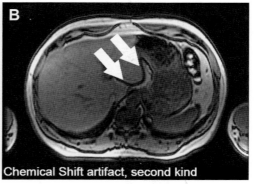

Fig. 14. A 32-year-old woman undergoing hepatobiliary MR imaging using two-dimensional T1-weighted in-phase (*A*) and opposed-phase (*B*) imaging at 3 T. Note the chemical shift artifact of the first kind on in-phase (*arrows*) and chemical shift artifact of the second kind on opposed-phase (*arrows*) imaging series.

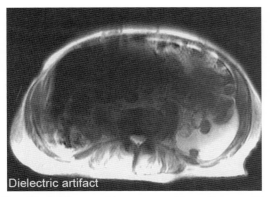

Fig. 15. A 75-year-old woman with ascites on T2-weighted imaging at 3 T. Note the dielectric artifact leading to detrimental signal loss in the midabdomen.

chemical shift; however, this also decreases image SNR.

Chemical shift artifact of the second kind, also known as India ink artifact, is not restricted to frequency-encoding direction, but can be seen throughout all pixels located along water/fat interfaces and originates from intravoxel water/fat phase cancellations (**Fig. 14**B). These cancellation phenomena and the extent of the resultant signal voids are not dependent on the underlying magnetic field strength, but rather the spatial resolution of the imaging sequence itself.

Inhomogeneity Artifacts

The increase in the Larmor frequency from 64 MHz to 128 MHz as the magnetic field is amplified from 1.5 T to 3 T also requires adjustment of the frequency spectrum of the B_1 transmit fields used at 3 T. The design of excitation and gradient

pulses, as well as RF coils, is complex because of resulting nonlinear power depositions and dielectric effects.[5] The B_1 inhomogeneity artifacts noted at 3 T are usually inconspicuous on T1-weighted gradient-echo imaging, but become more apparent on, and sometimes even detrimental to, T2-weighted fast spin-echo sequences (**Fig. 15**).[32] The increase in transmit field frequency to 128 MHz results in an inverse decrease in electromagnetic radiation wavelength. In combination with subsequent interactions with abdominal tissues and body fluids, with their high dielectric constants, a further decrease in electromagnetic radiation wavelength to less than the abdominal diameter occurs. Constructive and destructive interference effects of the resulting intra-abdominal standing waves lead to areas of brightening and darkening throughout the abdomen. High-field hepatobiliary MR imaging of larger patients, especially with ascites present, is affected by this artifact type.[33,34] Technically demanding approaches have been proposed to limit the extent of B_1 inhomogeneity artifacts such as multichannel RF transmission techniques as well as passive coil coupling methods, both focusing on homogenizing the B_1 transmit fields. A simpler approach uses dielectric pads, or RF cushions, which interfere with the interference patterns and thereby reduce the constructive and destructive signal alterations within the abdomen. These pads and cushions contain materials with high dielectric constants, such as ultrasound gel, in combination with highly concentrated manganese- and gadolinium-based solutions, which eliminate signal from the pad itself by shortening the relaxation times of their contents (**Fig. 16**).[5,35]

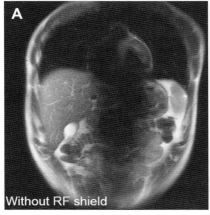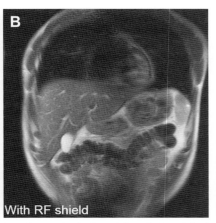

Fig. 16. A 65-year-old man with ascites on T2-weighted imaging at 3 T before (*A*) and after (*B*) placement of RF cushions, which interfere with the interference patterns and thereby reduce the constructive and destructive signal alterations within the abdomen.

SUMMARY

Clinical high-field MR for hepatobiliary imaging continues to evolve at a fast rate. Recent pre-contrast T1-weighted 3 T MR imaging using Dixon postprocessing techniques achieve tissue contrasts that are comparable with, or better than, 1.5 T imaging. However, challenges arising from amplified magnetic fields are not trivial and require a combination of numerous modifications to acquisition schemes established at 1.5 T, such as parallel acceleration and transition from two-dimensional to three-dimensional acquisitions. Substantial gains can be realized in postcontrast T1-weighted imaging at 3 T. The different relaxivities for various gadolinium chelates decrease only minimally as the magnetic field doubles; however, the hepatic T1 relaxation times are prolonged substantially, resulting in an apparent contrast gain on high-field MR studies.

T2-weighted hepatobiliary MR imaging using three-dimensional fast spin-echo sequences, in particular those used for MRCP, are particularly prone to dielectric artifacts and easily reach SAR limits, especially when used in larger patients and those with ascites. Possible solutions to reduce dielectric artifacts include the implementation of multiple transmit coil technology.

Diffusion-weighted echo-planar imaging at 3 T is especially susceptible to limitations by dielectric phenomena. Potential implementation of parallel acceleration represents a promising approach to reducing the occurrence of intra-abdominal standing wave effects.

REFERENCES

1. Boll DT, Merkle EM. Diffuse liver disease: strategies for hepatic CT and MR imaging. Radiographics 2009;29:1591–614.

2. Merkle EM, Dale BM. Abdominal MRI at 3.0 T: the basics revisited. AJR Am J Roentgenol 2006;186: 1524–32.

3. Schindera ST, Merkle EM, Dale BM, et al. Abdominal magnetic resonance imaging at 3.0 T what is the ultimate gain in signal-to-noise ratio? Acad Radiol 2006;13:1236–43.

4. de Bazelaire CM, Duhamel GD, Rofsky NM, et al. MR imaging relaxation times of abdominal and pelvic tissues measured in vivo at 3.0 T: preliminary results. Radiology 2004;230:652–9.

5. Soher BJ, Dale BM, Merkle EM. A review of MR physics: 3T versus 1.5T. Magn Reson Imaging Clin N Am 2007;15:277–90, v.

6. Boll DT, Marin D, Redmon GM, et al. Pilot study assessing differentiation of steatosis hepatis, hepatic iron overload, and combined disease using two-point Dixon MRI at 3 T: in vitro and in vivo results of a 2D decomposition technique. AJR Am J Roentgenol 2010;194:964–71.

7. Goldberg MA, Hahn PF, Saini S, et al. Value of T1 and T2 relaxation times from echoplanar MR imaging in the characterization of focal hepatic lesions. AJR Am J Roentgenol 1993; 160:1011–7.

8. Van Lom KJ, Brown JJ, Perman WH, et al. Liver imaging at 1.5 Tesla: pulse sequence optimization based on improved measurement of tissue relaxation times. Magn Reson Imaging 1991;9: 165–71.

9. Stanisz GJ, Odrobina EE, Pun J, et al. T1, T2 relaxation and magnetization transfer in tissue at 3T. Magn Reson Med 2005;54:507–12.

10. Takahashi M, Uematsu H, Hatabu H. MR imaging at high magnetic fields. Eur J Radiol 2003;46:45–52.

11. Weigel M, Hennig J. Contrast behavior and relaxation effects of conventional and hyperecho-turbo spin echo sequences at 1.5 and 3 T. Magn Reson Med 2006;55:826–35.

12. Hargreaves BA, Cunningham CH, Nishimura DG, et al. Variable-rate selective excitation for rapid MRI sequences. Magn Reson Med 2004;52:590–7.

13. Bernstein MA, Huston J III, Ward HA. Imaging artifacts at 3.0T. J Magn Reson Imaging 2006;24: 735–46.

14. Rohrer M, Bauer H, Mintorovitch J, et al. Comparison of magnetic properties of MRI contrast media solutions at different magnetic field strengths. Invest Radiol 2005;40:715–24.

15. Lin SP, Brown JJ. MR contrast agents: physical and pharmacologic basics. J Magn Reson Imaging 2007;25:884–99.

16. Vogl TJ, Kummel S, Hammerstingl R, et al. Liver tumors: comparison of MR imaging with Gd-EOB-DTPA and Gd-DTPA. Radiology 1996;200:59–67.

17. van den Brink JS, Watanabe Y, Kuhl CK, et al. Implications of SENSE MR in routine clinical practice. Eur J Radiol 2003;46:3–27.

18. Griswold M, Jakob P, Heidemann R, et al. Push-button PPA Reconstructions: GRAPPA. Proc Int Soc Magn Reson Med 2001;1:8.

19. Sodickson DK, Manning WJ. Simultaneous acquisition of spatial harmonics (SMASH): fast imaging with radiofrequency coil arrays. Magn Reson Med 1997;38:591–603.

20. Sodickson DK. Tailored SMASH image reconstructions for robust in vivo parallel MR imaging. Magn Reson Med 2000;44:243–51.

21. Sodickson DK, McKenzie CA. A generalized approach to parallel magnetic resonance imaging. Med Phys 2001;28:1629–43.

22. Dixon WT. Simple proton spectroscopic imaging. Radiology 1984;153:189–94.

23. Lee JK, Dixon WT, Ling D, et al. Fatty infiltration of the liver: demonstration by proton spectroscopic imaging. Preliminary observations. Radiology 1984; 153:195–201.

24. Rofsky NM, Lee VS, Laub G, et al. Abdominal MR imaging with a volumetric interpolated breath-hold examination. Radiology 1999;212:876–84.

25. Tsurusaki M, Semelka RC, Zapparoli M, et al. Quantitative and qualitative comparison of 3.0T and 1.5T MR imaging of the liver in patients with diffuse parenchymal liver disease. Eur J Radiol 2009;72: 314–20.

26. Parikh T, Drew SJ, Lee VS, et al. Focal liver lesion detection and characterization with diffusion-weighted MR imaging: comparison with standard breath-hold T2-weighted imaging. Radiology 2008; 246:812–22.

27. Bruegel M, Holzapfel K, Gaa J, et al. Characterization of focal liver lesions by ADC measurements using a respiratory triggered diffusion-weighted single-shot echo-planar MR imaging technique. Eur Radiol 2008;18:477–85.

28. Lewin JS, Duerk JL, Jain VR, et al. Needle localization in MR-guided biopsy and aspiration: effects of field strength, sequence design, and magnetic field orientation. AJR Am J Roentgenol 1996;166:1337–45.

29. Merkle EM, Nelson RC. Dual gradient-echo in-phase and opposed-phase hepatic MR imaging: a useful tool for evaluating more than fatty infiltration or fatty sparing. Radiographics 2006;26:1409–18.

30. Merkle EM. Pneumobilia: where to look for on hepatic MR imaging? Eur Radiol 2006;16: 2366–8.

31. Merkle EM, Dale BM, Thomas J, et al. MR liver imaging and cholangiography in the presence of surgical metallic clips at 1.5 and 3 Tesla. Eur Radiol 2006;16:2309–16.

32. Schick F. Whole-body MRI at high field: technical limits and clinical potential. Eur Radiol 2005;15: 946–59.

33. Collins CM, Liu W, Schreiber W, et al. Central brightening due to constructive interference with, without, and despite dielectric resonance. J Magn Reson Imaging 2005;21:192–6.

34. Alsop DC, Connick TJ, Mizsei G. A spiral volume coil for improved RF field homogeneity at high static magnetic field strength. Magn Reson Med 1998; 40:49–54.

35. Franklin KM, Dale BM, Merkle EM. Improvement in B1-inhomogeneity artifacts in the abdomen at 3T MR imaging using a radiofrequency cushion. J Magn Reson Imaging 2008;27:1443–7.

Functional Magnetic Resonance Imaging of the Liver: Parametric Assessments Beyond Morphology

Dow-Mu Koh, MD, MRCP, FRCR[a],*,
Anwar R. Padhani, FRCP, FRCR[b]

KEYWORDS
- Dynamic contrast-enhanced MR imaging
- Functional MR imaging • Apparent diffusion coefficient
- Liver imaging • MR spectroscopy

FUNCTIONAL MAGNETIC RESONANCE IMAGING OF THE LIVER

Magnetic resonance (MR) assessment of the liver has largely relied on visual assessment of unenhanced T1- and T2-weighted, as well as contrast-enhanced, images. These conventional imaging sequences form the backbone for the detection and characterization of liver diseases. However, structural alterations in the liver often occur late in the disease process, and the degree to which conventional imaging can assess earlier phases of disease evolution is limited. Thus, despite the success of conventional liver MR imaging techniques in daily clinical practice, there is growing interest in exploring and using functional imaging techniques to provide additional information.

Functional MR imaging techniques are designed to acquire information that reflects specific aspects of the disease pathophysiology. A key feature of these techniques is that they are quantitative, resulting in the derivation or calculation of quantitative parameters that can be used to describe and measure pathophysiologic derangements associated with diseases. The development of these techniques in the liver has been borne out of unmet clinical needs for the assessment of common conditions for which early diagnosis of disease state or treatment response would have a major effect on patient management.

This article provides a summary of the different functional MR imaging techniques currently in use in the clinic or for research applications. We discuss the more frequently used functional imaging techniques: dynamic contrast-enhanced (DCE) MR imaging, diffusion-weighted (DW) MR imaging, MR spectroscopy (MRS), in- and opposed-phase MR imaging, and T2*-weighted imaging. For each technique, the biologic underpinning for the technique is explained, its clinical application surveyed, and the challenges for its application enumerated. Developing and less frequently used techniques, such as MR elastography (MRE), blood oxygenation level dependent (BOLD) imaging, dynamic susceptibility contrast-enhanced (DSC) MR imaging, and diffusion-tensor (DT) imaging are reviewed. DCE MR imaging and MRE are covered in more depth elsewhere in this issue. The potential for combining information from different MR functional techniques is highlighted in the context of future developments. Challenges to widespread adoption of functional MR imaging and obstacles to the translation of such techniques to high field strengths are also discussed.

[a] Department of Radiology, Royal Marsden Hospital, Downs Road, Sutton SM2 5PT, UK
[b] Paul Strickland MRI Center, Mount Vernon Hospital, Rickmansworth Road, Northwood, Middlesex HA6 2RN, UK
* Corresponding author.
E-mail address: dmkoh@btinternet.com

Magn Reson Imaging Clin N Am 18 (2010) 565–585
doi:10.1016/j.mric.2010.07.002
1064-9689/10/$ — see front matter © 2010 Elsevier Inc. All rights reserved.

FUNCTIONAL MR IMAGING TECHNIQUES

Several functional MR imaging techniques can now be used for the evaluation of both malignant and nonmalignant conditions of the liver. These techniques are summarized in **Table 1**; each technique provides information on different aspects of the disease pathophysiology via quantitative measures. These techniques can be applied on

most modern-day MR imaging systems, and combinations of them can be realistically incorporated into a study protocol of approximately 30 to 45 minutes' duration. As these imaging techniques are increasingly used, there is a valuable opportunity to compare and correlate such biologically relevant information, acquired in a spatially and temporarily resolved way, to improve

Table 1
Functional MR imaging techniques that can be used in the liver for disease assessment

Functional MR Imaging Technique	Principles of MR Measurement	Typical Measurement Time	Biologic Property on Which Measurement is Based	Commonly Derived Quantitative Imaging Parameter	Pathophysiologic Correlates
More widely used					
DCE MR imaging	Gadolinium contrast-enhanced T1-weighted imaging at high temporal resolution (<4 s). Mathematical modeling of data	Less than 10 min (including precontrast and postcontrast T1 measurements)	Rate of contrast uptake in tissues, which is influenced by blood flow, contrast transfer rates, extracellular volume, and plasma volume fraction	Initial area under the gadolinium curve, transfer and rate constants (K^{trans}, k_{ep}), leakage space fraction (v_e), fractional plasma volume (V_p)	Vessel density, vascular permeability, perfusion, extravascular space, plasma volume
DW MR imaging	Single-shot spin-echo echo-planar imaging. Contrast medium not required	20 s to a few minutes	Differences in water diffusivity between tissues	Apparent diffusion coefficient. Use of biexponential data fitting can be used to estimate fast diffusion component, which may represent microcapillary perfusion	Tissue architecture (cell density, extracellular space tortuosity, cell membrane integrity), fluid viscosity, microcapillary perfusion
^{1}H MRS	Single-voxel or three-dimensional chemical-shift imaging. Metabolite assignment based on chemical shift effects	15–20 min	Cell membrane turnover/energetics, chemical composition of tissues	Quantified ratios of metabolites including choline, creatine, lipids, lactate, and others depending on echo time	Tumor grade, tumor proliferation, metabolic derangements
In- and opposed-phase MR imaging	2-point or 3-point Dixon technique T1-weighted imaging	Few minutes	Chemical shift resulting from presence of fat or iron within each image voxel	Quantified estimates of fat within image voxels	Hepatic steatosis
T2*-weighted imaging	Gradient-echo imaging	Few minutes	Iron in tissues results in shortening of the T2-relaxation time	Quantified estimates of iron within image voxels	Hepatic iron deposition

(continued on next page)

Table 1
(continued)

Functional MR Imaging Technique	Principles of MR Measurement	Typical Measurement Time	Biologic Property on Which Measurement is Based	Commonly Derived Quantitative Imaging Parameter	Pathophysiologic Correlates
Less widely used					
MRE	Modified phase-contrast gradient-echo sequence with cyclic motion-encoding gradients synchronized to the passive pneumatic driver	<1 min	Differences in the wavelengths of shear waves propagated through tissue depending on the stiffness or elasticity of tissue	Mean liver stiffness (in kPa)	Liver fibrosis Liver cirrhosis
DSC MR imaging	T2*-weighted MR imaging at high temporal resolution to measure first pass of gadolinium contrast passage through the liver	1–2 min	Blood volume and blood flow	Relative blood volume (rBV/rBF), Mean transit time (MTT)	Vessels density, Blood flow, Tumor grade
BOLD or intrinsic susceptibility weighted MR imaging	T2*-weighted imaging performed using different echo times to detect and quantify susceptibility effects	<5 min	Deoxyhemoglobin shows higher relaxivity than oxyhemoglobin. Measurements also reflect blood volume, perfusion and intrinsic tissue composition	Intrinsic tissue relation rates (R2* = 1/T2*)	Ferromagnetic property of tissues, Level of tissue oxygenation
DT imaging	Single-short echo-planar imaging in 6 or more diffusion gradient encoding directions	5–15 min	Degree of directionality of water diffusion	Apparent diffusion coefficient, relative anisotropy, fractional anisotropy, volume ratio	Tissue organization and structure

understanding of the biologic aberrations caused by diseases.

Among the various functional MR imaging techniques currently in use, DCE MR imaging[1] and DW MR imaging[2-4] are now widely applied clinically and in research. Although these 2 techniques have different biologic underpinnings, DW MR imaging has the advantages of being a quick examination (1–5 minutes) and there is no need for administration of an exogenous contrast medium. By contrast, DCE MR imaging requires meticulous technique for its implementation, and can require image registration and more complex data processing, which may not be widely available. ^{1}HMRS[5] has been used to evaluate hepatic steatosis[6,7] but the Dixon MR technique and its variants,[8] based on phase shifts between water and fat protons, is now increasingly used for fat quantification because of its relative ease of application. T2*-weighted imaging has been shown as an accurate method for estimating hepatic iron content. MRE[9,10] is a relatively new functional imaging technique that requires specific hardware (a pneumatic driver) for its deployment. However, the technique is already showing substantial promise for the evaluation of liver fibrosis.[11] Other functional imaging techniques, such as DSC MR imaging, DT imaging, and BOLD imaging have been investigated in the liver, but their roles for liver assessment are not fully defined.

PERFUSION MR IMAGING OF THE LIVER

Perfusion MR imaging refers to functional measurement of the microcirculation of the liver by applying the DCE MR imaging technique.

Biologic Basis for MR Measurements

Perfusion MR imaging of the liver tracks the passage of contrast medium through the liver tissue following intravenous injection. The temporal evolution of signal intensity change in the liver parenchyma or tumor is used to extract quantitative kinetic parameters that reflect the vascular compartment within each imaging voxel. Because of the limited spatial resolution of MR imaging, it is not possible to directly image microvessel blood flow. Instead, the signal measured at DCE MR imaging represents changes that occur on a global level as a consequence of microcirculatory changes within the liver.

Technical Considerations

Following intravenous contrast administration, repeated T1-weighted imaging is performed in the liver at a high temporal resolution (typically every 4 seconds or less) to track the passage of contrast through the liver, which is observed as change in the tissue signal intensity.[12] Typically, a T1-weighted three-dimensional (3D) spoiled gradient-echo technique is used, to which parallel imaging may be applied to reduce the scan time and improve temporal sampling. Motion correction can be performed prospectively using navigator techniques that track the diaphragm, and/or retrospectively by registration software; coronal data acquisition facilitates these procedures. A typical imaging sequence protocol is presented in **Table 2**.

By making assumptions about the vascular supply to the liver (eg, dual input, in keeping with the dual vascular supply of the liver from the hepatic artery [25%] and portal vein [75%] depending on the postprandial state) and the way contrast leaks from the intravascular compartment into the extracellular interstitial compartment (eg, a 2-compartment system), mathematical models can be used to derive quantitative indices that describe the behavior of hepatic vasculature. Examples of such indices

Table 2
Example of an imaging sequence used for perfusion MR imaging of the liver

MR Imaging Platform	1.5 T Avanto (Siemens, Erlangen, Germany)
Type of pulse sequence	3D FLASH
Image acquisition plane	Coronal
Repetition time	3.28 ms
Echo time	0.89 ms
Partition thickness	5 mm
Slices per slab	12
Matrix	128×128 interpolated
Phase encode direction	Right to left
Number of averages	1
Sensitivity encoding factor	2
Flip angle before contrast	2° and 18°
Flip angle after contrast	18°
Bandwidth	650 Hz/pixel
Radiofrequency spoiling	Yes
Temporal resolution	5 s per slab of 12 image sections
Precontrast scans	4 measurements of each flip angle averaged for calculation of native T1
Gadolinium injection	0.2 mmol/kg at 3 mL/s followed by 20 mL flush
Patient respiration	Sequential breath hold or quiet respiration
Postcontrast scans	A total of 80 consecutive measurements. Inject contrast only when the sixth measurement has completed
Scan sections to use for processing	Center 6–8 image sections only

include the inflow transfer constant (K^{trans}), leakage space (v_e), and outflow rate constant (k_{ep}) (**Fig. 1** provides an explanation of these terms). However, depending on the mathematical model applied, the quantitative parameters obtained may differ between kinetic models. More simplistic non–model-based approaches have also been successfully used in several studies and are further explained elsewhere in this issue. The non–model-based analysis techniques rely on comparing signal intensity before and after contrast to derive semiquantitative parametric estimates. For example, the hepatic perfusion index (HPI) can be calculated from the slope of the arterial perfusion divided by the sum of the slope of the arterial and portal perfusion. This value is typically about 0.30 in the normal liver, but is increased in metastases. The initial area under the gadolinium concentration curve (IAUGC) represents the integrated area under the gadolinium tissue enhancement curve usually in the first 60 or 120 seconds of contrast enhancement, which represents the leakage of contrast into the extracellular space, therefore indirectly reflecting tissue vasculature.

Clinical Applications of Perfusion MR Imaging in the Liver

Alterations in the vascular kinetics of the liver have been used as the basis for characterization of liver tumors, assessment of therapeutic response, and evaluation of cirrhosis.[12]

Liver metastases

Several studies have demonstrated that perfusion imaging is able to detect changes in the liver at risk of developing liver metastases. Totman and colleagues[13] showed that the non–model-based parameter HPI was increased in patients with overt metastases compared with patients without metastases (**Fig. 2**). It was also found that the increased HPI could help to identify patients with micrometastases.[14] In addition, perfusion maps could increase the sensitivity of metastatic detection in the liver because of better visualization of the enhanced tumor rim.[15,16]

Hepatocellular carcinoma

In a study by Abdullah and colleagues,[17] no significant difference was found in the HPI between colorectal metastases and hepatocellular carcinoma

Pre-treatment   Post-treatment

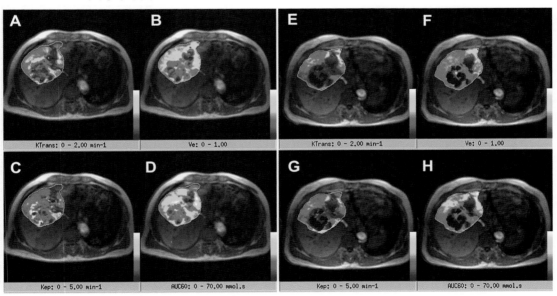

Fig. 1. A 54-year-old man with colorectal liver metastasis. Quantitative color scale parametric maps of K^{trans} (*A, E*), v_e (*B, F*), k_{ep} (*C, G*) and IAUGC60 (*D, H*) overlaid on corresponding T1-weighted axial image before (*A, B, C, D*) and at 14 days after treatment (*E, F, G, H*) using an antiangiogenic drug.* The color scale is as shown on images with low values in blue, intermediate values in yellow and red, and high values in white. Note reduction in all parameters within tumor after treatment but no significant change in tumor size. Posttreatment maps show absence of color within center of tumor in keeping with central devascularization and presumed necrosis.

---

*K^{trans} is the rate constant that describes contrast leakage into tissue, v_e is the extravascular extracellular space which the contrast medium distributes and k_{ep} is the rate constant of contrast wash out from tissue.

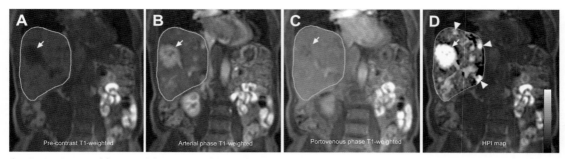

Fig. 2. A 46-year-old man with neuroendocrine liver metastases. Coronal (*A*) precontrast T1-weighted, (*B*) post-gadolinium contrast arterial phase T1-weighted, (*C*) portovenous phase T1-weighted, and (*D*) map of HPI overlaid on corresponding precontrast T1-weighted images. The liver is outlined in blue and a marker metastasis in the right lobe of the liver is marked by an arrow. This metastasis shows marked arterial enhancement in the arterial phase, becoming near isointense to the liver in the portovenous phase. The HPI (color scaled from 0 in black to 1 in white) is increased within the metastasis. Several other smaller metastases are also clearly visible on the HPI map (*arrowheads*).

(HCC) (n = 50). In another study (n = 30) using computed tomography (CT) perfusion, the blood flow, blood volume, and permeability surface area product (an index of vascular permeability) were found to be significantly higher in well-differentiated HCC compared with moderately or poorly differentiated variants, suggesting that the perfusion imaging may help to determine tumor grade.[18]

Assessment of treatment response

Quantitative and semiquantitative perfusion indices have been used to evaluate tumor response to treatment. Miyazaki and colleagues[19] applied HPI for assessing the efficacy of antiangiogenic therapy (**Fig. 3**). They found that HPI was measurably decreased by 15% at 28 days after antiangiogenic treatment in patients who responded to treatment using standard Response Evaluation Criteria in Solid Tumors (RECIST) size criteria. By model fitting, Chen and colleagues[20] found using the perfusion CT technique that the hepatic arterial fraction, hepatic artery perfusion, and hepatic blood volume all significantly decreased following chemoembolization of hepatic malignancy. Thus, the potential of using model-based approaches for assessing the effects of antiangiogenic or antivascular treatment is being evaluated.[21–23] In a study of patients receiving an antiangiogenic drug in a phase I clinical trial, Morgan and colleagues[24] found a significant negative correlation between the

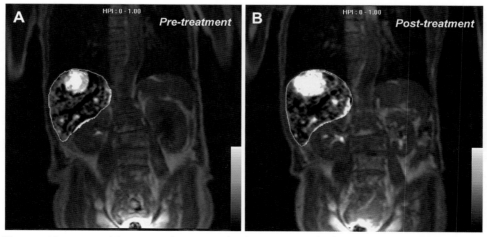

Fig. 3. 63-year-old women with metastatic neuroendocrine tumor to the liver. Coronal maps of HPI overlaid on precontrast T1-weighted images (*A*) before and (*B*) at 2 months after targeted radiolabeled therapy. The liver is outlined in blue. The metastasis in the right lobe of liver shows marked increase in HPI at the tumor rim, accompanied by slight increase in tumor size. The patient showed disease progression at the end of treatment.

percentage change in the inflow rate constant (K_i) and the dose of the drug administered.

Liver cirrhosis

Increase in hepatic artery perfusion and decrease in portal venous perfusion have been shown in various CT and MR perfusion studies.[25–28] The HPI has been shown to increase in cirrhotic liver.

Thus, MR liver perfusion imaging provides unique functional information about the microcirculation of the liver parenchyma and focal liver lesions. However, most published studies are from single institutions with small study cohorts.[21] Hence, there is a cogent need for further validation by conducting such studies in larger populations across multicenter sites.

DW MR IMAGING OF THE LIVER

DW MR imaging is emerging as a powerful technique for the evaluation of hepatic diseases. DW MR imaging is a robust imaging technique that can be implemented on most modern MR imaging platforms. Widely available vendor software applications make it possible to obtain quantitative data with relative ease.

Biologic Basis for MR Measurements

The mechanism of contrast of DW MR imaging is based on differences in the mobility of water protons between tissues. Water diffusion is a thermally driven process characterized by random motion of water molecules. However, in biologic tissues, the motion of such molecules is modified by their interaction with cell membranes and macromolecules. Hence, water diffusion in tissues reflects the tortuosity of the extracellular space, tissue cellularity, integrity of cell membranes, and fluid viscosity.[2]

Cellular tissues show lesser degrees of signal attenuation with increasing diffusion weighting (b-values), and hence are conspicuous on DW MR imaging, thus facilitating their detection. By quantitative evaluation, cellular tissues usually return lower apparent diffusion coefficients (ADC), indicating impeded water diffusivity. However, because DW MR imaging discriminates tissues by water diffusion, the technique is not specific for malignancy.

Technical and Imaging Considerations

A detailed discussion of the technical aspects of DW MR imaging is beyond the scope of this article. The reader is referred to published works related to the topic.[2,3,29] A typical imaging sequence protocol is presented in **Table 3**.

High-quality DW MR images can be attained by free-breathing image acquisition using the single-shot echo-planar imaging technique. The free-breathing technique is highly versatile, and can be effectively implemented on most imaging platforms at 1.5T.[2,30] Furthermore, such imaging is quick to perform and can be completed within 3 to 6 minutes. As an extension, some prefer to perform DW MR imaging of the liver with

Table 3
A typical imaging sequence used for DW MR imaging of the liver

MR Imaging Platform	1.5T Avanto (Siemens, Erlangen, Germany)
Type of pulse sequence	Single-shot spin-echo echo-planar imaging
Scan orientation	Axial
Respiration	Free-breathing
Repetition time	5000 ms
Echo time	68 ms
Partition thickness	6 mm
Matrix	128×128
Phase encode direction	Anterior to posterior
Number of averages	4
Sensitivity encoding factor	GRAPPA 2
Field of view	380 mm
b-values	0, 100, 750
Receiver bandwidth	1780 Hz
Fat suppression	Spectral attenuated inversion recovery

respiratory triggering to further overcome the effects of respiratory motion. However, this can significantly increase acquisition times because images can only be acquired in part of the respiratory cycle. Another technique is to perform breath-hold DW MR imaging. Such acquisitions are quick to perform (typically less than 1 minute), but at the expense of signal/noise ratio and the number of b-values that can be accommodated for the measurement.

As the T2-relaxation time of the liver is short, the b-values used for liver imaging typically range between 0 and 800 s/mm^2 to ensure sufficient signal/noise is attained at higher b-values. To allow accurate calculation of the ADC, 2 or more b-values should be used.

Clinical Applications of DW MR Imaging in the Liver

DW MR imaging has been applied to evaluate both oncological and nononcological conditions of the liver.

Diffuse liver disease

The use of DW MR imaging for diffuse liver disease is being investigated. Several studies have shown that the ADC values of cirrhotic liver are significantly lower than those of normal liver.[31–38] Koinuma and colleagues[34] showed that, although there was a negative correlation between ADC values and the fibrosis score, no relationship was found between ADC values and the grade of inflammation. In another study,[37] the ADC value was found to be significantly lower for patients with moderate to severe liver fibrosis compared with those without, or with mild, liver fibrosis. Luciani and colleagues[39] used a more

sophisticated method of applying the principles of intravoxel incoherent motion to estimate the capillary perfusion of the liver using DW MR imaging. They found that the perfusion fraction was significantly reduced in patients with liver cirrhosis. One of the problems of using DW MR imaging for prospective evaluation of liver fibrosis is the substantial overlap of ADC values between normal and abnormal liver, and also between the various grades of liver fibrosis. The recommended thresholds to be applied for discriminating liver fibrosis also vary significantly between studies, in part because of differences in technique and b-values used. Thus, although promising, the value of ADC for ascertaining the degree of liver fibrosis requires further validation in larger patient cohorts.

Detection of focal liver lesions

DW MR imaging has proved valuable for the detection of focal live lesions by visual assessment of the b-value images. Applying a small diffusion weighting (eg, b = 50 s/mm^2), suppresses the high signal from intrahepatic vasculature, allowing focal liver lesions to be readily detected (**Fig. 4**). Several studies have shown that DW MR imaging is superior to conventional T2-weighted MR imaging for lesion detection.[40–43] DW MR imaging also improved the detection of liver metastases compared with superparamagnetic iron oxide nanoparticle–enhanced MR imaging[44] or manga-fodipir trisodium– enhanced MR imaging[45] on its own. However, most solid hepatic lesions show variable degrees of high signal impeded diffusion on DW MR imaging. Hence, qualitative assessment alone does not allow reliable discrimination between different solid lesions.

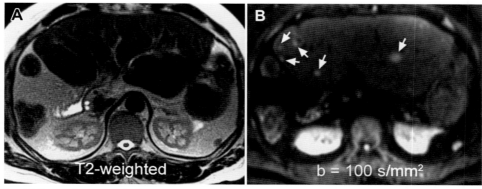

Fig. 4. A middle-aged man with liver metastases and previous right hepatectomy. Axial (A) T2-weighted MR imaging and (B) DW MR image acquired at b-value of 100 s/mm^2. Application of the diffusion weighting suppresses signal from the intrahepatic vasculature, allowing the liver metastases to be clearly identified (*arrows*).

Lesion characterization

Given the limitations of qualitative visual assessment of DW MR images, quantitative ADC value of liver lesions has been proposed as a method to distinguish between benign and malignant liver lesions. In several studies, benign liver lesions were found to return higher ADC values compared with malignant liver lesions.[40,42,46–50] Despite considerable heterogeneity of the imaging techniques across these studies, the ADC thresholds found helpful in distinguishing between benign and malignant lesions were remarkably similar $(1.47-1.63 \times 10^{-3} \text{ mm}^2/\text{s})$, with reportedly high sensitivity (74%–100%) and specificity (77%–100%) when applied.[51] Hepatic hemangiomas returned the highest ADC values among the solid liver lesions,[51] which, when observed, can add confidence to its identification (**Fig. 5**). However, there is considerable overlap in the ADC values of benign and malignant solid hepatic lesions reported in the literature. A problematic area is the identification and characterization of HCC in patients with liver cirrhosis. This problem arises because liver cirrhosis and nodular regeneration also reduce water diffusivity, thus diminishing the contrast and ADC difference between HCC and the background cirrhotic changes[52,53]

Assessment of tumor response and disease prognostication

ADC values have been shown to increase in liver metastases that respond to chemotherapy, and this can be observed as early as 7 days after the commencement of treatment.[54] Thus, quantitative ADC has the potential to be an important early response biomarker (**Fig. 6**). There is no consensus yet on the percentage increase in mean or median tumor ADC that is regarded as significant. One method of defining the significance of ADC change is to establish the measurement reproducibility; any ADC measurement that increases or decreases beyond the limits of measurement reproducibility is regarded as significant.[55]

In patients with HCC receiving sorefinib, an anti-angiogenic treatment, ADC has been reported to initially decrease and then subsequently increase.[56] The mechanism underlying the decrease in ADC observed is not understood but vascular normalization and reduction of extracellular space may be contributory. The tumor ADC value may also be a predictive biomarker to cytotoxic chemotherapy. Liver metastases that show higher pretreatment ADC values have been found to be associated with poor response to chemotherapy treatment.[54,57]

MRS

The use of MRS in the liver is still not widespread because of the considerable technical expertise required for its implementation and for data analysis. However, MRS provides the opportunity to study metabolic signatures in diffuse liver disease and tumors. By focusing on different nuclei at MRS studies, information that reflects cellular energetics and metabolism are derived and quantified.

Biologic Basis for MRS Measurements

When placed within a magnetic field, certain nuclei (eg, ^{1}H, ^{13}C, and ^{31}P) contained in human tissues demonstrate characteristic resonant frequencies. Depending on the local microenvironment, different protons associated with a molecule resonate at slightly different frequencies that are expressed as the chemical shift. Chemical shifts are usually very small (eg, measured in Hz) compared with the resonant frequency of the nuclei (eg, MHz), and can be expressed in parts per million (ppm). By observing chemical shifts in

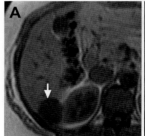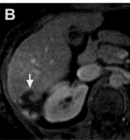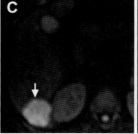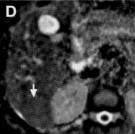

Fig. 5. A 58-year-old women with breast cancer. Axial (A) T1-weighted, (B) postgadolinium portovenous phase fat-suppressed T1-weighted, (C) DW MR imaging at b-value of 750 s/mm² and (D) ADC map. The hemangioma in the right lobe of liver (*arrows*) show typical peripheral nodular enhancement on T1-weighted imaging after contrast administration (B). The hemangioma shows high signal impeded diffusion on the DW MR imaging (C) and appears mildly hyperintense to the liver on the ADC map (D).

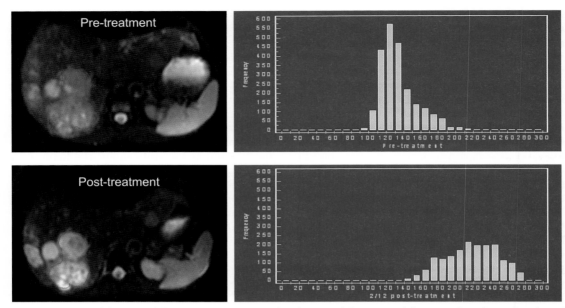

Fig. 6. A 53-year-old man with liver metastases treated with a novel therapy. Axial DW MR imaging at b-value of 750 s/mm² obtained before and at the end of treatment shows marginal reduction in size of a target lesion (outlined in red) but not amounting to a partial response. ADC histograms (ADC displayed in units of $\times 10^{-5}$ mm²/s) showed a large increase (>50%) in the median ADC value of tumor from 125×10^{-5} mm²/s to 220×10^{-5} mm²/s and a clear shift of the histogram to the right in keeping with treatment response. The patient showed continued disease stabilization by tumor size measurement at 6 months after treatment.

tissues, it is possible to infer information about the chemical microenvironment in which these molecules reside, and also about the interaction of these molecules (eg, J-coupling through chemical bonds) with others. In this way, metabolic profiles of the tissues can be obtained, characterized, and quantified.

Measurement Considerations

Among the different nuclei that can be studied using MRS in the body, hydrogen (^{1}H) is the most abundant and can be studied on any clinical MR system without hardware modifications. However, the wide occurrence of this nucleus in water and fat also means that that signal associated with other chemical compounds (eg, choline) may be obscured if water and fat signals are not satisfactorily suppressed during measurements. By contrast, MRS evaluating other nuclei has potentially higher metabolic specificity (eg, ^{31}P detection of metabolites such as phosphomonesterase [PME], phosphodiesterase [PDE], inorganic phosphate, phosphocreatine, and ATP), but at the expense of sensitivity. However, MRS measurements of nuclei other than ^{1}H require special MR coils tuned to selected frequencies, which are usually not readily available.

To perform a successful ^{1}H MRS examination in the liver, meticulous care needs to be exercised both at image acquisition and data processing. Because of respiratory motion, ^{1}H MRS is usually performed using single-voxel measurements where voxel sizes of approximately 3×3×3 cm are used to obtained data in approximately 5 to 6 minutes. Images may be acquired in quiet respiration but navigator-controlled respiratory triggered acquisition should be considered where technically feasible. Two techniques are most widely used: stimulated-echo acquisition mode (STEAM) and point-resolved spectroscopy (PRESS); the former is less sensitive to J-coupling effects but results in lower signal/noise ratio. The choice of echo time determines the visibility of the metabolite of interest. For example, in the evaluation of liver fat, a shorter echo time may be appropriate to estimate the fat/water ratio, whereas a longer echo time (eg, >120 milliseconds) may be preferred for choline quantification because better suppression of the lipid signal can be achieved. A typical single-voxel ^{1}H MRS imaging protocol is as shown in **Table 4**.

More recently, multivoxel ^{1}H MRS has been developed to further improve the accuracy of liver MRS but at the expense of increased data acquisition times.[58,59] Correction for T2-relaxation of water and fat signal and tissue T1 relaxation time is also necessary to ensure accurate quantification

Table 4
A typical ^{1}H MRS imaging sequence used to evaluate the liver

MR Imaging Platform	Avanto (Siemens, Erlangen, Germany)
Type of pulse sequence	PRESS
Respiration	Quiet respiration/navigator controlled
Volume shimming	Gradient recalled echo shim
Repetition time	1500 ms
Echo time	135 ms (tumor study), 35 ms (steatosis study)
Voxel size	20×20×20 mm
Number of signal acquisitions	50–192
Vector length	1024
Water suppression	Chemical-shift-selective saturation
Water reference	8 signal acquisitions without water suppression

of signal. In malignant tissues, the choline/water ratio is often estimate.

Although MRS techniques have been applied both intracranially and extracranially for several years, these techniques have not found a place in routine clinical use. The main impediments to their wider applications are the lack of standardization, reproducibility within and between institutions, and the need for significant technical expertise for postprocessing of the imaging data. Furthermore, the use of ^{31}P MRS would require multinuclear capability on MR platforms to be enabled, which incurs addition costs to machine hardware. The future clinical uptake of MRS techniques in the liver relies on addressing these challenges.

Clinical Applications of MRS in the Liver

MRS has been applied to the evaluation of diffuse liver disease, including hepatic steatosis, and for the characterization of focal liver lesions.

Diffuse liver diseases

MRS has been most widely applied on clinical MR systems for the evaluation of hepatic steatosis. The importance of hepatic steatosis has been recognized because of the morbidity and mortality associated with nonalcoholic fatty liver disease. Initial studies evaluating fat/water ratio by ^{1}H MRS relied on single-voxel measurements. Such measurements were found to have good correlations with liver fat content determined at histopathology (**Fig. 7**).[6] In a recent study by Lee and colleagues,[60] ^{1}H MRS was found to have 80% sensitivity and 80% specificity for the diagnosis of hepatic steatosis of 5% or more. Single-voxel ^{1}H MRS measurements have been shown to be accurate and have good intraindividual reproducibility.[7,61] More recently, multivoxel ^{1}H MRS has been developed to further improve the accuracy of liver fat averaged over multiple voxels.[58,59] ^{1}H MRS has also been applied to evaluate hepatic steatosis in the general population.[7]

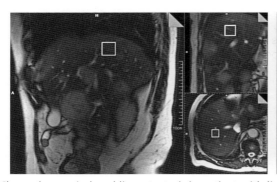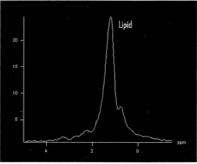

Fig. 7. Chemotherapy induced liver steatosis in patient with liver metastases. ^{1}H MRS study using a single-voxel PRESS technique acquired with navigator-controlled respiratory triggering and water suppression using chemical-shift-selective saturation (CHESS) shows a characteristic lipid peak at 1.4 ppm. The percentage fat within the voxel may be estimated by comparing the peaks of the water and fat spectra acquired without water suppression.

The use of ^{31}P MRS to study metabolism in the liver is more limited to research applications, although centers engaged in such work are enthusiastic about its potentials. ^{31}P MRS has been used to study the energetics of the liver associated with chronic liver disease.[62] Increase in PDE, decrease in PME, and increase in the PME/PDE ratio have been documented in patients with liver cirrhosis and chronic hepatitis.[62,63] Readers should refer to recent review articles for a wider discussion of the role of ^{31}P MRS for the evaluation of hepatic metabolism and function in a variety of diffuse liver diseases.[64,65]

Focal liver lesion

The use of MRS for the evaluation of focal liver lesions has been limited to single-center studies in selected cohorts.[66] With ^{1}H MRS, the diagnosis of malignant liver lesions has relied on the identification of choline signature (**Fig. 8**), which is nonspecific. ^{1}H MRS has been found to have limited sensitivity and specificity for the diagnosis of malignant liver lesions.[66] MRS has a potential role to play for the evaluation of tumor response to treatment, but this requires further investigations. In a study in patients with HCC, the total choline and choline/lipid ratios were found to reduce following transcatheter arterial chemoembolization (TACE) of the tumor.[67]

IN- AND OPPOSED-PHASE MR IMAGING

In- and opposed-phase MR imaging are widely used to demonstrate and quantify intravoxel fat, and rely on differences in the precessional frequencies of protons associated with fat and water in tissues. Consequently, a signal drop is observed within a voxel containing fat and water when the MR measurement is made at an echo time at which a phase difference in the transverse magnetization is observed between the precessing fat and water protons. The relative ease of application makes the technique an attractive option for the quantification of hepatic steatosis.

Implementation of in- and opposed-phase MR imaging can be simply achieved using a dual-echo gradient-echo technique. Using this 2-point Dixon technique, with images acquired when water and fat are in phase and out of phase, the quantity of fat within each image voxel can be readily calculated (**Fig. 9**). However, there are potential disadvantages of using such an approach. First, the phase shifts associated with fat and water protons may be misregistered, which can lead to errors in fat quantification if robust phase correction algorithms are not applied. Second, there is a tendency to overestimate the fat content, especially when the percentage of fat within the voxel is low (<10%).[68] Third, the technique is sensitive to magnetic field inhomogeneity that can result from iron deposition.[69] Another approach is the iterative decomposition of water and fat with echo asymmetry and least-squared estimations (IDEAL) gradient-echo technique.[70–73] The IDEAL technique acquires images with different phase shifts between fat and water protons and reportedly has less sensitivity to inhomogeneity of the local magnetic field. There are other variations in techniques that exploit the differences in the signal phase of water and fat for the quantification of hepatic steatosis (eg, 3-point Dixon technique),[74–76] which may be of interest to some readers but are not discussed here. MR imaging quantification of liver fat and iron are discussed elsewhere in this issue.

T2*-WEIGHTED IMAGING

T2*-weighted gradient-echo imaging, as well as T2-weighted imaging, have been applied for the

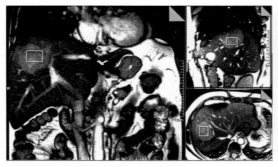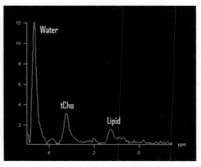

Fig. 8. 48-year-old man with metastatic melanoma to the liver. ^{1}H MRS study using a single-voxel (3×2×2 cm) PRESS technique with navigator-controlled respiratory triggering (echo time 135 milliseconds) and water suppression using CHESS with 50 acquisitions. Note the presence of choline (3.2 ppm) and lipid within the tumor. The amount of choline present may be estimated, as in this case, by comparing with an internal reference (water), or by comparing with results obtained using an external reference (eg, phantom).

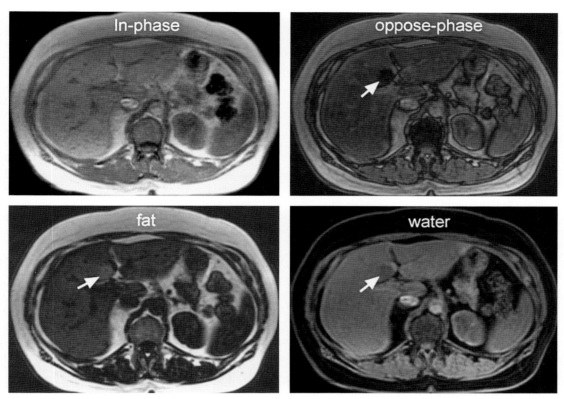

Fig. 9. In-phase and opposed-phase T1-weighted imaging acquired using a 2-point Dixon gradient-echo technique. The implementation allows for the derivation of fat and water images, from which the proportion of water and fat within imaging voxels can be estimated. There is a general signal decrease in the liver parenchyma on the opposed-phase image compared with the in-phase image, indicating fatty infiltration. However, a more focal area of more intense signal drop is observed in the left lobe of the liver (*arrow*). This appears because of a higher signal on the fat image and lower signal on the water image, consistent with focal fatty infiltration. The proportion of fat in this area was estimated to be about 20%.

quantification of liver iron deposition. Iron deposition in tissues, in the form of ferritin or hemosiderin, results in shortening of the T2 and T2* relaxation time, which can be measured using spin-echo or gradient-echo sequences. One method of quantifying liver iron content is by measuring the signal intensity ratio of the liver compared with a reference tissue (eg, paraspinal muscle). However, quantification based on signal intensity ratios may be less accurate, particularly in the presence of severe iron overload or liver cirrhosis,[77,78] but this experience is not universal.[79] Increasingly, liver iron quantification is performed by direct measurement of tissue R2 or R2* relaxation rates (which are the reciprocal of the T2 and T2* relaxation times) using multiecho spin-echo or gradient-echo sequences.

In patients with thalassemia major, measurement of liver R2 and R2* has been shown to have a strong correlation ($r = 0.98$ and $r = 0.97$) with biopsy measured liver iron content.[80] In the same study, the reproducibility between examinations was better for R2 measurements than for R2* measurements.[80] In another study comparing R2, R2*, and signal intensity ratio–based measurements, R2 measurements were found to be the most accurate, particularly in patients with severe iron overload.[78] These imaging techniques have also been successfully used for the quantification of hepatic iron content in patients with hemochromatosis[79,81] and other chronic liver diseases.

OTHER FUNCTIONAL MR IMAGING TECHNIQUES
MRE

MRE is a recent innovation that relies on the use of motion-encoded shear waves generated by a pneumatic driver placed on the external abdominal wall, which are propagated through target organs of interest. By measuring the wavelengths of the shear waves within a tissue, it is possible to calculate the tissue viscoelasticity, which is usually expressed in units of kilopascals (kPa). Several studies have shown the value of MRE in diagnosing and grading the severity of liver cirrhosis.[82–85] In one study, the sensitivity and specificity of MRE in detecting liver fibrosis of all grades was greater than 95%.[83] Unlike DW MR imaging, which seems to be insensitive to early stages of liver cirrhosis, MRE has been shown to be sensitive for the detection of early grades of liver fibrosis. The reader is referred to another article in this issue for a further discussion of the technique.

DSC MR Imaging

DSC MR imaging is underpinned by observing the first-pass passage of contrast through tissues, and is observed as transient signal loss on T2*-weighted MR imaging. From these imaging data, mathematical modeling using a γ-variate fit can be used to derive the hepatic blood volume, hepatic blood flow, and mean transit time. Although the technique has been used widely and successfully in the brain, its application in the liver is more limited. In one study of 17 patients with histologically proven HCC before and after TACE, serial changes in tumor perfusion measured using gadolinium-enhanced imaging on hepatic blood volume maps were correlated with vascularity on hepatic angiography.[86] Hyperperfusion was noted in most of the tumors on hepatic blood volume maps before TACE and moderate to marked hypoperfusion following TACE.[86]

BOLD Imaging

BOLD imaging has been applied both intracranially and extracranially, but experience of the technique in the liver is more limited. The basis for MR imaging contrast is on the difference in the relaxivity of oxygenated and deoxygenated hemoglobin. Deoxygenated hemoglobin shows increased susceptibility effects and higher longitudinal relaxation rate, R2* (which is the reciprocal of the longitudinal relaxation time T2*). Thus, the measured tissue R2* indirectly reflects tissue oxygenation/hypoxia and tissue blood volume. Using a VX-2 (a fast-growing, transplantable, squamous cell carcinoma) tumor model in rabbits, Rhee and colleagues[87] showed that there was a significant reduction in the tumor's apparent transverse relaxation time from 55 milliseconds before embolization to 41 milliseconds after embolization ($P<.01$). This reduction in T2* corresponded to a decrease in hepatic tumor oxygenation. Recently O'Connor and colleagues[88] reported the use of oxygen-enhanced T1 imaging. The transverse relaxation rate, R1, was shown to increase in the tumor when oxygen was administered to patients. Furthermore, there was matching between the degree of tumor oxygenation and tumor perfusion measured using DCE MR imaging. Nevertheless, the use of BOLD imaging in the liver requires further investigation (**Fig. 10**).

DT Imaging

DT imaging is a DW MR imaging technique that explores differences in the directionality of water diffusion in tissues. Isotropic diffusion (ie, equal water diffusion in all directions of measurements) is typically observed in tumor tissues. However, anisotropic diffusion (ie, diffusion that is dominant in 1 direction compared with another) can provide addition information about tissue microstructure. Taouli and colleagues[89] showed the feasibility of using this technique and noted that, compared with conventional DW MR imaging, hepatic ADC measured by DT imaging was not significantly different between the 2 techniques. In an investigation in patients with chronic liver disease, the ADC derived from DT imaging was not superior to those derived from conventional DW MR imaging for the detection of liver fibrosis.[38] Thus, the clinical role of DT imaging in the liver has yet to be determined.

MULTIPARAMETRIC IMAGING

Given that each functional MR imaging technique provides a unique insight into a particular aspect of altered pathophysiology in diseased state, there is now the opportunity to compare and correlate parametric maps derived using more than 1 functional MR technique. Such correlative imaging comparison is not confined to within MR-derived information, but can also be extended to CT or positron emission tomography–derived data. By combining the information derived from several imaging techniques, it is possible to gain a multifaceted insight into the phenotypic expression of diseases.

There is emerging evidence that a multiparametric imaging approach is valuable in many areas regarding imaging assessment. In oncology, multiparametric imaging can be used to cross-validate observations between imaging techniques, thereby enhancing the understanding of diseases. A multiparametric approach also helps in the characterization of tumor phenotypes and aids the interpretation of biologic transformation of tumors in response to treatment. In radiotherapy planning, optimal definition of the target tumor volume is necessary for accurate targeted treatment by newer therapeutic options such as

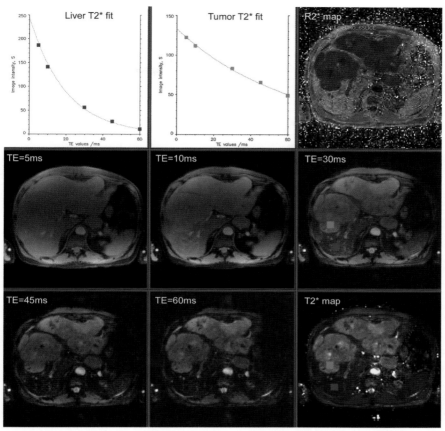

Fig. 10. A 61-year-old man with metastatic colorectal cancer. BOLD-MR images are acquired using a spoiled gradient recalled echo (GRE) sequence (repetition time 100 milliseconds; echo time 5–65 milliseconds; fractional anisotropy, 25°). Quantitative T2* times and R2* relaxation rates are calculated by monoexponential fitting of changing signal intensity with increasing echo times. These data are shown for the normal liver (blue region of interest; R2*, 20.8/s) and tumor (red region of interest; R2* = 55.1/s). Parametric quantitative T2* and R2* maps are shown. Interpretation of liver and tumor T2* and R2* requires perfusion information as discussed in **Fig. 11.**

intensity-modulated radiotherapy or Gamma knife surgery. Combining the functional imaging information derived from different techniques may enable better definition of the target volume according to the underlying biology. In drug development, multiparametric assessment provides the means to noninvasively track different biologic changes in response to drug administration, thus providing pharmacodynamic data to aid pharmaceutical decision making. An example of a multiparametric study of a patient with liver metastases is shown in **Fig. 11**.

The framework for such multiparametric comparison of imaging techniques is still in development, although there is clearly increasing interest in exploring such correlative information. In the early endeavors in interpreting multiparametric datasets, it would be helpful if the imaging observations could be validated by histopathology, so that confidence may be gained for rational interpretation of the observations. Nevertheless, it should also be recognized that histopathologic validation may not always be possible and that histopathology may not provide definitive information because of sampling bias. Noninvasive imaging can interrogate entire diseased tissue volumes and may provide a better global perspective of the disease compared with histologic sampling. Thus, corroborative evidence of pathologic alterations derived from multimodality imaging may potentially be even more relevant and important to understanding tissue alterations in diseased states across the entire diseased volume.

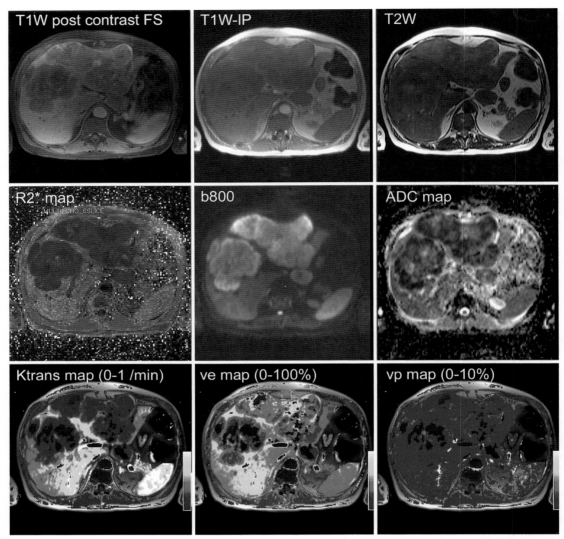

Fig. 11. 61-year-old man with metastatic colorectal cancer. (*Top row*) T1-weighted postcontrast with fat suppression, T1-weighted opposed-phase, and T2-weighted images. (*Middle row*) R2* map, diffusion weight MR imaging (b800) and ADC map. (*Bottom row*) T1-weighted DCE MR images depicting transfer constant (K^{trans}), leakage space (v$_e$), and fractional plasma volume (v$_p$). Areas where there is missing color information are zero enhancing pixels that do not always correlate spatially with presumed necrotic, high-ADC pixels. Fast R2* values in the normal liver despite high-fraction plasma blood volume indicate marked deoxygenation of red blood cells. In contrast, slow R2* in tumors seems to indicate better oxygenation compared with normal liver.

FUTURE DEVELOPMENTS AND CHALLENGES

One of the key challenges in the development of multiparametric imaging, and functional MR imaging as a whole, is the lack of standardization in image acquisition and data analysis.[90] To some extent, the lack of standardization has resulted from MR vendor–driven innovations, which have had commercial motives to emphasize and create differences between imaging platforms, rather than to encourage similarities and harmonization between MR systems. However, there is now recognition within the industry and research organizations of the need to move and work toward more standardized functional MR imaging methods.

Functional MR techniques yield quantitative parametric data, but many of these are still regarded as prebiomarkers because they do not yet fulfill the robust criteria that regulatory bodies set out for an imaging biomarker. Hence, more work is needed to ensure systematic validation of these imaging techniques in well-designed prospective studies, particularly in those in which there is tissue collection or sampling; and in those in which important clinical end-points (eg, time to disease progression or disease survival) are assessed.

There is a need to develop suitable quality assurance and quality-control programs associated with each of these functional MR imaging techniques. These programs would ensure that the quantitative metrics associated with each technique can be reliably measured, and that processes are in place to check individual system performance. This includes the design, testing, and adoption of phantoms that can be distributed widely to check MR scanner performance.

There is also a need to develop and standardize software for data analysis. Most MR vendors have proprietary software that work with data acquired on their own individual MR systems, but may not handle data acquired from other MR platforms. There are also differences in how data are analyzed between MR systems. For example, data obtained from DCE MR imaging studies may be processed using different kinetic models and different physiologic assumptions embedded in individual software, which yield different quantitative metrics, making it difficult to compare results derived from one software application with another.

More studies are needed that address the measurement reproducibility of functional MR measurements, and the radiologist should become familiar with the ethos of the roadmap of imaging biomarker development. To date, there have been many published papers investigating the usefulness of individual functional imaging techniques, but few have addressed measurement reproducibility within individual studies or across studies. However, understanding measurement reproducibility is critical because it creates confidence that a change in a measured biomarker value is likely to be real in an individual, rather than as a result of instrumental, biologic, or observer variations.

Functional MR imaging studies generate large imaging datasets that have significant effects on informatics, data storage, and data retrieval. A typical DCE MR imaging study generates 500 to 3000 images, and this number increases significant with multiparametric studies. Multiparametric and multimodality imaging datasets have implications for radiological workflow, because systems will need to be designed to accommodate the simultaneous display of different functional data, which allow the user to compare the findings with relative ease. Such development would be necessary to ensure the success and adoption of a multiparametric approach to disease assessment.

Currently, most functional imaging studies in the liver are conducted on clinical MR scanners at a field strength of 1.5T. There is a desire and drive to translate these methods to higher field strengths; however, the introduction of functional MR imaging techniques in the liver at 3.0T has not been easy, with some techniques proving more difficult than others. The variations in scanner design, and technical implementations across 3.0T MR systems from different manufacturers, make it difficult to recommend a generalized approach to problem solving. For example, using DW MR imaging, there are substantial variations in the eddy current performance across different 3.0T MR scanners, which makes it difficult to obtain consistent high-quality DW MR images of liver on all MR platforms. Thus, many functional MR imaging studies of the liver at 3.0T are still being evaluated within research rather than clinical arenas.

SUMMARY

Functional MR imaging techniques provide unique quantitative information that reflects specific aspects of tumor biology. Some of these techniques are now being used for the diagnosis of diseases, assessment of disease severity, and monitoring of treatment response. Combinations of such imaging techniques are also being investigated in clinical trials and drug development to elucidate the mechanistic actions of drugs and observe drug effects. However, there are still impediments to the widespread adoption of functional MR techniques in the liver, even for those that have substantial evidence for their use. Technical performance, standardization, and quality assurance are keys to imaging biomarker development, and the radiological community should work in concert to bring these technologies to the forefront for clinical and research practice.

ACKNOWLEDGMENTS

We would like to acknowledge David Collins, Keiko Miyazaki, and Michael Germuska from the Institute of Cancer Research (UK), for their invaluable help and contributions to the manuscript.

REFERENCES

1. Padhani AR, Choyke PL. New techniques in oncologic imaging. New York: Taylor & Francis; 2006.

2. Koh DM, Collins DJ. Diffusion-weighted MRI in the body: applications and challenges in oncology. AJR Am J Roentgenol 2007;188:1622–35.

3. Patterson DM, Padhani AR, Collins DJ. Technology insight: water diffusion MRI–a potential new biomarker of response to cancer therapy. Nat Clin Pract Oncol 2008;5:220–33.

4. Thoeny HC, De Keyzer F. Extracranial applications of diffusion-weighted magnetic resonance imaging. Eur Radiol 2007;17:1385–93.

5. Payne GS, Leach MO. Applications of magnetic resonance spectroscopy in radiotherapy treatment planning. Br J Radiol 2006;79(1):S16–26.

6. Longo R, Pollesello P, Ricci C, et al. Proton MR spectroscopy in quantitative in vivo determination of fat content in human liver steatosis. J Magn Reson Imaging 1995;5:281–5.

7. Szczepaniak LS, Nurenberg P, Leonard D, et al. Magnetic resonance spectroscopy to measure hepatic triglyceride content: prevalence of hepatic steatosis in the general population. Am J Physiol Endocrinol Metab 2005;288:E462–8.

8. Dixon WT. Simple proton spectroscopic imaging. Radiology 1984;153:189–94.

9. Rouviere O, Yin M, Dresner MA, et al. MR elastography of the liver: preliminary results. Radiology 2006; 240:440–8.

10. Ehman RL. Science to practice: can MR elastography be used to detect early steatohepatitis in fatty liver disease? Radiology 2009;253:1–3.

11. Huwart L, Sempoux C, Salameh N, et al. Liver fibrosis: noninvasive assessment with MR elastography versus aspartate aminotransferase-to-platelet ratio index. Radiology 2007;245:458–66.

12. Thng CH, Koh TS, Collins DJ, et al. Perfusion MR imaging of the liver. World J Gastroenterol 2010;16: 1598–604.

13. Totman JJ, O'Gorman RL, Kane PA, et al. Comparison of the hepatic perfusion index measured with gadolinium-enhanced volumetric MRI in controls and in patients with colorectal cancer. Br J Radiol 2005;78:105–9.

14. Tsushima Y, Blomley MJ, Yokoyama H, et al. Does the presence of distant and local malignancy alter parenchymal perfusion in apparently disease-free areas of the liver? Dig Dis Sci 2001;46:2113–9.

15. Meijerink MR, van Waesberghe JH, van der Weide L, et al. Total-liver-volume perfusion CT using 3-D image fusion to improve detection and characterization of liver metastases. Eur Radiol 2008;18:2345–54.

16. Miyazaki M, Tsushima Y, Miyazaki A, et al. Quantification of hepatic arterial and portal perfusion with dynamic computed tomography: comparison of maximum-slope and dual-input one-compartment model methods. Jpn J Radiol 2009;27:143–50.

17. Abdullah SS, Pialat JB, Wiart M, et al. Characterization of hepatocellular carcinoma and colorectal liver metastasis by means of perfusion MRI. J Magn Reson Imaging 2008;28:390–5.

18. Sahani DV, Holalkere NS, Mueller PR, et al. Advanced hepatocellular carcinoma: CT perfusion of liver and tumor tissue—initial experience. Radiology 2007;243:736–43.

19. Miyazaki K, Collins DJ, Walker-Samuel S, et al. Quantitative mapping of hepatic perfusion index using MR imaging: a potential reproducible tool for assessing tumour response to treatment with the antiangiogenic compound BIBF 1120, a potent triple angiokinase inhibitor. Eur Radiol 2008;18:1414–21.

20. Chen G, Ma DQ, He W, et al. Computed tomography perfusion in evaluating the therapeutic effect of transarterial chemoembolization for hepatocellular carcinoma. World J Gastroenterol 2008;14: 5738–43.

21. O'Connor JP, Jackson A, Parker GJ, et al. DCE-MRI biomarkers in the clinical evaluation of antiangiogenic and vascular disrupting agents. Br J Cancer 2007;96:189–95.

22. Mross K, Drevs J, Muller M, et al. Phase I clinical and pharmacokinetic study of PTK/ZK, a multiple VEGF receptor inhibitor, in patients with liver metastases from solid tumours. Eur J Cancer 2005;41:1291–9.

23. Thomas AL, Morgan B, Horsfield MA, et al. Phase I study of the safety, tolerability, pharmacokinetics, and pharmacodynamics of PTK787/ZK 222584 administered twice daily in patients with advanced cancer. J Clin Oncol 2005;23:4162–71.

24. Morgan B, Thomas AL, Drevs J, et al. Dynamic contrast-enhanced magnetic resonance imaging as a biomarker for the pharmacological response of PTK787/ZK 222584, an inhibitor of the vascular endothelial growth factor receptor tyrosine kinases, in patients with advanced colorectal cancer and liver metastases: results from two phase I studies. J Clin Oncol 2003;21:3955–64.

25. Annet L, Materne R, Danse E, et al. Hepatic flow parameters measured with MR imaging and Doppler US: correlations with degree of cirrhosis and portal hypertension. Radiology 2003;229:409–14.

26. Leggett DA, Kelley BB, Bunce IH, et al. Colorectal cancer: diagnostic potential of CT measurements of hepatic perfusion and implications for contrast enhancement protocols. Radiology 1997;205: 716–20.

27. Miles KA, Hayball MP, Dixon AK. Functional images of hepatic perfusion obtained with dynamic CT. Radiology 1993;188:405–11.

28. Koh TS, Thng CH, Hartono S, et al. Dynamic contrast-enhanced CT imaging of hepatocellular carcinoma in cirrhosis: feasibility of a prolonged dual-phase imaging protocol with tracer kinetics modeling. Eur Radiol 2009;19:1184–96.

29. Bammer R. Basic principles of diffusion-weighted imaging. Eur J Radiol 2003;45:169–84.

30. Koh DM, Takahara T, Imai Y, et al. Practical aspects of assessing tumors using clinical diffusion-weighted imaging in the body. Magn Reson Med Sci 2007;6:211–24.

31. Girometti R, Furlan A, Bazzocchi M, et al. [Diffusion-weighted MRI in evaluating liver fibrosis: a feasibility study in cirrhotic patients]. Radiol Med 2007;112:394–408 [in Italian].

32. Girometti R, Furlan A, Esposito G, et al. Relevance of b-values in evaluating liver fibrosis: a study in healthy and cirrhotic subjects using two single-shot spin-echo echo-planar diffusion-weighted sequences. J Magn Reson Imaging 2008;28:411–9.

33. Aube C, Racineux PX, Lebigot J, et al. [Diagnosis and quantification of hepatic fibrosis with diffusion weighted MR imaging: preliminary results]. J Radiol 2004;85:301–6 [in French].

34. Koinuma M, Ohashi I, Hanafusa K, et al. Apparent diffusion coefficient measurements with diffusion-weighted magnetic resonance imaging for evaluation of hepatic fibrosis. J Magn Reson Imaging 2005;22:80–5.

35. Lewin M, Poujol-Robert A, Boelle PY, et al. Diffusion-weighted magnetic resonance imaging for the assessment of fibrosis in chronic hepatitis C. Hepatology 2007;46:658–65.

36. Boulanger Y, Amara M, Lepanto L, et al. Diffusion-weighted MR imaging of the liver of hepatitis C patients. NMR Biomed 2003;16:132–6.

37. Taouli B, Tolia AJ, Losada M, et al. Diffusion-weighted MRI for quantification of liver fibrosis: preliminary experience. AJR Am J Roentgenol 2007;189:799–806.

38. Taouli B, Chouli M, Martin AJ, et al. Chronic hepatitis: role of diffusion-weighted imaging and diffusion tensor imaging for the diagnosis of liver fibrosis and inflammation. J Magn Reson Imaging 2008;28:89–95.

39. Luciani A, Vignaud A, Cavet M, et al. Liver cirrhosis: intravoxel incoherent motion MR imaging–pilot study. Radiology 2008;249:891–9.

40. Parikh T, Drew SJ, Lee VS, et al. Focal liver lesion detection and characterization with diffusion-weighted MR imaging: comparison with standard breath-hold T2-weighted imaging. Radiology 2008;246:812–22.

41. Bruegel M, Gaa J, Waldt S, et al. Diagnosis of hepatic metastasis: comparison of respiration-triggered diffusion-weighted echo-planar MRI and five t2-weighted turbo spin-echo sequences. AJR Am J Roentgenol 2008;191:1421–9.

42. Bruegel M, Holzapfel K, Gaa J, et al. Characterization of focal liver lesions by ADC measurements using a respiratory triggered diffusion-weighted single-shot echo-planar MR imaging technique. Eur Radiol 2008;18:477–85.

43. Zech CJ, Herrmann KA, Dietrich O, et al. Black-blood diffusion-weighted EPI acquisition of the liver with parallel imaging: comparison with a standard T2-weighted sequence for detection of focal liver lesions. Invest Radiol 2008;43:261–6.

44. Nasu K, Kuroki Y, Nawano S, et al. Hepatic metastases: diffusion-weighted sensitivity-encoding versus SPIO-enhanced MR imaging. Radiology 2006;239:122–30.

45. Koh DM, Brown G, Riddell AM, et al. Detection of colorectal hepatic metastases using MnDPDP MR imaging and diffusion-weighted imaging (DWI) alone and in combination. Eur Radiol 2008;18(5):903–10.

46. Namimoto T, Yamashita Y, Sumi S, et al. Focal liver masses: characterization with diffusion-weighted echo-planar MR imaging. Radiology 1997;204:739–44.

47. Ichikawa T, Haradome H, Hachiya J, et al. Diffusion-weighted MR imaging with a single-shot echoplanar sequence: detection and characterization of focal hepatic lesions. AJR Am J Roentgenol 1998;170:397–402.

48. Kim T, Murakami T, Takahashi S, et al. Diffusion-weighted single-shot echoplanar MR imaging for liver disease. AJR Am J Roentgenol 1999;173:393–8.

49. Taouli B, Vilgrain V, Dumont E, et al. Evaluation of liver diffusion isotropy and characterization of focal hepatic lesions with two single-shot echo-planar MR imaging sequences: prospective study in 66 patients. Radiology 2003;226:71–8.

50. Gourtsoyianni S, Papanikolaou N, Yarmenitis S, et al. Respiratory gated diffusion-weighted imaging of the liver: value of apparent diffusion coefficient measurements in the differentiation between most commonly encountered benign and malignant focal liver lesions. Eur Radiol 2008;18:486–92.

51. Taouli B, Koh DM. Diffusion-weighted MR imaging of the liver. Radiology 2010;254:47–66.

52. Nasu K, Kuroki Y, Tsukamoto T, et al. Diffusion-weighted imaging of surgically resected hepatocellular carcinoma: imaging characteristics and relationship among signal intensity, apparent diffusion coefficient, and histopathologic grade. AJR Am J Roentgenol 2009;193:438–44.

53. Muhi A, Ichikawa T, Motosugi U, et al. High-b-value diffusion-weighted MR imaging of hepatocellular lesions: estimation of grade of malignancy of hepatocellular carcinoma. J Magn Reson Imaging 2009;30:1005–11.

54. Cui Y, Zhang XP, Sun YS, et al. Apparent diffusion coefficient: potential imaging biomarker for prediction and early detection of response to chemotherapy in hepatic metastases. Radiology 2008;248:894–900.

55. Koh DM, Blackledge M, Collins DJ, et al. Reproducibility and changes in the apparent diffusion coefficients of solid tumours treated with combretastatin A4 phosphate and bevacizumab in a two-centre phase I clinical trial. Eur Radiol 2009;19:2728–38.

56. Schraml C, Schwenzer NF, Martirosian P, et al. Diffusion-weighted MRI of advanced hepatocellular carcinoma during sorafenib treatment: initial results. AJR Am J Roentgenol 2009;193:W301–7.

57. Koh DM, Scurr E, Collins D, et al. Predicting response of colorectal hepatic metastasis: value of pretreatment apparent diffusion coefficients. AJR Am J Roentgenol 2007;188:1001–8.

58. Sijens PE, Smit GP, Borgdorff MA, et al. Multiple voxel 1H MR spectroscopy of phosphorylase-b kinase deficient patients (GSD IXa) showing an accumulation of fat in the liver that resolves with aging. J Hepatol 2006;45:851–5.

59. Thomsen C, Becker U, Winkler K, et al. Quantification of liver fat using magnetic resonance spectroscopy. Magn Reson Imaging 1994;12:487–95.

60. Lee SS, Park SH, Kim HJ, et al. Non-invasive assessment of hepatic steatosis: prospective comparison of the accuracy of imaging examinations. J Hepatol 2010;52:579–85.

61. Machann J, Thamer C, Schnoedt B, et al. Hepatic lipid accumulation in healthy subjects: a comparative study using spectral fat-selective MRI and volume-localized 1H-MR spectroscopy. Magn Reson Med 2006;55:913–7.

62. Menon DK, Sargentoni J, Taylor-Robinson SD, et al. Effect of functional grade and etiology on in vivo hepatic phosphorus-31 magnetic resonance spectroscopy in cirrhosis: biochemical basis of spectral appearances. Hepatology 1995;21:417–27.

63. van Wassenaer-van Hall HN, van der Grond J, van Hattum J, et al. 31P magnetic resonance spectroscopy of the liver: correlation with standardized serum, clinical, and histological changes in diffuse liver disease. Hepatology 1995;21:443–9.

64. Dagnelie PC, Leij-Halfwerk S. Magnetic resonance spectroscopy to study hepatic metabolism in diffuse liver diseases, diabetes and cancer. World J Gastroenterol 2010;16:1577–86.

65. Sijens PE. Parametric exploration of the liver by magnetic resonance methods. Eur Radiol 2009;19:2594–607.

66. Kuo YT, Li CW, Chen CY, et al. In vivo proton magnetic resonance spectroscopy of large focal hepatic lesions and metabolite change of hepatocellular carcinoma before and after transcatheter arterial chemoembolization using 3.0-T MR scanner. J Magn Reson Imaging 2004;19:598–604.

67. Soper R, Himmelreich U, Painter D, et al. Pathology of hepatocellular carcinoma and its precursors using proton magnetic resonance spectroscopy and a statistical classification strategy. Pathology 2002;34:417–22.

68. Kim H, Taksali SE, Dufour S, et al. Comparative MR study of hepatic fat quantification using single-voxel proton spectroscopy, two-point Dixon and three-point IDEAL. Magn Reson Med 2008;59:521–7.

69. Westphalen AC, Qayyum A, Yeh BM, et al. Liver fat: effect of hepatic iron deposition on evaluation with opposed-phase MR imaging. Radiology 2007;242:450–5.

70. Reeder SB, Pineda AR, Wen Z, et al. Iterative decomposition of water and fat with echo asymmetry and least-squares estimation (IDEAL): application with fast spin-echo imaging. Magn Reson Med 2005;54:636–44.

71. Costa DN, Pedrosa I, McKenzie C, et al. Body MRI using IDEAL. AJR Am J Roentgenol 2008;190:1076–84.

72. Reeder SB, McKenzie CA, Pineda AR, et al. Water-fat separation with IDEAL gradient-echo imaging. J Magn Reson Imaging 2007;25:644–52.

73. Reeder SB, Hargreaves BA, Yu H, et al. Homodyne reconstruction and IDEAL water-fat decomposition. Magn Reson Med 2005;54:586–93.

74. Szumowski J, Coshow WR, Li F, et al. Phase unwrapping in the three-point Dixon method for fat suppression MR imaging. Radiology 1994;192:555–61.

75. Szumowski J, Coshow W, Li F, et al. Double-echo three-point-Dixon method for fat suppression MRI. Magn Reson Med 1995;34:120–4.

76. Coombs BD, Szumowski J, Coshow W. Two-point Dixon technique for water-fat signal decomposition with B0 inhomogeneity correction. Magn Reson Med 1997;38:884–9.

77. Angelucci E, Giovagnoni A, Valeri G, et al. Limitations of magnetic resonance imaging in measurement of hepatic iron. Blood 1997;90:4736–42.

78. Christoforidis A, Perifanis V, Spanos G, et al. MRI assessment of liver iron content in thalassamic patients with three different protocols: comparisons and correlations. Eur J Haematol 2009;82:388–92.

79. Gandon Y, Olivie D, Guyader D, et al. Non-invasive assessment of hepatic iron stores by MRI. Lancet 2004;363:357–62.

80. Wood JC, Enriquez C, Ghugre N, et al. MRI R2 and R2* mapping accurately estimates hepatic iron concentration in transfusion-dependent thalassemia and sickle cell disease patients. Blood 2005;106:1460–5.

81. Kaltwasser JP, Gottschalk R, Schalk KP, et al. Non-invasive quantitation of liver iron-overload by magnetic resonance imaging. Br J Haematol 1990;74:360–3.

82. Huwart L, Peeters F, Sinkus R, et al. Liver fibrosis: non-invasive assessment with MR elastography. NMR Biomed 2006;19:173–9.

83. Yin M, Talwalkar JA, Glaser KJ, et al. Assessment of hepatic fibrosis with magnetic resonance elastography. Clin Gastroenterol Hepatol 2007;5:1207–13 e1202.

84. Asbach P, Klatt D, Hamhaber U, et al. Assessment of liver viscoelasticity using multifrequency MR elastography. Magn Reson Med 2008;60:373—9.

85. Klatt D, Asbach P, Rump J, et al. In vivo determination of hepatic stiffness using steady-state free precession magnetic resonance elastography. Invest Radiol 2006;41:841—8.

86. Tsui EY, Chan JH, Cheung YK, et al. Evaluation of therapeutic effectiveness of transarterial chemoembolization for hepatocellular carcinoma: correlation of dynamic susceptibility contrast-enhanced echoplanar imaging and hepatic angiography. Clin Imaging 2000;24:210—6.

87. Rhee TK, Larson AC, Prasad PV, et al. Feasibility of blood oxygenation level-dependent MR imaging to monitor hepatic transcatheter arterial embolization in rabbits. J Vasc Interv Radiol 2005;16:1523—8.

88. O'Connor JP, Naish JH, Parker GJ, et al. Preliminary study of oxygen-enhanced longitudinal relaxation in MRI: a potential novel biomarker of oxygenation changes in solid tumors. Int J Radiat Oncol Biol Phys 2009;75:1209—15.

89. Taouli B, Martin AJ, Qayyum A, et al. Parallel imaging and diffusion tensor imaging for diffusion-weighted MRI of the liver: preliminary experience in healthy volunteers. AJR Am J Roentgenol 2004;183:677—80.

90. Guiu B, Loffroy R, Hillon P, et al. Magnetic resonance imaging and spectroscopy for quantification of hepatic steatosis: urgent need for standardization! J Hepatol 2009;51:1082—3 [author reply: 1083—4].

Tumors of the Liver and Intrahepatic Bile Ducts: Radiologic—Pathologic Correlation

Rachel B. Lewis, MD[a,b,c,*], Grant E. Lattin Jr, MD[a,c],
Hala R. Makhlouf, MD, PhD[d], Angela D. Levy, MD[e]

KEYWORDS

• Liver • Hepatic neoplasms • Magnetic resonance imaging

Primary tumors of the liver can be broadly classified pathologically based on their cell of origin. Epithelial tumors arise from hepatocytes or biliary epithelium and include the benign neoplasms or tumor-like lesions focal nodular hyperplasia (FNH), hepatocellular adenoma (HCA), and biliary cystadenoma; in addition to the malignant neoplasms hepatocellular carcinoma (HCC), fibro-lamellar carcinoma, and intrahepatic cholangiocarcinoma (ICC). Nonepithelial tumors consist of lymphoma and mesenchymal tumors, including cavernous hemangioma, angiomyolipoma, solitary fibrous tumor (SFT), angiosarcoma, and hepatic epithelioid hemangioendothelioma. Characteristic findings on MR imaging can be seen in many cases. In this article we review the MR imaging appearance of these tumors with pathologic correlation.

BENIGN TUMORS
Epithelial

Focal nodular hyperplasia
Clinical and pathologic features

FNH is the second most common benign hepatic tumor following hemangioma, accounting for 8% of primary hepatic tumors.[1] It is classified as a regenerative lesion rather than a neoplasm. It is thought to represent a hyperplastic response to a congenital or acquired arterial malformation. FNH with histologic characteristics of both FNH and HCA and atypical pathologic and imaging characteristics for FNH, such as heterogeneity and lack of a central scar, were previously categorized as telangiectatic FNH. Because of recent molecular evidence, they are now recognized as a subset of HCA.[2]

The authors have nothing to disclose.
The views expressed in this article are those of the authors and do not necessarily reflect the official policy or position of the Department of the Navy, Department of Defense, nor the United States government.
[a] Department of Radiologic Pathology, Armed Forces Institute of Pathology, 6825 16th Street NW, Washington, DC 20306-6000, USA
[b] Department of Radiology, National Naval Medical Center, 8901 Rockville Pike, Bethesda, MD 20889, USA
[c] Department of Radiology and Nuclear Medicine, Uniformed Services University of the Health Sciences, 4301 Jones Bridge Road, Bethesda, MD 20814, USA
[d] Division of Hepatic and Gastrointestinal Pathology, Armed Forces Institute of Pathology, 6825 16th Street NW, Washington, DC 20306-6000, USA
[e] Department of Radiology, Georgetown University Hospital, 3800 Reservoir Road NW, Washington, DC 20007, USA
* Corresponding author. Department of Radiologic Pathology, Armed Forces Institute of Pathology, 6825 16th Street NW, Washington, DC 20306-6000.
E-mail address: rachel.lewis@med.navy.mil

Magn Reson Imaging Clin N Am 18 (2010) 587–609
doi:10.1016/j.mric.2010.08.010
1064-9689/10/$ — see front matter. Published by Elsevier Inc.

Approximately 89% to 94% of FNH occur in women with a mean age at diagnosis of 38 years.[3,4] The majority of patients are asymptomatic. In the remainder, abdominal pain and palpable mass are the most common symptoms. Reports of hemorrhage or rupture of FNH are extremely rare.

FNH are named for their nodular architecture, subdivided by fibrous septa that coalesce into a central or eccentric stellate scar. They are nonencapsulated, but sharply marginated with a lobulated contour. Prominent vessels cover their surface. Hemorrhage and necrosis are rare because their growth is usually proportional to their vascular supply.[1] Their size ranges from 1 mm to 19 cm in diameter, with a mean of 5 cm.[3] Approximately 20% are multiple and there are reported associations with other vascular malformations and neoplasms, including cavernous hemangiomas, which are present in 20% of patients with FNH.[4]

Microscopically, FNH consist of hyperplastic hepatocytes that are arranged in two-cell thick hepatic plates separated by sinusoids containing endothelial cells and Kupffer cells. The fibrous septa contain numerous vessels, particularly thick-walled arteries with fibromuscular hyperplasia and intimal fibrosis, in addition to an inflammatory infiltrate.[5] Bile ductules are present at the junction of the fibrous septa and hepatocytes; however, they do not connect to the intrahepatic bile ducts.

MR imaging features

The diagnosis of FNH can be made with confidence when all typical MR imaging features are present on unenhanced and intravenous contrast-enhanced sequences (**Fig. 1**). These include isointensity or hypointensity on T1-weighted sequences (90% to 100% of cases) and slight hyperintensity or isointensity on T2-weighted sequences (99% to 100% of cases) with homogeneous signal intensity except for a central scar.[6–10] The scar is hyperintense on T2-weighted sequences because of the presence of vascular channels, bile ductules, and myxomatous tissue.[1] After the administration of intravenous gadolinium, FNH typically demonstrate moderate-to-strong homogeneous arterial enhancement, with slight hyperintensity or isointensity to background liver in the portal venous and equilibrium phases (95% to 99% of cases).[7,8] The central scar demonstrates initial relative hypointensity during the arterial phase of contrast enhancement, and subsequent delayed enhancement from the progressive accumulation of contrast within the fibrous tissue.[1] Prominent peripheral draining veins or a dominant draining vein may be observed surrounding the lesion on equilibrium phase images (see **Fig. 1D**).

Atypical imaging features are found in 21% to 57% of FNH.[7,11,12] A central scar may not be visualized in up to 50% of cases, particularly in lesions less than 3 cm in diameter.[6,7] Rarely, the scar may demonstrate low T2 signal intensity (1%) or lack of enhancement (1% to 2%) simulating fibrolamellar carcinoma.[7,8,11] Other atypical features include hypoenhancement during any phase of contrast-enhanced imaging, heterogeneous signal intensity from hemorrhage, high T1 signal intensity from sinusoidal dilatation or steatosis, and a peripheral pseudocapsule of low T1 and high T2 signal intensity from adjacent compressed liver.[11]

Liver-specific MR imaging contrast agents can be helpful in the diagnosis of FNH. Superparamagnetic iron oxide (SPIO) particles taken up by Kupffer cells lower the signal intensity of FNH on T2-weighted and T2*-weighted sequences, although usually to a slightly less extent than normal liver, and improve visualization of the central scar.[13] Hepatobiliary agents, such as mangafodipir or delayed imaging with gadobenate dimeglumine, result in isointensity or hyperintensity on T1-weighted images because FNH contains functioning hepatocytes and biliary ductules (see **Fig. 1E**). In one study of gadobenate dimeglumine, 97% of FNH were hyperintense or isointense compared with 100% of HCA being hypointense on a 1 to 3 hour delayed T1 sequence.[8] The central scar, hypointense during the hepatobiliary phase, was also better delineated.

Differential diagnosis

Focal hepatic lesions that may have a central scar or scar-like fibrosis include hemangioma, fibrolamellar carcinoma and HCC. Giant hemangiomas may contain focal fibrosis that simulates a central scar (discussed below). This is usually larger and more hyperintense on T2-weighted sequences compared with the scar of FNH and the contrast enhancement pattern of hemangiomas is distinctive. The scar of fibrolamellar carcinoma contains calcification in 55% and is typically hypointense on T2-weighted sequences. Both fibrolamellar carcinoma and HCC tend to be more heterogeneous than FNH because they commonly have intratumoral hemorrhage and necrosis.

Hypervascular liver lesions such as HCA and HCC may also be considered in the differential diagnosis of FNH, particularly when a central scar is not visualized. The distinction between these tumors is discussed in the following section on HCA.

Hepatocellular adenoma

Clinical and pathologic features

HCA is a rare benign neoplasm that most often arises in the setting of hormonal or metabolic

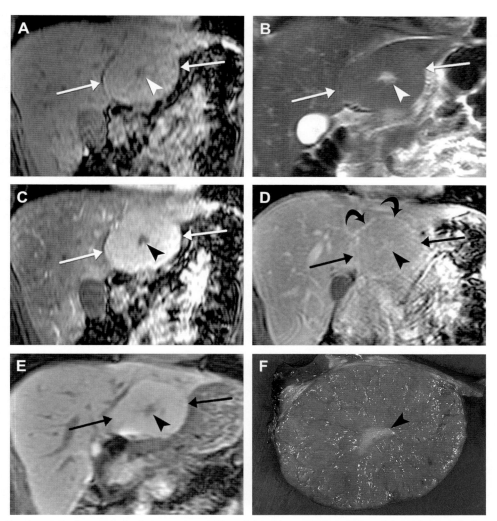

Fig. 1. Focal nodular hyperplasia. Fat-suppressed T1-weighted image (*A*) and T2-weighted image (*B*) shows a circumscribed mass (*arrows*) isointense to normal liver with a low T1, high T2 signal intensity central scar (*arrowhead*). Fat-suppressed T1-weighted images (*C–E*) during the intravenous administration of gadobenate dimeglumine show homogeneous hyperintensity of the mass (*arrows*) during the arterial phase (*C*) with the exception of the hypointense central scar (*arrowhead*). During the equilibrium phase (*D*), the mass (*arrows*) is isointense to liver and there is delayed enhancement of the central scar (*arrowhead*). Prominent draining vessels are present around the periphery (*curved arrows*). (*E*) A three-hour delayed hepatobiliary phase image shows isointensity of the mass (*arrows*) with a well-delineated central scar (*arrowhead*). (*F*) Photograph of the cut surface of the resected specimen reveals a nodular mass with a central stellate scar (*arrowhead*).

stimulation. The most common cause is oral contraceptives, with an annual incidence of 3 to 4 per 100,000 in women on long-term contraceptives, compared with 1 per million in women who have not taken oral contraceptives or have taken them for less than 2 years.[14] Risk increases with the duration of use and potency of oral contraceptives and appears to be lower with second and third generation lower dose formulations.[15] Other risk factors for HCA include anabolic steroid use, pregnancy, gynecologic tumors, glycogen storage

diseases (particularly type Ia, von Gierke disease), and galactosemia. Sporadic cases have been reported in men and women without any risk factors, but are rare.

Similar to FNH, HCA are usually found in women of childbearing age, with most in the third to fourth decades of life. The majority of patients are symptomatic, complaining of acute, episodic, or chronic abdominal pain, or a palpable mass. Only 5% to 10% of lesions are incidentally discovered.[5] Twenty five percent present with tumor rupture and subcapsular or intraperitoneal hemorrhage, which occurs in lesions 5 cm or greater in diameter.[16] Besides hemorrhage, the other main worrisome complication of HCA is malignant transformation to HCC, with a frequency of 4% to 9% in surgical series, found in lesions over 4 cm in diameter.[16,17]

The majority, 70% to 80%, of HCAs are solitary. Multiple lesions are often seen with anabolic steroid use and glycogen storage diseases. An entity called liver adenomatosis has been described consisting of greater than 10 adenomas in patients without hormonal risk factors or glycogen storage disease. However, this may not warrant a separate classification, since many of the cases described have been in women on oral contraceptives and other than the number of lesions, there is no difference in imaging or pathology.[18–20]

On sectioning, HCAs are typically well circumscribed round or oval masses 5 to 15 cm in diameter with a variegated appearance from areas of hemorrhage, necrosis, and infarction. They are usually unencapsulated, but a thin fibrous capsule is sometimes present. Histologically, they are composed of a trabecular pattern of normal appearing hepatocytes that may have increased cytoplasmic fat and glycogen. Thin-walled arteries supply the parenchyma but without other elements of portal triads including bile ducts or significant connective tissue support, which may predispose to hemorrhage.[2] Degenerative changes are commonly seen on histology, including infarction, hemorrhage, peliosis, and sinusoidal dilatation.[2]

MR imaging features

The appearance of HCA on MR imaging is quite variable, reflecting the various gross pathologic features. Focal areas of high T1 signal are present in 45% to 77% of HCAs, which correspond to steatosis, hemorrhage, or peliosis on pathologic correlation (**Fig. 2**).[21–23] With steatosis, signal intensity loss on chemical shift imaging is seen. On T2-weighted sequences, 47% to 74% of HCAs are predominantly hyperintense with only 4% to 10% hypointense.[21–23] Heterogeneity is present on T1- or T2-weighted sequences in 51% to 94%, correlating pathologically with hemorrhagic necrosis and peliosis.[21–23] A capsule is seen on MR imaging

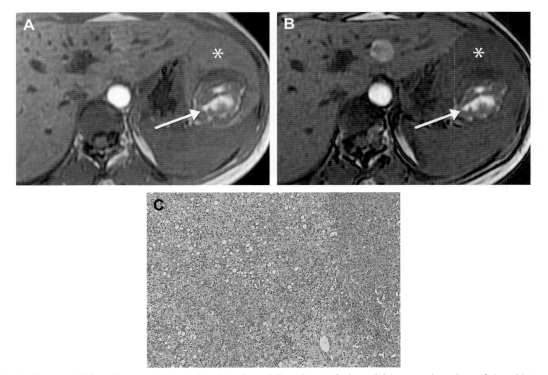

Fig. 2. Hepatocellular adenoma. T1-weighted in-phase (*A*) and out-of-phase (*B*) images show loss of signal intensity in the mass (*asterisk*) in (*B*), compatible with steatosis. Areas of high signal intensity in both images (*arrow*) represent subacute hemorrhage. (*C*) Photomicrograph (original magnification, ×40; hematoxylin-eosin [H-E] stain) of the corresponding specimen demonstrates tumor cells (*left*) that are paler than the normal hepatocytes (*right*) with many tumor cells containing fat vacuoles.

in 17% to 31% of cases, which demonstrates low T1 and variable T2 signal intensity.[21,23]

During the administration of intravenous gadolinium, 96% of HCAs demonstrate marked arterial enhancement (**Fig. 3**).[8] Signal intensity in the portal venous and equilibrium phases is more varied and HCAs may be hyperintense, isointense, or hypointense although the majority of HCAs appear isointense in the equilibrium phase.[8] Contrast enhancement may be heterogeneous or homogeneous. Kupffer cells are reduced in number and function so adenomas rarely show uptake of SPIO particles.[24]

Differential diagnosis

FNH, HCC, hypervascular metastases, as well as HCA should be considered in the differential diagnosis of hypervascular hepatic lesions. In a study by Arrivé and colleagues,[21] 88% of adenomas had heterogeneous signal, T1 hyperintensity or a peripheral rim, which distinguish them from FNH. Conversely, the demonstration of a central scar-like area of fibrosis is unusual in HCA. However, the MR imaging features of FNH without a central scar are similar to homogeneous HCA without hemorrhage, fat or

necrosis, particularly seen in smaller lesions. Delayed imaging with gadobenate dimeglumine may be helpful in these cases. Fibrolamellar carcinoma is more common in men than HCA and may be distinguished by a central scar, lobulated margins, and malignant features. There is tremendous overlap in the features of HCA and HCC. Biopsy is often performed for HCAs not requiring surgical resection. MR elastography, which measures the stiffness of tissue, may help differentiate benign tumors, including HCA, from malignant tumors since benign hepatic tumors demonstrate lower shear stiffness, based on preliminary results.[25] Hypervascular metastases are usually multiple, markedly hyperintense on T2-weighted sequences, and rarely contain fat and hemorrhage.

Biliary cystadenoma and cystadenocarcinoma
Clinical and pathologic features

Biliary cystadenomas are rare cystic neoplasms, accounting for less than 5% of intrahepatic cysts of bile duct origin in a surgical series.[26] Other biliary derived cysts include simple hepatic cysts, polycystic liver disease, choledochal cysts, and biliary hamartomata. Biliary cystadenocarcinomas

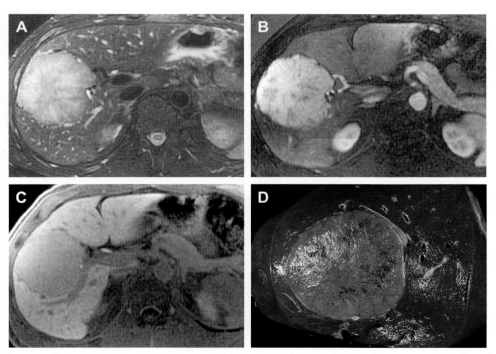

Fig. 3. Hepatocellular adenoma. (*A*) Fat-suppressed T2-weighted image shows a heterogeneously hyperintense mass in the right lobe. Arterial phase (*B*) and two-hour delayed (*C*) images after the administration of gadobenate dimeglumine show immediate heterogeneous hyperintensity of the mass and hypointensity during the hepatobiliary phase. (*D*) Photograph of the cut specimen demonstrates a sharply marginated mass with focal areas of hemorrhage.

are the malignant counterpart of cystadenomas, and are discussed together with cystadenomas because of overlapping pathologic and imaging features. Biliary cystadenomas are most commonly found in middle-aged women, with an average age of 38 to 45 years and female preponderance of 93% to 96%.[27,28] Biliary cystadenocarcinomas occur on average at a slightly older age, 56 years, and are relatively more common in men than women compared with cystadenomas (62% of cystadenocarcinomas are found in women).[29] Clinical symptoms are nonspecific, including abdominal pain and palpable mass. Jaundice can be seen when there is biliary obstruction.

The majority of biliary cystadenomas and cystadenocarcinomas are intrahepatic, but occur occasionally in the extrahepatic bile ducts and gallbladder.[27–29] They are encapsulated, multilocular cystic masses with a smooth outer contour. The cyst contents vary and may be clear, mucinous, bilious, hemorrhagic, or mixed fluid.[27] Biliary cystadenocarcinomas are more likely than cystadenomas to demonstrate papillary excrescences and polypoid masses in the cyst cavities.[5]

Benign columnar or cuboidal epithelial cells line the cyst locules of cystadenomas. Similar benign appearing epithelium is found in addition to malignant epithelial cells in over 90% of biliary cystadenocarcinomas, supporting the theory of a progression between the two.[29] A layer of mesenchymal tissue that resembles ovarian stroma usually surrounds the epithelium. The ovarian-like stroma is only seen in women, and may confer a better prognosis in cases of cystadenocarcinoma.[27]

MR imaging features

Cystadenomas and cystadenocarcinomas are multilocular cystic masses on imaging (**Fig. 4**). MR imaging allows characterization of the cyst contents, although the signal varies with protein concentration and age of hemorrhage. In general, compared with muscle, mucinous fluid is isointense on T1-weighted sequences and hyperintense on T2-weighted sequences, serous fluid has low T1 and high T2 signal intensity, and hemorrhage can be identified by high T1 signal intensity or fluid-fluid levels. A low T2 signal intensity outer capsule may be seen, likely from hemorrhage within the wall.[27,30] With contrast administration, there is enhancement of the cyst wall and septa. Although the imaging findings overlap, the presence of enhancing mural nodules is suggestive of biliary cystadenocarcinoma, and their absence favors biliary cystadenoma.[27,30] No imaging finding correlates with the presence of ovarian-like stroma.[27]

Magnetic resonance cholangiopancreatography (MRCP) can help define the relationship of the cyst

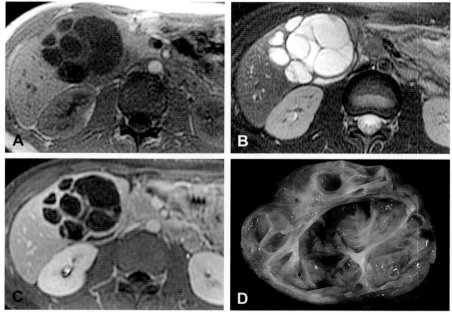

Fig. 4. Biliary cystadenoma. T1-weighted (*A*) and fat-suppressed T2-weighted (*B*) images show a cystic mass with multiple septa dividing locules of low T1 and high T2 signal intensity. (*C*) Intravenous gadolinium contrast enhanced fat-suppressed T1-weighted image shows enhancement of the cyst wall and septa. (*D*) Photograph of the cut surface of the resected specimen shows a multiloculated cystic mass.

to the bile ducts. Dilatation of the peripheral bile ducts may be seen from obstruction. Rarely, biliary cystadenomas or cystadenocarcinomas may communicate with or prolapse into a bile duct.[31]

Differential diagnosis

The differential diagnosis of a hepatic complex cystic mass is broad. Infectious causes, including pyogenic abscess, amebic abscess, and hydatid cysts are a main consideration. Clinical and laboratory data, including amebic and echinococcal serologies, can help distinguish these. Helpful MR imaging findings include low signal intensity, nonenhancing walls of the daughter cysts, or non-enhancing membranes within a hydatid cyst. Pyogenic and amebic abscesses are not encapsulated, have ill-defined enhancing margins, and often have a rim of edema between central areas of necrosis and adjacent normal liver. Cystic hepatic neoplasms, including mesenchymal hamartoma and undifferentiated embryonal cell sarcoma, are usually found in children. Cystic metastases are often multiple and there is a clinical history of known primary. Hepatocellular carcinoma may have a cystic appearance when there is significant necrosis after treatment.

Nonepithelial

Cavernous hemangioma

Clinical and pathologic features

Cavernous hemangioma is the most common benign hepatic tumor with a reported prevalence of 1% up to 20%.[32,33] It can occur at any age and demonstrates a female predominance, with a female-to-male ratio of 2:1 to 5:1.[34] The vast majority are incidentally found. Patients with large lesions may present with abdominal pain or symptoms from mass effect on adjacent structures. Rare complications include intratumoral hemorrhage, rupture with hemoperitoneum, and unusual hematologic manifestations such as erythrocytosis from secretion of erythropoietin and Kasabach-Merritt syndrome, which consists of a consumptive coagulopathy, thrombocytopenia, and hemolytic anemia.

Cavernous hemangiomas are well-circumscribed and vary from less than 1 cm to over 30 cm in size.[5] Ten to twenty percent are multiple and there is a re-ported association with focal nodular hyperplasia.[4] Microscopically, a honeycomb appearance is generated by numerous blood filled spaces, each lined by a single layer of flat endothelial cells in contrast to hepatic peliosis, which is characterized by blood-filled spaces without an endothelial lining. They can be quite heterogeneous, containing areas of recent or organized thrombus, fibrosis, and, rarely, calcification. Fibrosis is typically central but

can involve the entire lesion, referred to as a sclerosed or hyalinized hemangioma.[5]

MR imaging features

On imaging, hepatic cavernous hemangiomas have smooth well-defined margins and are round or lobular in shape. They are hypointense on T1-weighted sequences except for regions of hyperintensity in the rare occasion of hemorrhage. Hemangiomas have high T2 signal intensity approaching that of cerebrospinal fluid and show even higher signal intensity on long TE T2-weighted sequences. They may not be completely homogeneous, with nodules or septa of low T2 signal intensity in 80% of cases, corresponding to fibrosis on pathology.[35] Additionally, many giant hemangiomas, variably defined as greater than 4 cm up to greater than 12 cm in diameter, contain a central cleft of cystic degeneration or liquefaction that compared with the remainder of the lesion is hypointense on T1-weighted sequences and hyperintense on T2-weighted sequences (**Fig. 5**).[36]

During the administration of intravenous gadolinium contrast agents, a pattern of early peripheral discontinuous nodular enhancement with progressive centripetal complete or incomplete filling-in has 84% sensitivity, 100% specificity, and 95% accuracy for the diagnosis of hemangioma.[37] The signal intensity of the enhancing areas parallels aortic enhancement (see **Fig. 5B** and **C**). The fibrous septa and central clefts of large hemangiomas do not enhance (see **Fig. 5C**). Another frequent enhancement pattern is early homogeneous hyperenhancement, which is often called flash-filling. In a study of 154 hemangiomas by Semelka and colleagues,[38] 23% displayed that pattern; all were less than 1.5 cm in diameter.

Completely sclerosed hemangiomas demonstrate extensive fibrosis, resulting in atypical imaging findings. Volume loss from fibrosis may cause adjacent retraction of the hepatic capsule.[39] T2 signal may be less hyperintense and there may be a lack of early enhancement with delayed slight peripheral enhancement.[34] Increased fibrosis with volume loss and capsular retraction can also be seen in hemangiomas in the setting of progressive cirrhosis.[40]

Differential diagnosis

There is no differential diagnosis for cavernous hemangiomas that demonstrate a classic pattern of contrast enhancement. The imaging features of lesions with rapid homogeneous enhancement overlap with other hypervascular liver tumors, including HCC, HCA, and hypervascular metastases. One helpful finding in differentiating a flash-filling hemangioma from a hypervascular metastasis

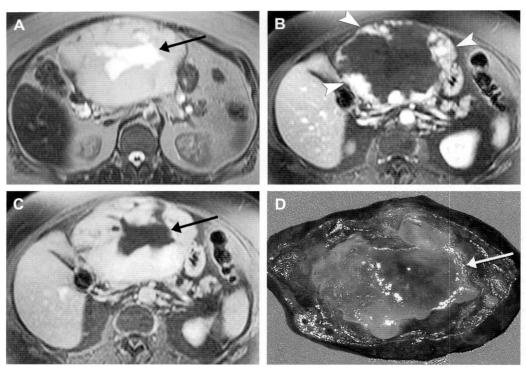

Fig. 5. Giant cavernous hemangioma. (*A*) T2-weighted image shows a large hyperintense mass arising from the left hepatic lobe with central stellate high T2 signal intensity (*arrow*). Intravenous gadolinium contrast-enhanced, fat-suppressed images show peripheral nodular discontinuous enhancement (*arrowheads*) in the portal venous phase (*B*) with progressive filling in on the delayed image (*C*). The central scar-like region (*arrow*) does not enhance. (*D*) Photograph of the cut surface of the resected specimen reveals spongy hemorrhagic tissue with a central myxoid area (*arrow*).

is hyperintensity of a hemangioma on the delayed phase. Metastases often demonstrate heterogeneous or peripheral washout.

Angiomyolipoma

Clinical and pathologic features

Angiomyolipoma is a benign tumor composed of smooth muscle, fat, and thick-walled blood vessels. It rarely occurs in the liver, with over 200 cases reported in medical literature.[41] The average age of presentation is 50 years (range 10 to 79) with a female predominance.[42] The majority are sporadic, although 6% to 10% occur in patients with tuberous sclerosis.[42,43] Conversely, 13% of patients with tuberous sclerosis have hepatic angiomyolipomas, which are usually multiple and associated with multiple bilateral renal angiomyolipomas.[44] Patients either have nonspecific symptoms such as abdominal discomfort or mass or the lesion is an incidental finding, although intraperitoneal rupture and malignant transformation rarely occur.[45,46]

Angiomyolipomas are well-circumscribed non-encapsulated round or ovoid masses that vary in size from less than 1 cm to 36 cm in diameter.[42] The cut surface is yellow to tan in color and focal areas of hemorrhage or necrosis may be present. Microscopic findings are diverse since the relative proportion of smooth muscle cells, mature adipose tissue, and blood vessels varies widely. The myoid component usually predominates and consists of spindle cells, epithelioid cells, and intermediate ovoid or short spindle cells. The fat component varies from scattered cells involving less than 10% of the tumor in 30% of cases to greater than 70% in 10% of cases.[43] The vascular component includes both a rich capillary network in addition to multiple tortuous thick-walled vessels with occasional calcification.

MR imaging features

Hepatic angiomyolipomas demonstrate a spectrum of appearances on MR imaging, reflecting their varied histologic composition. They may be hyperintense, hypointense, or heterogeneous with hyperintense and hypointense areas on T1-weighted sequences, depending on the amount and distribution of fat.[46–49] Areas of macroscopic fat demonstrate peripheral low signal (etching artifact or India ink artifact) on out-of-phase sequences and diffusely decreased signal intensity with fat-suppression sequences (**Fig. 6**). Areas of microscopic fat demonstrate diffuse loss of signal on out of phase sequences.[50] Fat signal intensity may not be present in lesions with minimal pathologic fat composition.[51] On T2-weighted sequences, hepatic angiomyolipomas are homogeneously or heterogeneously hyperintense. With gadolinium, most hepatic angiomyolipomas demonstrate hyperenhancement during the arterial phase and may be hyperintense, isointense, or hypointense during the portal venous and delayed phases.[46–48,51]

Differential diagnosis

HCA, HCC, myelolipoma, and fat-containing metastases, such as liposarcoma and malignant teratoma, can contain fat and soft tissue components and their MR imaging appearance may be difficult to distinguish from angiomyolipomas.

Solitary fibrous tumor
Clinical and pathologic features

SFT is a rare hepatic neoplasm that is similar to tumors arising in the pleura, mediastinum, and other sites. It occurs in adults, with a mean age of 57 years and a 2:1 female-to-male ratio.[52] Clinical presentation varies from asymptomatic to abdominal discomfort or fullness due to mass effect.[53]

SFT is typically a large well-circumscribed intrahepatic or pedunculated firm mass with a nodular or smooth surface. When sectioned, these tumors are gray to white in color with a whorled appearance and may contain central hemorrhage or necrosis.[5,52] Bundles of spindle cells with either a haphazard arrangement or a storiform pattern are present microscopically.[5,52] The majority of SFTs are benign in biologic behavior but malignant transformation may occur. The true incidence of malignant transformation is not known owing to the low number of reported tumors. With slightly greater than 50 tumors appearing in the literature to date, to the authors' knowledge there is only one reported case of a primary hepatic SFT with distant metastases.[54]

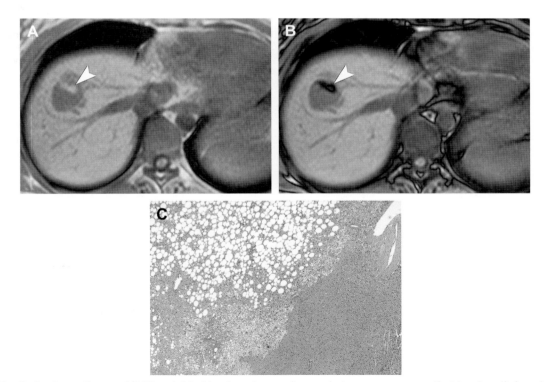

Fig. 6. Angiomyolipoma. (*A*) T1-weighted in-phase image shows a heterogeneous mass that is primarily hypointense with a focus of high signal intensity (*arrowhead*). (*B*) T1-weighted out-of-phase image shows etching artifact of the areas of high signal intensity on the in-phase image (*arrowhead*) consistent with macroscopic fat. (*C*) Photomicrograph (original magnification, ×40; H-E stain) of the corresponding specimen demonstrates components of smooth muscle cells, fat cells, and blood vessels.

MR imaging features

When evaluated by MR imaging, SFT of the liver is characteristically hypointense on T1-weighted sequences, variably hypointense or hyperintense on T2-weighted sequences and demonstrates heterogeneous enhancement following the administration of intravenous contrast.[55,56] Contrast enhancement may be avid and progressive, increasing through the arterial and venous phases resulting in increased enhancement in the delayed phase (**Fig. 7**).[57] The marked enhancement of some tumors is thought to be due to prominent vascularity.[57]

Differential diagnosis

The imaging findings of a large, solitary, well-demarcated, heterogeneous mass are largely nonspecific. Progressive delayed enhancement can be seen with fibrotic lesions, including ICC, the sclerosing type of HCC and epithelioid hemangioendothelioma in addition to SFT. Vascular lesions such as cavernous hemangioma and angiosarcoma also demonstrate progressive enhancement, although the typical early peripheral discontinuous nodular enhancement pattern of a hemangioma distinguishes it from SFT.

MALIGNANT TUMORS
Epithelial

Hepatocellular carcinoma and precursor lesions
Clinical and pathologic features

HCC is the most common primary liver malignancy in adults. It is the fifth most common cancer in the world, although there is striking geographic variation depending on the prevalence of major risk factors. Hepatitis B virus infection and aflatoxin B1 contribute to the high incidence in Africa and parts of Asia, whereas hepatitis C virus infection is the main risk factor in Japan.[58] The incidence of HCC in the United States has more than doubled in the past two decades, primarily related to an epidemic of hepatitis C virus infection from the 1960s to the 1980s.[59] Other predisposing factors include cirrhosis of any cause, such as heavy alcohol consumption, hemachromatosis, hereditary tyrosinemia, and alpha-1-antitrypsin disease. Obesity and diabetes are also related to HCC through nonalcoholic fatty liver disease. Between 15% and 50% of patients in the United States have no known risk factor.[59]

The incidence of HCC increases with age, with a mean age of diagnosis of 65 years in the United

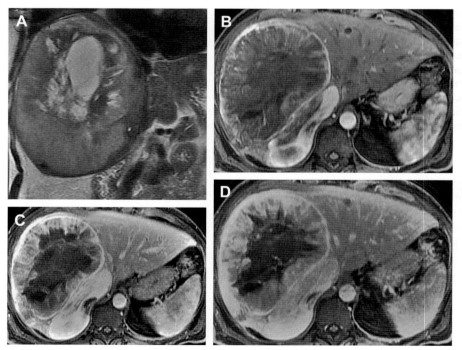

Fig. 7. Solitary fibrous tumor. (*A*) T2-weighted image shows a large heterogeneous mass with marked increased signal intensity centrally corresponding to regions of necrosis. Dynamic intravenous gadolinium-enhanced, fat-suppressed T1-weighted images show a multilobulated mass with avid peripheral enhancement in the arterial phase (*B*) that increases centripetally in the portal venous phase (*C*) and persists in the equilibrium phase (*D*).

States. In countries where hepatitis B virus is endemic, HCC occurs at an earlier age, often before 40.[58] Three quarters of patients are male, which may relate to higher rates of known risk factors and androgen receptors often present on the tumors.[5] Clinical symptoms vary widely. Most patients present with abdominal pain, weight loss, and hepatomegaly, often with a palpable mass. Decompensated cirrhosis may be the only indication of HCC, likely from neoplastic portal or hepatic vein thrombosis. Rarely, HCC can cause obstructive jaundice, spontaneous rupture with hemoperitoneum, or paraneoplastic syndromes, including hypertrophic osteoarthropathy. Serum alpha-fetoprotein is reportedly elevated in 70% to 90% of patients; however, it is usually normal or minimally elevated in patients with small HCCs (defined as >2 cm in diameter).[5,60] The sensitivity and specificity of serum alpha-fetoprotein as a screening test vary widely depending on the cutoff value (<20 ng/mL is most commonly used) in addition to other factors, and higher quality studies are needed to determine its utility.[61,62]

HCC may arise from a single cell or group of hepatocytes or may develop in a stepwise pattern in cases of cirrhosis from a regenerative nodule through a spectrum of low-grade and high-grade dysplastic nodules. A regenerative nodule is a localized proliferation of hepatocytes and support stroma with normal blood supply and no atypia. Low-grade and high-grade dysplastic nodules demonstrate increasing nuclear to cytoplasmic ratios, nuclear atypia, distortion of the normal plate architecture, and increasing arterial supply. These changes are more advanced in well-differentiated HCC, which are also associated with mitotic figures and invasion of the stroma or portal tracts. There are several histologic growth patterns of HCC,

with a trabecular pattern being most common (**Fig. 8A**). The fibrolamellar pattern, which has abundant stroma, has distinct clinical and pathologic features and is discussed separately.

A single mass with or without satellite nodules is the most common gross appearance of HCC. It also may arise as multiple discrete nodules throughout the liver or more rarely diffuse infiltration. Large tumors are often heterogeneous and a mosaic appearance may be seen from areas of steatosis, hemorrhage, cholestasis, fibrosis, and necrosis (see **Fig. 8B**). They are soft tumors because of a lack of desmoplasia except for fibrolamellar and rare scirrhous variants. A fibrous capsule is common in lesions over 1.5 cm in diameter.[60] Vascular invasion is found in close to three quarters, usually involving the portal or hepatic veins. Bile duct invasion is much more infrequent, seen in about 3%.[5] Intrahepatic, lung, regional lymph nodes, bone, and adrenal gland are the most common sites of metastatic disease.

MR imaging features

MR imaging has the highest combination of sensitivity and specificity for HCC compared with other imaging modalities, at 81% and 85%, respectively.[61] However, sensitivity is less for smaller tumors that may be similar in appearance to cirrhotic nodules. Regenerative nodules and low-grade dysplastic nodules demonstrate variable T1 signal intensity, low T2 signal intensity and are isointense or slightly hypointense with intravenous gadolinium enhancement. High-grade dysplastic nodules are usually less than 2 cm in diameter and can display slightly higher T2 signal intensity and arterial phase enhancement with portal venous phase washout, similar to small HCC.[60,63] Small HCC are usually well

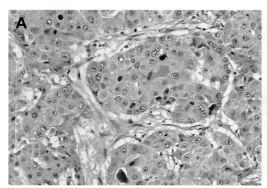
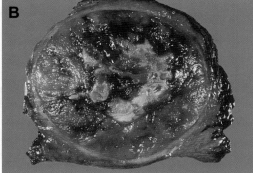

Fig. 8. Pathologic features of hepatocellular carcinoma. (*A*) Photomicrograph (original magnification, ×200; H-E stain) of a bile producing, moderately differentiated hepatocellular carcinoma with a trabecular growth pattern. (*B*) Photograph of the cut surface of a hepatocellular carcinoma shows an encapsulated mass and a variegated appearance with areas of fat and hemorrhage.

differentiated and demonstrate variable T1 signal intensity, slightly high T2 signal intensity, and homogeneous intense arterial phase enhancement with portal venous phase washout.[63] Small HCC also may have a nodule-in-a-nodule appearance, indicating that it is arising within a larger regenerative or dysplastic nodule.

The appearance of large HCCs is quite variable. The most common pattern is hypointensity on T1-weighted sequences, hyperintensity on T2-weighted sequences and diffuse heterogeneous immediate enhancement (**Fig. 9**).[64] Hyperintense T1 signal can be seen, from intratumoral fat, copper, or glycogen, and is more common in low-grade tumors.[65] A mosaic pattern of varying signal intensities on unenhanced and enhanced sequences is frequent, reflecting the heterogeneous pathologic appearance. A tumor capsule, more common in larger tumors, usually demonstrates low T1 and T2 signal intensity and delayed enhancement. In capsules over 4 mm in thickness, inner low T2 and outer high T2 signal intensity layers may be seen from layers of inner fibrous tissue and outer compressed vessels and bile ducts.[65] Evidence of invasiveness is frequent in larger tumors, including extracapsular extension, satellite nodules (**Fig. 10**), vascular invasion, and metastatic disease. Tumor thrombus can be distinguished from bland thrombus by expansion

of the lumen and contiguity to and similar imaging characteristics with the primary tumor, including on T2, postcontrast and diffusion-weighted sequences.[66,67]

In addition to gadolinium chelates, several other intravenous contrast agents have been studied in the diagnosis of HCC. After the administration of SPIO particles, HCC is typically hyperintense on T2- and T2*-weighted sequences although some well-differentiated tumors may demonstrate uptake and be isointense or hypointense.[63] To improve sensitivity, some investigators advocate a double-contrast protocol of SPIO particles and a gadolinium chelate because of their synergistic effects.[68] Combined extracellular and hepatocellular agents, including gadoxetic acid, may also improve sensitivity.[69] Larger prospective studies are needed to determine the best screening method.

Differential diagnosis

In patients with cirrhosis, arterial enhancing lesions are not uncommon and, in addition to HCC, they may represent dysplastic nodules or transient arterial enhancement from arterioportal shunts or obstructed distal parenchymal portal veins. In one study, 93% of arterial enhancing lesions less than or equal to 2 cm in diameter and not seen on other phases of enhancement or unenhanced sequences

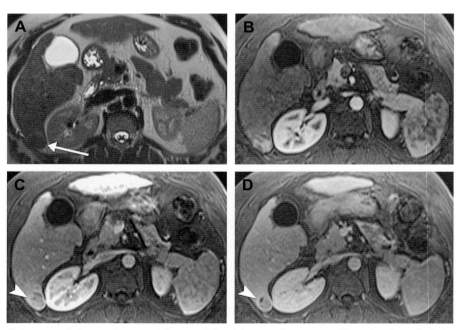

Fig. 9. Small hepatocellular carcinoma. (*A*) T2-weighted image shows a small predominantly isointense mass (*arrow*). Dynamic intravenous gadolinium-enhanced, fat-suppressed T1-weighted images show heterogeneous hyperenhancement in the arterial phase (*B*) and central washout with peripheral capsular enhancement (*arrowhead*) in the portal venous phase (*C*) and equilibrium phase (*D*).

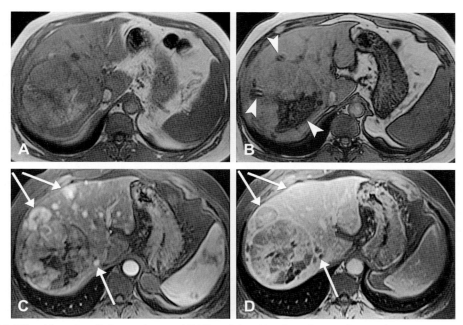

Fig. 10. Multifocal hepatocellular carcinoma. (*A*) T1-weighted in-phase image shows a heterogeneous mass containing areas of hyperintensity, isointensity, and hypointensity. (*B*) T1-weighted out-of-phase image shows multiple areas of etching artifact from macroscopic fat (*arrowheads*). Intravenous gadolinium-enhanced, fat-suppressed T1-weighted images show heterogeneous enhancement of the dominant mass as well as multiple additional hyperenhancing masses (*arrows*) in the arterial phase (*C*) with central washout and peripheral capsular enhancement in the portal venous phase (*D*).

were nonneoplastic.[70] Confluent fibrosis can appear mass-like and have hyperintense T2 signal intensity, although it typically is wedge-shaped, demonstrates delayed enhancement, may be associated with capsular retraction, and is commonly centrally located, in the anterior and medial segments of the liver.[67]

In patients without cirrhosis, the differential diagnosis of small HCCs includes other arterial enhancing masses such as flash-filling hemangiomas, FNH, HCA, and hypervascular metastasis. The differential of a large, encapsulated, heterogeneous mass includes HCC, HCA, SFT, and hepatic sarcomas.

Fibrolamellar carcinoma

Clinical and pathologic features

Fibrolamellar carcinoma is a distinct variant of HCC seen in young patients usually without previous liver disease.[71] It has an equal gender distribution with a mean age of presentation of 23 years.[72] Presenting symptoms range from abdominal pain, hepatomegaly, and palpable mass to, more rarely, gynecomastia or venous thrombosis.[72] Serum alpha-fetoprotein levels are generally not elevated in contrast to patients with HCC; however, mild elevation may occur in approximately 10% of patients.[5]

The gross appearance of fibrolamellar carcinoma is usually a nonencapsulated but well-demarcated solitary mass. Less frequent morphologic appearances include a mass with peripheral satellite lesions, bilobed mass, or diffuse multifocal disease.[72] Two thirds occur in the left lobe.[5] Fibrolamellar carcinoma is characterized histologically by prominent fibrous lamellae (**Fig. 11**) supporting groups of tumor cells that contain a coarse eosinophilic granular cytoplasm attributable to the

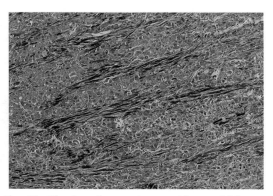

Fig. 11. Fibrolamellar carcinoma. Masson trichrome stain shows bands of blue staining fibrous lamellae in between sheets of rounded and polyhedral cells that are deeply eosinophilic staining.

presence of abundant mitochondria.[5] The fibrous tissue may coalesce into a central scar, which commonly contains calcification.

MR imaging features

On MR imaging, fibrolamellar carcinoma is large, lobulated mass that is characteristically hypointense to isointense and hyperintense to isointense on T1- and T2-weighted sequences, respectively.[72,73] A central scar usually demonstrates low T1 and T2 signal intensity because of its fibrous content. Calcification of the scar is better evaluated by CT scan. Following the intravenous administration of gadolinium, there is heterogeneous enhancement in the arterial and portal venous phases becoming more homogeneous in the delayed phase (**Fig. 12**).[72] The central scar most commonly does not enhance and will appear more conspicuous on the delayed phase. Rarely, high T2 signal and delayed enhancement can be seen in scars with increased vascularity.[72]

Differential diagnosis

In a young adult patient without underlying hepatic disease or other risk factors, the main differential considerations for fibrolamellar carcinoma are FNH and HCA. FNH typically demonstrates homogeneous enhancement apart from the central scar and the scar is hyperintense on T2-weighted

sequences and usually smaller than that of fibrolamellar carcinoma.[73] HCA usually does not have a central scar and, unlike fibrolamellar carcinoma, often contains areas of high T1 signal intensity.

Intrahepatic cholangiocarcinoma
Clinical and pathologic features

Defined as an adenocarcinoma originating from the intrahepatic bile ducts, ICC is the second most common primary liver malignancy. Risk factors encompass the spectrum of biliary conditions leading to chronic inflammation, including chronic parasitic infection, recurrent pyogenic cholangitis, hepatolithiasis, primary sclerosing cholangitis, and congenital anomalies, including choledochal cysts and Caroli disease. The most significant worldwide risk factors are parasitic infection and intrahepatic stone formation.[5] Clinical features in a series from the *Atlas of Tumor Pathology*[5] (AFIP) showed a nearly 3:1 male-to-female ratio with presenting symptoms of upper abdominal pain and ascites, weight loss, jaundice, weakness, and nausea and vomiting, in decreasing frequency.

ICC is a nonencapsulated, firm or hard tumor that varies from white to tan in color. Necrosis and hemorrhage rarely occur. The patterns of growth may be characterized as mass-forming, periductal infiltrating, or intraductal.[74,75] Microscopic features

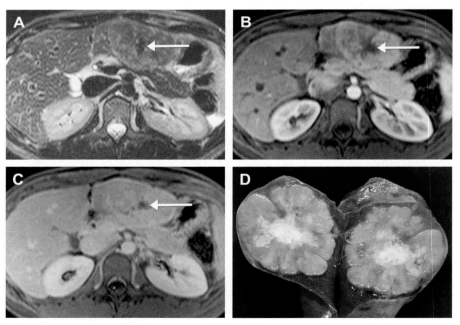

Fig. 12. Fibrolamellar carcinoma. (*A*) Fat-suppressed T2-weighted image shows an isointense mass in the left hepatic lobe containing a hypointense central scar (*arrow*). Dynamic intravenous gadolinium contrast-enhanced, fat-suppressed T1-weighted images during arterial (*B*) and equilibrium (*C*) phases show early heterogeneous enhancement with progressive increased homogeneity (*arrow*). (*D*) Photograph of the cut surface of the bivalved resected specimen shows a white fibrous central scar arising within a solitary mass.

include cells that are arranged in tubules, nests, acini, or trabeculae, and may mimic adenocarcinomas originating outside of the liver. Generally, ICC is well-differentiated and consists of cuboidal to columnar epithelium with moderate cytoplasm that varies from clear to mildly granular and eosinophilic.[5] It is hypovascular and may have a marked fibrous component.

MR imaging features

The MR imaging features of ICC differ according to its pattern of growth. Mass-forming ICC is irregularly marginated and demonstrates hyperintense T2 and hypointense T1 signal intensity. Following the administration of intravenous contrast, irregular peripheral enhancement may be observed with gradual centripetal filling that persists into the delayed phase of imaging owing to the fibrous composition (**Fig. 13**).[75] Encasement of hepatic vessels without thrombosis and hepatolithiasis are not uncommon findings.[75] Transient hepatic intensity differences and capsular retraction may also be observed.[74,76]

Pure periductal infiltrating tumors are rare in ICC in contrast to hilar cholangiocarcinoma, but often are found in a combined pattern with the mass-forming variant.[75] Periductal ICC grows along a narrowed or dilated duct, causing peripheral ductal dilatation.[74,75] MRCP can be helpful in identifying the ductal irregularity and dilatation.

The intraductal variant rarely occurs in the intrahepatic ducts. It may appear on MR imaging as duct dilatation with or without a visible polypoid mass.[74] T2 sequences are helpful in identifying intraductal filling defects and associated ductal dilatation. Both periductal and intraductal enhancement may be seen with each of these respective growth patterns.

Differential diagnosis

The differential diagnosis of hepatic masses and mass-like lesions with delayed phase enhancement includes scirrhous HCC, metastatic disease, immature abscess, confluent hepatic fibrosis, and SFT. Scirrhous HCC versus ICC is an important preoperative distinction due to differences in surgical management and prognosis. Both of these tumors demonstrate arterial phase peripheral enhancement with progressive centripetal filling. However, scirrhous HCC is usually homogeneously hypointense on the hepatobiliary phase imaging following the administration of gadobenate dimeglumine compared with ICC which demonstrates a peripheral washout pattern.[77]

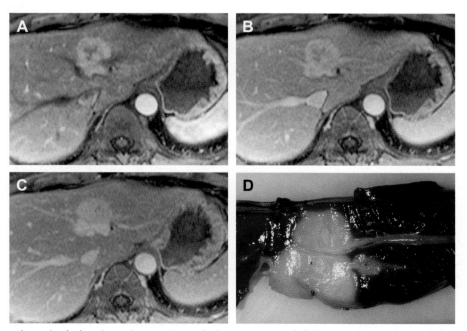

Fig. 13. Intrahepatic cholangiocarcinoma. Dynamic intravenous gadolinium contrast-enhanced, fat-suppressed T1-weighted images show peripheral enhancement in the arterial phase (*A*) with gradually increasing centripetal enhancement and retention of contrast at 60 seconds (*B*) and 5 minutes (*C*) post injection. (*D*) Photograph of the resected gross specimen shows a white mass encompassing an intrahepatic vein.

Nonepithelial

Angiosarcoma
Clinical and pathologic features
Although the most common primary mesenchymal hepatic malignancy, angiosarcoma is rare. It is a high-grade vascular neoplasm of spindled or epithelioid endothelial cells. Early cases were attributable to environmental exposures to vinyl chloride, Thorotrast, arsenic, and anabolic steroids, but they are now generally considered to be idiopathic or secondary to cirrhosis.[78] There is an association with hemochromatosis and neurofibromatosis type 1.[79] The peak incidence is in the sixth decade of life with a male predominance.[5] Clinical symptoms include hepatomegaly, ascites, jaundice, pain, and, rarely, an acute abdomen with hemoperitoneum.

Grossly, angiosarcoma is a grayish white tumor mass or multiple nodules ranging in size from a few millimeters to several centimeters with hemorrhagic foci and cavities of blood. There are four main morphologic patterns: multiple nodules, a dominant mass, a combination of a mass and nodules, or diffuse infiltration without definable mass.[78] Microscopically, an aggressive pattern is observed with endothelial cells growing along sinusoids, portal venous branches, and terminal hepatic venules.[5] Sinusoidal growth eventually results in irregular cavity walls lined by tumor cells filled with blood, whereas invasion of the peripheral portal and hepatic venous systems results in luminal obstruction leading to hemorrhage, infarction, and necrosis.[5]

MR imaging features
Angiosarcoma is often hypointense on T1-weighted sequences and hyperintense on T2-weighted sequences, although areas of high T1 signal intensity and heterogeneous T2 signal intensity or fluid levels may be present owing to intratumoral hemorrhage (**Fig. 14**).[80] Rim enhancement is seen early following the administration of intravenous contrast with delayed centripetal enhancement. Enhancement is heterogenous in the arterial phase with progressive enhancement on the delayed phase that is frequently irregular, ring-shaped, or bizarre in morphology, and is distinguishable from the more nodular peripheral enhancement of hemangiomas.[78]

Differential diagnosis
Given that angiosarcoma can present as a dominant mass or multiple nodules, the differential diagnosis includes more common neoplasms such as metastatic disease and HCC. Persistent delayed enhancement, intratumoral hemorrhage and the presence of splenic or pulmonary metastasis are findings suggestive of angiosarcoma.[78] Hemangioma may be a consideration within the differential diagnosis as well. With only 10 to 20 new cases of angiosarcoma diagnosed in the United States annually, hemangiomas are approximately 10,000 times more common than angiosarcomas.[79] Although angiosarcomas may rarely mimic hemangiomas, they usually appear more heterogeneous and can be distinguished from the characteristic peripheral discontinuous nodular enhancement seen in hemangiomas.[81] Mass-forming ICCs may also mimic angiosarcoma with peripheral arterial phase enhancement and progressive centripetal filling. Bile duct dilatation, if present, favors cholangiocarcinoma.[79]

Epithelioid hemangioendothelioma
Clinical and pathologic features
Epithelioid hemangioendothelioma is a rare low-grade malignant vascular tumor of endothelial origin. It has a variable clinical course. There is

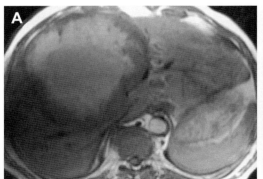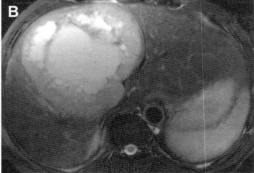

Fig. 14. Angiosarcoma. (*A*) T1-weighted image shows a hypointense mass containing a large area of high signal intensity compatible with hemorrhage. (*B*) Fat-suppressed T2-weighted image shows a hyperintense mass with central higher signal intensity hemorrhage.

an increased female to male incidence with 62% of cases occurring in women within a series of 137 tumors studied at the AFIP.[82] Age range varied from 12 to 86 years of age with a mean of 47 years and highest incidence in the 30- to 40-year range. Clinical features vary from asymptomatic (42% of cases in the AFIP series) to severe and include nausea, periodic vomiting, anorexia, weakness, jaundice, pain, and hepatosplenomegaly. Other less common findings include hemoperitoneum, liver failure or a Budd-Chiari—like syndrome.[5]

The gross appearance of epithelioid hemangioendothelioma is a tan to white tumor nodule with firm consistency that may be hyperemic along its margin. These nodules vary from several millimeters to centimeters in size and may coalesce in a subcapsular location with associated capsular retraction.[83] Histologically, the nodules consist of central relatively fibrous hypocellular stroma with marginal active proliferation of epithelioid and dendritic cells.[83] The nodules are ill-defined and demonstrate multiacinar involvement, growing along and invading sinusoids, portal venous branches, and terminal hepatic venules.[5]

MR imaging features

The characteristic imaging morphology is multifocal nodules in a subcapsular distribution that may coalesce, associated with capsular retraction or venous invasion. Epithelioid hemangioendothelioma is hypointense on T1-weighted sequences and heterogeneously hyperintense on T2-weighted sequences. A pattern described as the bright-dark ring sign consists of a peripheral rim of high T1 and low T2 signal intensity which may be from peripheral thrombosed vascular channels (**Fig. 15**).[84]

Following the administration of intravenous gadolinium, a multilayered appearance may be seen with central hypointensity surrounded by a ring of increased enhancement and an outer hypointense rim.[83] These alternating areas of signal intensity correlate with a hypocellular central stroma surrounded by hyperemic tissue secondary to cell proliferation with a thin avascular rim due to sinusoid and small vessel invasion.[83] The central fibrous portion demonstrates delayed enhancement.[84] Well-defined peripheral tumors that have a portal or hepatic venous branch

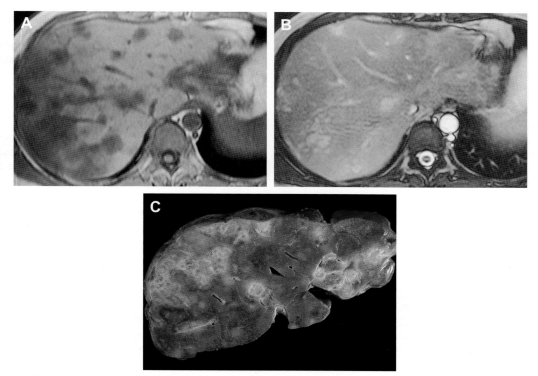

Fig. 15. Epithelioid hemangioendothelioma. (A) T1-weighted image shows multiple subcapsular masses and coalescent nodular masses, many with central low and peripheral relatively higher signal intensity. (B) T2-weighted image shows central high and peripheral relatively lower signal intensity of the nodules. (C) Photograph of the resected gross specimen shows multiple fibrotic masses and coalescent nodules with capsular hepatic retraction.

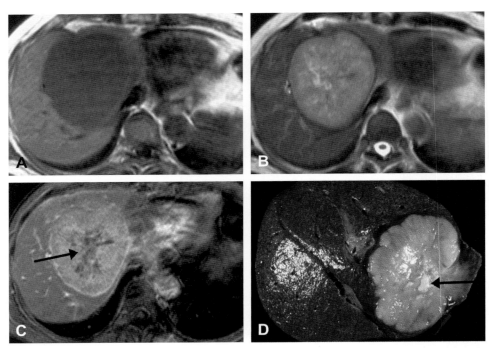

Fig. 16. Primary hepatic lymphoma, diffuse large B-cell type. T1-weighted (*A*) and T2-weighted (*B*) images show a large solitary mass that is T1 hypointense and heterogeneously hyperintense on the T2-weighted image. (*C*) Intravenous gadolinium contrast enhanced fat suppressed T1-weighted image shows peripheral rim enhancement and central hypointensity due to necrosis (*arrow*). (*D*) Photograph of the cut surface of the resected specimen shows a well-demarcated white-tan tumor with a central stellate necrotic area (*arrow*).

tapering or terminating at its periphery have been observed in epithelioid hemangioendothelioma, referred to as the lollipop sign.[85]

Differential diagnosis
Epithelioid hemangioendothelioma may be confused for metastatic disease, cholangiocarcinoma, angiosarcoma, sclerosing HCC, abscess, cirrhosis, or venooclusive disease. Although many of these diagnoses may show increasing enhancement through the delayed phase of imaging, a multinodular morphology in a subcapsular location with capsular retraction can help to narrow the differential. Lesions in this distribution with concentric rings of varying signal intensity favors epithelioid hemangioendothelioma.

Primary hepatic lymphoma
Clinical and pathologic features
Primary hepatic lymphoma defined by its origin within or confinement to the liver is a rare malignancy with secondary involvement of the liver much more common. A higher incidence is seen in patients that are immunocompromised, such as transplant recipients and patients with increased exposure to viruses such as Epstein Barr virus, HIV, or hepatitis viruses.[86] Most patients are middle aged men with nonspecific

symptoms such as abdominal pain or discomfort, weight loss, fever, and hepatomegaly.[87]

Generally an aggressive disease, primary hepatic lymphoma has been treated with varying combinations of surgery, radiotherapy, and chemotherapy. When resected, the gross specimen consists of bulky solitary or multiple nodules that are white to yellow in color. Depending on the cause, a variety of cell types such as small B-cell, large B-cell, and T-cell, in addition to virus-specific proliferative findings, may be present. The majority are large B-cell lymphomas.[5]

MR imaging features
Primary hepatic lymphoma usually presents as a solitary mass compared with secondary lymphoma, which is more frequently diffuse or multifocal.[86] Other patterns include multifocal masses or diffuse infiltration. It is usually hypointense and hyperintense on T1- and T2-weighted sequences, respectively.[88,89] However, slightly increased T1 signal intensity and low T2 signal intensity have also been reported.[86,89] With administration of gadolinium contrast agents, patchy enhancement in the arterial phase with progressive portal venous enhancement has been described.[90] There may be prominent perilesional rim

Table 1
Summary of MR imaging features of hepatic tumors

	Precontrast[a]		Postcontrast		Helpful Features
	T1	T2	Arterial	Portal Venous or Delayed	
Focal Nodular Hyperplasia Central Scar	Iso to hypo Hypo	Iso to hyper Hyper	Hyper Hypo	Iso to hyper Hyper	Homogeneity except for central scar
Hepatocellular Adenoma	Variable	Iso to hyper	Hyper	Variable	Often heterogeneous, may have hemorrhage, steatosis, capsule
Cavernous Hemangioma Central Scar	Hypo Hypo	Hyper Hyper	Peripheral nodular Hypo	Centripetal filling Hypo	Small may be flash-filling, enhancement parallels blood pool
Angiomyolipoma	Variable	Hyper	Hyper	Variable	Contains variable amount of fat
Solitary Fibrous Tumor	Hypo	Variable	Heterogeneous	Progressive	Large well-circumscribed mass
Hepatocellular Carcinoma Capsule	Variable Hypo	Hyper Hypo	Hyper Hypo	Hypo Hyper	Small HCC may be homogeneous, larger HCC may have a mosaic pattern, capsule, vascular invasion
Fibrolamellar Carcinoma Central Scar	Hypo to iso Hypo	Iso to hyper Hypo	Heterogeneous Hypo	Increasingly homogeneous Hypo	Low signal scar on all sequences, no internal fat
Intrahepatic Cholangiocarcinoma	Hypo	Hyper	Peripheral	Gradual centripetal	Biliary dilatation, capsular retraction
Angiosarcoma	Hypo	Hyper	Rim, heterogeneous	Irregular centripetal	Hemorrhage, splenic metastasis
Epithelioid Hemangioendothelioma	Hypo with hyper rim	Hyper with hypo rim	Concentric rings	Delayed central	Subcapsular location, capsular retraction
Primary Hepatic Lymphoma	Hypo	Hyper	Rim, heterogeneous	Progressive	No specific features

Abbreviations: Hyper, hyperintense; Hypo, hypointense; Iso, isointense.
[a] Signal intensity of lesion in comparison to liver parenchyma and signal intensity of scar in comparison to remainder of the lesion.

enhancement, attributed to adjacent vasculitis.[90] Central heterogeneous signal and enhancement may also be present depending on the degree of necrosis, fibrosis, and vascularity (**Fig. 16**).[89,90]

Differential diagnosis

Secondary hepatic lymphoma may be easier to diagnose than primary hepatic lymphoma given evidence of extrahepatic nodal disease. The differential diagnosis for primary hepatic lymphoma is quite broad, including other primary and secondary hepatic malignancies, as well as infectious and inflammatory processes. As a result, biopsy is often required with immunohistochemistry for diagnosis.

SUMMARY

Primary hepatic tumors demonstrate diverse clinical and pathologic features. When typical imaging features are present (**Table 1**), the MR imaging appearance may be diagnostic, such as FNH and cavernous hemangioma, or suggestive of the diagnosis, such as biliary cystadenoma or cystadenocarcinoma, angiomyolipoma, HCC in the background of cirrhosis, fibrolamellar carcinoma, ICC, or epithelioid hemangioendothelioma. In many cases, however, biopsy is required for diagnosis and treatment planning. Newer MR imaging contrast agents and techniques may prove to further narrow the imaging differential diagnosis.

REFERENCES

1. Buetow PC, Pantongrag-Brown L, Buck JL, et al. Focal nodular hyperplasia of the liver: radiologic-pathologic correlation. Radiographics 1996;16(2): 369–88.
2. Bioulac-Sage P, Balabaud C, Bedossa P, et al. Pathological diagnosis of liver cell adenoma and focal nodular hyperplasia: Bordeaux update. J Hepatol 2007;46(3):521–7.
3. Nguyen BN, Flejou JF, Terris B, et al. Focal nodular hyperplasia of the liver: a comprehensive pathologic study of 305 lesions and recognition of new histologic forms. Am J Surg Pathol 1999;23(12):1441–54.
4. Vilgrain V, Uzan F, Brancatelli G, et al. Prevalence of hepatic hemangioma in patients with focal nodular hyperplasia: MR imaging analysis. Radiology 2003; 229(1):75–9.
5. Ishak KG, Goodman ZD, Stocker JT. Tumors of the liver and intrahepatic bile ducts. Atlas of Tumor Pathology—Third Series. Washington, DC: American Registry of Pathology; 2001.
6. Ba-Ssalamah A, Schima W, Schmook MT, et al. Atypical focal nodular hyperplasia of the liver: imaging features of nonspecific and liver-specific MR

contrast agents. AJR Am J Roentgenol 2002; 179(6):1447–56.
7. Grazioli L, Morana G, Federle MP, et al. Focal nodular hyperplasia: morphologic and functional information from MR imaging with gadobenate dimeglumine. Radiology 2001;221(3):731–9.
8. Grazioli L, Morana G, Kirchin MA, et al. Accurate differentiation of focal nodular hyperplasia from hepatic adenoma at gadobenate dimeglumine-enhanced MR imaging: prospective study. Radiology 2005;236(1):166–77.
9. Lee MJ, Saini S, Hamm B, et al. Focal nodular hyperplasia of the liver: MR findings in 35 proved cases. AJR Am J Roentgenol 1991;156(2):317–20.
10. Mahfouz AE, Hamm B, Taupitz M, et al. Hypervascular liver lesions: differentiation of focal nodular hyperplasia from malignant tumors with dynamic gadolinium-enhanced MR imaging. Radiology 1993;186(1):133–8.
11. Ferlicot S, Kobeiter H, Tran Van Nhieu J, et al. MRI of atypical focal nodular hyperplasia of the liver: radiology-pathology correlation. AJR Am J Roentgenol 2004;182(5):1227–31.
12. Vilgrain V, Flejou JF, Arrive L, et al. Focal nodular hyperplasia of the liver: MR imaging and pathologic correlation in 37 patients. Radiology 1992;184(3): 699–703.
13. Precetti-Morel S, Bellin MF, Ghebontni L, et al. Focal nodular hyperplasia of the liver on ferumoxides-enhanced MR imaging: features on conventional spin-echo, fast spin-echo and gradient-echo pulse sequences. Eur Radiol 1999; 9(8):1535–42.
14. Rooks JB, Ory HW, Ishak KG, et al. Epidemiology of hepatocellular adenoma. The role of oral contraceptive use. JAMA 1979;242(7):644–8.
15. Lindgren A, Olsson R. Liver damage from low-dose oral contraceptives. J Intern Med 1993;234(3): 287–92.
16. Deneve JL, Pawlik TM, Cunningham S, et al. Liver cell adenoma: a multicenter analysis of risk factors for rupture and malignancy. Ann Surg Oncol 2009; 16(3):640–8.
17. Micchelli ST, Vivekanandan P, Boitnott JK, et al. Malignant transformation of hepatic adenomas. Mod Pathol 2008;21(4):491–7.
18. Brancatelli G, Federle MP, Vullierme MP, et al. CT and MR imaging evaluation of hepatic adenoma. J Comput Assist Tomogr 2006;30(5):745–50.
19. Grazioli L, Federle MP, Ichikawa T, et al. Liver adenomatosis: clinical, histopathologic, and imaging findings in 15 patients. Radiology 2000;216(2): 395–402.
20. Lewin M, Handra-Luca A, Arrive L, et al. Liver adenomatosis: classification of MR imaging features and comparison with pathologic findings. Radiology 2006;241(2):433–40.

21. Arrivé L, Flejou JF, Vilgrain V, et al. Hepatic adenoma: MR findings in 51 pathologically proved lesions. Radiology 1994;193(2):507—12.

22. Chung KY, Mayo-Smith WW, Saini S, et al. Hepato-cellular adenoma: MR imaging features with pathologic correlation. AJR Am J Roentgenol 1995; 165(2):303—8.

23. Paulson EK, McClellan JS, Washington K, et al. Hepatic adenoma: MR characteristics and correlation with pathologic findings. AJR Am J Roentgenol 1994;163(1):113—6.

24. Paley MR, Mergo PJ, Torres GM, et al. Characterization of focal hepatic lesions with ferumoxides-enhanced T2-weighted MR imaging. AJR Am J Roentgenol 2000;175(1):159—63.

25. Venkatesh SK, Yin M, Glockner JF, et al. MR elastography of liver tumors: preliminary results. AJR Am J Roentgenol 2008;190(6):1534—40.

26. Ishak KG, Willis GW, Cummins SD, et al. Biliary cystadenoma and cystadenocarcinoma: report of 14 cases and review of the literature. Cancer 1977; 39(1):322—38.

27. Buetow PC, Buck JL, Pantongrag-Brown L, et al. Biliary cystadenoma and cystadenocarcinoma: clinical-imaging-pathologic correlations with emphasis on the importance of ovarian stroma. Radiology 1995; 196(3):805—10.

28. Devaney K, Goodman ZD, Ishak KG. Hepatobiliary cystadenoma and cystadenocarcinoma. A light microscopic and immunohistochemical study of 70 patients. Am J Surg Pathol 1994;18(11): 1078—91.

29. Lauffer JM, Baer HU, Maurer CA, et al. Biliary cystadenocarcinoma of the liver: the need for complete resection. Eur J Cancer 1998;34(12):1845—51.

30. Lewin M, Mourra N, Honigman I, et al. Assessment of MRI and MRCP in diagnosis of biliary cystadenoma and cystadenocarcinoma. Eur Radiol 2006;16(2): 407—13.

31. Choi BI, Lim JH, Han MC, et al. Biliary cystadenoma and cystadenocarcinoma: CT and sonographic findings. Radiology 1989;171(1):57—61.

32. Karhunen PJ. Benign hepatic tumours and tumour like conditions in men. J Clin Pathol 1986;39(2): 183—8.

33. Gandolfi L, Leo P, Solmi L, et al. Natural history of hepatic haemangiomas: clinical and ultrasound study. Gut 1991;32(6):677—80.

34. Vilgrain V, Boulos L, Vullierme MP, et al. Imaging of atypical hemangiomas of the liver with pathologic correlation. Radiographics 2000;20(2):379—97.

35. Ros PR, Lubbers PR, Olmsted WW, et al. Hemangioma of the liver: heterogeneous appearance on T2-weighted images. AJR Am J Roentgenol 1987; 149(6):1167—70.

36. Choi BI, Han MC, Park JH, et al. Giant cavernous hemangioma of the liver: CT and MR imaging in 10 cases. AJR Am J Roentgenol 1989;152(6): 1221—6.

37. Whitney WS, Herfkens RJ, Jeffrey RB, et al. Dynamic breath-hold multiplanar spoiled gradient-recalled MR imaging with gadolinium enhancement for differentiating hepatic hemangiomas from malignancies at 1.5 T. Radiology 1993;189(3):863—70.

38. Semelka RC, Brown ED, Ascher SM, et al. Hepatic hemangiomas: a multi-institutional study of appearance on T2-weighted and serial gadolinium-enhanced gradient-echo MR images. Radiology 1994;192(2):401—6.

39. Doyle DJ, Khalili K, Guindi M, et al. Imaging features of sclerosed hemangioma. AJR Am J Roentgenol 2007;189(1):67—72.

40. Brancatelli G, Federle MP, Blachar A, et al. Hemangioma in the cirrhotic liver: diagnosis and natural history. Radiology 2001;219(1):69—74.

41. Xu AM, Zhang SH, Zheng JM, et al. Pathological and molecular analysis of sporadic hepatic angiomyolipoma. Hum Pathol 2006;37(6):735—41.

42. Nonomura A, Mizukami Y, Kadoya M. Angiomyolipoma of the liver: a collective review. J Gastroenterol 1994;29(1):95—105.

43. Tsui WM, Colombari R, Portmann BC, et al. Hepatic angiomyolipoma: a clinicopathologic study of 30 cases and delineation of unusual morphologic variants. Am J Surg Pathol 1999;23(1):34—48.

44. Fricke BL, Donnelly LF, Casper KA, et al. Frequency and imaging appearance of hepatic angiomyolipomas in pediatric and adult patients with tuberous sclerosis. AJR Am J Roentgenol 2004;182(4): 1027—30.

45. Dalle I, Sciot R, de Vos R, et al. Malignant angiomyolipoma of the liver: a hitherto unreported variant. Histopathology 2000;36(5):443—50.

46. Zhou YM, Li B, Xu F, et al. Clinical features of hepatic angiomyolipoma. Hepatobiliary Pancreat Dis Int 2008;7(3):284—7.

47. Ahmadi T, Itai Y, Takahashi M, et al. Angiomyolipoma of the liver: significance of CT and MR dynamic study. Abdom Imaging 1998;23(5):520—6.

48. Hogemann D, Flemming P, Kreipe H, et al. Correlation of MRI and CT findings with histopathology in hepatic angiomyolipoma. Eur Radiol 2001;11(8):1389—95.

49. Takayama Y, Moriura S, Nagata J, et al. Hepatic angiomyolipoma: radiologic and histopathologic correlation. Abdom Imaging 2002;27(2):180—3.

50. Balci NC, Akinci A, Akun E, et al. Hepatic angiomyolipoma: demonstration by out of phase MRI. Clin Imaging 2002;26(6):418—20.

51. Yoshimura H, Murakami T, Kim T, et al. Angiomyolipoma of the liver with least amount of fat component: imaging features of CT, MR, and angiography. Abdom Imaging 2002;27(2):184—7.

52. Moran CA, Ishak KG, Goodman ZD. Solitary fibrous tumor of the liver: a clinicopathologic and

immunohistochemical study of nine cases. Ann Diagn Pathol 1998;2(1):19—24.

53. Perini MV, Herman P, D'Albuquerque LA, et al. Solitary fibrous tumor of the liver: report of a rare case and review of the literature. Int J Surg. 2008;6(5):396—9.

54. Yilmaz S, Kirimlioglu V, Ertas E, et al. Giant solitary fibrous tumor of the liver with metastasis to the skeletal system successfully treated with trisegmentectomy. Dig Dis Sci 2000;45(1):168—74.

55. Kandpal H, Sharma R, Gupta SD, et al. Solitary fibrous tumour of the liver: a rare imaging diagnosis using MRI and diffusion-weighted imaging. Br J Radiol 2008;81(972):e282—6.

56. Obuz F, Secil M, Sagol O, et al. Ultrasonography and magnetic resonance imaging findings of solitary fibrous tumor of the liver. Tumori 2007;93(1):100—2.

57. Moser T, Nogueira TS, Neuville A, et al. Delayed enhancement pattern in a localized fibrous tumor of the liver. AJR Am J Roentgenol 2005;184(5): 1578—80.

58. Llovet JM, Burroughs A, Bruix J. Hepatocellular carcinoma. Lancet 2003;362(9399):1907—17.

59. El-Serag HB. Epidemiology of hepatocellular carcinoma in USA. Hepatol Res 2007;37(Suppl 2): S88—94.

60. Terminology of nodular hepatocellular lesions. International Working Party. Hepatology 1995;22(3): 983—93.

61. Colli A, Fraquelli M, Casazza G, et al. Accuracy of ultrasonography, spiral CT, magnetic resonance, and alpha-fetoprotein in diagnosing hepatocellular carcinoma: a systematic review. Am J Gastroenterol 2006;101(3):513—23.

62. Gupta S, Bent S, Kohlwes J. Test characteristics of alpha-fetoprotein for detecting hepatocellular carcinoma in patients with hepatitis C. A systematic review and critical analysis. Ann Intern Med 2003; 139(1):46—50.

63. Hanna RF, Aguirre DA, Kased N, et al. Cirrhosis-associated hepatocellular nodules: correlation of histopathologic and MR imaging features. Radiographics 2008;28(3):747—69.

64. Kelekis NL, Semelka RC, Worawattanakul S, et al. Hepatocellular carcinoma in North America: a multi-institutional study of appearance on T1-weighted, T2-weighted, and serial gadolinium-enhanced gradient-echo images. AJR Am J Roentgenol 1998;170(4):1005—13.

65. Kadoya M, Matsui O, Takashima T, et al. Hepatocellular carcinoma: correlation of MR imaging and histopathologic findings. Radiology 1992;183(3):819—25.

66. Catalano OA, Choy G, Zhu A, et al. Differentiation of malignant thrombus from bland thrombus of the portal vein in patients with hepatocellular carcinoma: application of diffusion-weighted MR imaging. Radiology 2010;254(1):154—62.

67. Willatt JM, Hussain HK, Adusumilli S, et al. MR. Imaging of hepatocellular carcinoma in the cirrhotic liver: challenges and controversies. Radiology 2008; 247(2):311—30.

68. Hanna RF, Kased N, Kwan SW, et al. Double-contrast MRI for accurate staging of hepatocellular carcinoma in patients with cirrhosis. AJR Am J Roentgenol 2008;190(1):47—57.

69. Ahn SS, Kim MJ, Lim JS, et al. Added value of gadoxetic acid-enhanced hepatobiliary phase MR imaging in the diagnosis of hepatocellular carcinoma. Radiology 2010;255(2):459—66.

70. Holland AE, Hecht EM, Hahn WY, et al. Importance of small (< or = 20-mm) enhancing lesions seen only during the hepatic arterial phase at MR imaging of the cirrhotic liver: evaluation and comparison with whole explanted liver. Radiology 2005;237(3):938—44.

71. Craig JR, Peters RL, Edmondson HA, et al. Fibrolamellar carcinoma of the liver: a tumor of adolescents and young adults with distinctive clinico-pathologic features. Cancer 1980;46(2):372—9.

72. McLarney JK, Rucker PT, Bender GN, et al. Fibrolamellar carcinoma of the liver: radiologic-pathologic correlation. Radiographics 1999;19(2):453—71.

73. Ichikawa T, Federle MP, Grazioli L, et al. Fibrolamellar hepatocellular carcinoma: imaging and pathologic findings in 31 recent cases. Radiology 1999; 213(2):352—61.

74. Choi BI, Lee JM, Han JK. Imaging of intrahepatic and hilar cholangiocarcinoma. Abdom Imaging 2004;29(5):548—57.

75. Chung YE, Kim MJ, Park YN, et al. Varying appearances of cholangiocarcinoma: radiologic-pathologic correlation. Radiographics 2009;29(3):683—700.

76. Leyendecker JR, Gakhal M, Elsayes KM, et al. Fat-suppressed dynamic and delayed gadolinium-enhanced volumetric interpolated breath-hold magnetic resonance imaging of cholangiocarcinoma. J Comput Assist Tomogr 2008;32(2): 178—84.

77. Jeon TY, Kim SH, Lee WJ, et al. The value of gadobenate dimeglumine-enhanced hepatobiliary-phase MR imaging for the differentiation of scirrhous hepatocellular carcinoma and cholangiocarcinoma with or without hepatocellular carcinoma. Abdom Imaging 2010;35:337—45.

78. Koyama T, Fletcher JG, Johnson CD, et al. Primary hepatic angiosarcoma: findings at CT and MR imaging. Radiology 2002;222(3):667—73.

79. Buetow PC, Buck JL, Ros PR, et al. Malignant vascular tumors of the liver: radiologic-pathologic correlation. Radiographics 1994;14(1):153—66 [quiz: 67—8].

80. Yu RS, Chen Y, Jiang B, et al. Primary hepatic sarcomas: CT findings. Eur Radiol 2008;18(10): 2196—205.

81. Peterson MS, Baron RL, Rankin SC. Hepatic angiosarcoma: findings on multiphasic contrast-enhanced helical CT do not mimic hepatic hemangioma. AJR Am J Roentgenol 2000;175(1):165–70.

82. Makhlouf HR, Ishak KG, Goodman ZD. Epithelioid hemangioendothelioma of the liver: a clinicopathologic study of 137 cases. Cancer 1999;85(3):562–82.

83. Miller WJ, Dodd GD 3rd, Federle MP, et al. Epithelioid hemangioendothelioma of the liver: imaging findings with pathologic correlation. AJR Am J Roentgenol 1992;159(1):53–7.

84. Economopoulos N, Kelekis NL, Argentos S, et al. Bright-dark ring sign in MR imaging of hepatic epithelioid hemangioendothelioma. J Magn Reson Imaging 2008;27(4):908–12.

85. Alomari AI. The lollipop sign: a new cross-sectional sign of hepatic epithelioid hemangioendothelioma. Eur J Radiol 2006;59(3):460–4.

86. Avlonitis VS, Linos D. Primary hepatic lymphoma: a review. Eur J Surg 1999;165(8):725–9.

87. Lei KI. Primary non-Hodgkin's lymphoma of the liver. Leuk Lymphoma 1998;29(3–4):293–9.

88. Weissleder R, Stark DD, Elizondo G, et al. MRI of hepatic lymphoma. Magn Reson Imaging 1988;6(6):675–81.

89. Maher MM, McDermott SR, Fenlon HM, et al. Imaging of primary non-Hodgkin's lymphoma of the liver. Clin Radiol 2001;56(4):295–301.

90. Coenegrachts K, Vanbeckevoort D, Deraedt K, et al. Mri findings in primary non-Hodgkin's lymphoma of the liver. JBR-BTR. 2005;88(1):17–9.

Index

Magn Reson Imaging Clin N Am 18 (2010) 611–614
doi:10.1016/S1064-9689(10)00085-1

mri.theclinics.com

Moving?

Make sure your subscription moves with you!

To notify us of your new address, find your **Clinics Account Number** (located on your mailing label above your name), and contact customer service at:

Email: journalscustomerservice-usa@elsevier.com

800-654-2452 (subscribers in the U.S. & Canada)
314-447-8871 (subscribers outside of the U.S. & Canada)

Fax number: 314-447-8029

Elsevier Health Sciences Division
Subscription Customer Service
3251 Riverport Lane
Maryland Heights, MO 63043

*To ensure uninterrupted delivery of your subscription, please notify us at least 4 weeks in advance of move.

ELSEVIER